PUBLIC HEALTH AND PREVENTIVE MEDICINE IN CANADA

C. P. Shah

Fourth Edition

PUBLIC HEALTH AND PREVENTIVE MEDICINE IN CANADA

Chandrakant P. Shah
MD, DCH, MRCP (Glas), FRCPC, SM (Hyg), FACPM, FAAP

Professor
Department of Public Health Sciences
Department of Health Administration
Department of Paediatrics
and
Department of Family and Community Medicine
Faculty of Medicine
and
Faculty of Social Work
Faculty of Nursing
University of Toronto
and
Active Staff, The Hospital for Sick Children,
Courtesy Staff, St. Michael's Hospital
Staff Physician, Anishnawbe Health Toronto

Fourth Edition
Copyright © 1998
Printed in Canada

Dr. C.P. Shah
31 Newgate Road, Toronto, Ontario, M6B 3G6, CANADA
or email: c.shah@utoronto.ca

Printed by University of Toronto Press

ISBN 0-9694044-3-3

Canadian Cataloguing in Publication Data

Shah, Chandrakant P. (Chandrakant Padamshi), 1936-
Public health and preventive medicine in Canada

4th ed.
Includes bibliographical references and index.
ISBN 0-9694044-3-3

1. Public Health - Canada
2. Medical Care - Canada
3. Medicine, Preventive - Canada. I. Title

RA449.S48 1998   362.1'0971   C98-900672-7

Printed for Dr. C.P. Shah by University of Toronto Press in support of
the University's Scholarly Publishing Programme.

FOREWORD

It is a pleasure to be invited to write the foreword to the fourth edition of *Public Health and Preventive Medicine in Canada*, written by my long time colleague and friend, Chandrakant Shah. Previous editions have proven to be a valued resource for undergraduate and graduate students in the health sciences and professions since publication of the first edition some ten years ago. It is noteworthy that an adaptation in French has been published under the direction of Dr. Fernand Turcotte of Laval University, also a friend and long time colleague in academic public health and preventive medicine.

In producing this textbook, Dr. Shah has undertaken a monumental task, one might even say a lifelong task, because of the range of subject matter to be encompassed and the need to update the contents continuously in order to reflect the rapidly changing health care field. No such undertaking can hope, of course, to deal exhaustively with all aspects of such an eclectic and dynamic field, but this book makes a valiant and worthwhile effort. Chandrakant Shah is to be warmly commended for meeting the challenge in such a comprehensive and readable manner.

John E. F. Hastings, MD, DPH, FRCP(C)
Professor Emeritus, Community Health and Health Administration,
Faculty of Medicine, University of Toronto
President, Canadian Public Health Association

Toronto
May 28, 1998

PREFACE TO THE FOURTH EDITION

The pleasure of authoring a textbook comes from teaching and writing about a subject that one enjoys and finds exciting. The first edition of this book was targeted toward undergraduate students in medicine. However, due to lack of any comprehensive works on the health status of Canadians and Canada's health care system, this book has become the de facto textbook for both undergraduate and graduate courses for many different disciplines in the health sciences, such as medicine, nursing, health record administrators, and chiropractors, an exciting development for me as an author. It was also a great pleasure to me when my long-time friend and colleague Dr. Fernand Turcotte, professor at Laval University, translated the previous edition in French, which was published by the Laval University Press in 1995.

The purpose of this book is to help readers learn about their role as health care professionals, administrators, or policy makers within the health care system by understanding the extent of health and disease and of the functioning of the health care system in Canada. It is also intended for anyone interested in participating in the ongoing debate on health care issues by providing the fundamentals of health and health care of Canadians.

Preparing this fourth edition has been challenging for two reasons. First, drastic changes have taken place in the health care system across Canada over the past four years. Strapped with increasing debts and the poor performance of the economy in the early 1990s, governments at all levels were capping or reducing their health care budgets. This was achieved by restructuring and reforming the health care system and increasingly divesting themselves from health care and social services, thus allowing the private sector to take over some of those services they had previously provided. Second, a large number of population-based studies on health status are now being carried out by many provinces and by the federal government. Many of these studies are not easily accessible and publication dates lag far behind the study dates. I have tried to overcome these difficulties by using the Internet to research the latest available information. In this edition I have included lists of Web sites, along with information on how to access common data sources for the Canadian health care system.

There are some deliberate omissions in this book as far as certain details are concerned, because excellent textbooks already exist on subjects such as biostatistics and epidemiology. Even so, the first two chapters of this book are dense and synoptic in nature, and are not intended to replace any standard textbooks on the subjects covered. Elsewhere, details are omitted because of different legislation in different Canadian jurisdictions. However, the general principles are covered. Anyone who wishes to study a particular topic in greater depth is encouraged to consult one of several comprehensive textbooks of community health that are available.

In preparation for the fourth edition, a number of colleagues, teachers, and students were asked to provide comments on improving this book, and I am happy to say that their input was very constructive. As a result, all the chapters have been updated with current information, some have been completely rewritten, and new sections have been added. Nonetheless, caution has been taken so the book does not become too voluminous. An Appendix C outlines educational objectives and a detailed index is provided and lists relevant page numbers for quick reference.

I am indebted to many individuals across the country for their support and comments. This list by no means includes everyone who has made contributions, but I offer thanks to Drs. M. Wills, P. Gully, L. Panaro, E. Vayda, R. Deber, P. Williams, C. McCourt, J. Spika, D. Wigle, J. Levy, K. Young, and B. Choi, and to P. Rich and J.Whitehead. Special thanks to Dr. R. Upsur and K. Masnyk for their contributions to many chapters, and to Drs. C. Gardner, S. Galeo, and C. Inch, for their help on the chapter dealing with the health of special groups and to Dr. M. Schweigert for the chapter on occupational health. I am indebted to M. Koch for her editorial help, C. Blackburn for indexing, B. Patel and T. Lou for the initial design and preparation of graphic materials, and C.Woods for proofreading. The typing, with endless revisions and working with endnotes, was done by T. Lou, D. Ngyuen, E. Park, and S. Lang. Formatting and the production of camera-ready copy was done by D. O'Shaughnessy. I thank B. Ostrandler and the staff of the University of Toronto Press for their help during the printing process. As co-authors in previous editions, my son Sunil provided me with valuable guidance in all phases of the preparation of the book and his brother, Rajiv, helped set the standard for summary at the end of each chapter. I thank Dr. J. Hastings for writing the foreword and Dr. F. Turcotte for adapting and translating the previous edition of this book in French and for committing to do the same for this edition. I would also like to extend my gratitude to the many teachers who have adopted this book as a textbook for their courses and to my students who have challenged and inspired me. Finally, I thank my wife, Sudha, for her patience and silent endurance throughout this entire process.

C.P. Shah
University of Toronto
Toronto, Ontario
July 1998

Dedicated to those who have enriched my life
My children Rajiv, Sunil, and Kausha, my brothers and their wives,
Yogesh and Kailas, Praful and Jyoti, Suman and Sharda, Chiman and
Lilam and my close friends, Manju and Ravi, Anjali and Ashwin,
Asha and Pankaj, Ruxmani and Vitthal and my colleagues,
Mary Jane, Mary, Harvey and Sylvia

Contents

Part Two
Health of Canadians

Chapter 11
Periodic Health Examinations 275

Part Three
Canada's Health Care System

Chapter 12
Evolution of National Health Insurance 283

Chapter 16
Regulation of Health Care Professionals 413

Chapter 17
Canadian Health Care into the 21st Century 431

Appendices and Index

Tables

Figures

Part One

Health and Disease

Concepts, Determinants, and Promotion of Health

Many diseases have been controlled or almost eradicated in Canada with the advent of better living conditions, the availability of antibiotics, and public health intervention such as immunization, new technology, and universal health care. Mortality in the population has been drastically reduced and life span has increased. Chronic diseases, however, have emerged as an important health concern. With these changes, our concepts of health and disease have changed. The focus of health care is shifting toward disease prevention, health promotion, and "caring" rather than "curing". In this chapter we describe modern concepts of health and disease or illness, the determinants of health and disease in the population, death and dying, and newer approaches to promoting and maintaining the health of the population.

1. CONCEPTS OF HEALTH AND DISEASE

1.1. CONTEMPORARY DEFINITIONS OF HEALTH

Health is multidimensional: it is not merely the presence or absence of disease but also has social, psychological, and cultural determinants and consequences. In 1948, the World Health Organization (WHO) was the first to acknowledge the multidimensional nature of health. The WHO defined health as: "A complete state of physical, mental and social well-being and not merely the absence of illness" (1). More recently, the WHO has developed a new definition of health that recognizes the inextricable links between an individual and his or her environment. This is a "socioecological" definition. As such, **health** is defined as: "The ability to identify and to realize aspirations, to satisfy needs, and to change or cope with the environment. Health is therefore a resource for everyday life, not the objective of living. Health is a positive concept emphasizing social and personal resources, as well as physical capacities" (2). Measures of health must incorporate these distinct dimensions of human experience. Determinants of health are more than biological. Health, therefore, involves more than just bodily integrity; it encompasses social and political concerns and the relationship of individuals to the environment in which they live. From this perspective, health is not just the responsibility of the traditional "health care" sector, but of all sectors, institutions, and organizations that may influence the well-being of individuals and communities.

Furthermore, the "new" definition of health provides the foundation for the developing concept of "health promotion" that was defined in the First International Conference on Health Promotion, held in Ottawa in 1986. (The conference declaration is known as the "Ottawa Charter for Health Promotion.") The definition of health promotion is "The process of enabling people to increase control over, and to improve, their health" (2). Health promotion efforts attempt to increase the degree of control that individuals and communities have over their health and the determinants of health.

1.2. CONCEPTS OF DISEASE AND ITS CONSEQUENCES

The strength of the current broad definition of health is that it includes psychosocial as well as biophysical dimensions. **Disease** refers to abnormal, medically defined changes in the structure or functioning of the human body, while **illness** (or sickness) refers to the individual's experience or subjective perception of lack of physical or mental well-being and consequent inability to function normally in social roles.

Disease and illness have their consequences; a useful systemic taxonomy was developed by Wood (3) for the WHO. He defines three concepts that refer to distinct and important dimensions of human experience in the context of disease. **Impairment** is defined as any loss or abnormality of psychological, physiological, or anatomical structure or function. **Disability** is any restriction or lack of ability to perform an activity in a manner or within the range considered normal for a human being. **Handicap** is defined as the disadvantage for a given individual, arising out of impairment and disability, that limits or prevents the fulfilment of a role that is normal (depending on age, sex, and social and cultural factors) for that individual as determined by society. Consequently, impairment refers to changes in the individual's body, disability to changes in what the individual can and cannot do, and handicap to changes in the individual's relationship with the physical and social environment. According to Wood, handicap can only be truly understood through sociologic enquiry. These concepts are linked dynamically in the following way:

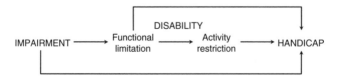

The relationships between impairment, disability, and handicap are not necessarily direct. Disability and handicap may result from impairment and handicap may be the outcome of disability, but these are not necessarily the case. Nor is there any necessary relationship between the severity of impairment and disability and the extent of handicap experienced. For example, a study of people with multiple sclerosis found that the psychosocial handicaps they experienced were not related to the severity of the underlying disease (4). Similarly, a study of individuals with chronic respiratory disease found that clinical measures of lung function were not good predictors of disability and that there was considerable variation in the extent of handicap associated with a given level of disability (5). This highlights the fact that these relationships are mediated by social, cultural and other factors.

The conceptual distinctions made in this scheme point to the many ways in which the well-being of people with various kinds of disorders may be improved. Clinical medicine has as its focus the limitation of impairment; rehabilitation is concerned with limiting disability and maximizing independent functioning, and social welfare mechanisms modify the disadvantage experienced by people with impairments and disabilities. For many people with chronic and disabling disorders, minimizing the social impact of their disease is the primary route to improving the well-being of both patient and family.

Illness behaviour can be defined as any activity undertaken by individuals who perceive they have a potential health problem for the purpose of defining their state of health and undertaking an appropriate remedy. The study of illness behaviour addresses the following question: In the presence of signs and symptoms, what will a person do, and why? This often, but not always, involves the use of medical care. Illness behaviour is significant because it determines the volume of professional services used, as they are currently provided by the health care system.

Research shows that most of the signs and symptoms that people experience are not brought to the attention of a medical professional but are dealt with in alternative ways. This phenomenon is known as the clinical iceberg and means that there is a permanent and irreducible gap between the need for medical care and the demand for it. The clinical iceberg is important for two reasons. First, many people tolerate symptoms that may be painful or otherwise distressing but may well respond to medical treatment. Second, cases of a particular disorder presenting for medical treatment may not be representative of cases of the disorder in the population. It is crucial to distinguish between factors related to the onset of the illness and factors related to the seeking of medical care. Illness behaviour depends on the level of medical knowledge, the perception of the costs and benefits associated with a medical consultation, and the influence of lay-referral networks.

One of the most important factors is cultural variation in perception of illness. People of differing cultural backgrounds interpret signs and symptoms in different ways. What may be regarded as part of the normal pattern of everyday life by one cultural group may indicate illness to another. There are also cultural differences in managing health problems of various kinds. Some cultural groups have highly developed systems of ethno-medicine; traditional and professional healers may be consulted according to the nature of the problem and whether or not it is recognized by scientific medicine. Culture is likely to play an important role in the formation and expression of health beliefs. The beliefs about health and illness held by individuals and groups are now seen as being very important with respect to the seeking of medical care, patient-practitioner communication, patient responses to consultation, and the degree of patient compliance with medical advice.

Compliance is the extent to which an individual follows the advice given by a health care provider or health educator. Compliance is a major factor in determining the success or failure of treatment regimens and lifestyle change directed toward improving health. Whether the individual will follow the advice depends upon many factors, including the nature of the health problem, the type, length, and cost of the regimen, the personality of the individual, and the pattern of communication between the provider and the individual. Although patient compliance with therapeutic regimens depends upon the severity, duration, and outcome of a disease, it is not always predictable. With lifestyle changes that require major effort and do not produce immediate benefits, such as smoking cessation, compliance rates are lower. Patients with psychiatric illness often have low compliance rates. Compliance improves when the care provider does not have a condescending attitude toward the patient, does not use professional jargon, and provides enough time for queries.

There are some general assumptions about the rate of adherence to a treatment regimen among the patient population. The rule of one third states that about one third of patients totally comply with treatment, one third partially complies, and the remaining third does not comply. Models that explain or predict the likelihood of compliance with health education efforts are described later in this chapter in the section on Health Education.

1.3. THEORIES OF DISEASE CAUSATION

Just as definitions of health have changed over time, so have theories about the nature and causes of disease. Recently the role ascribed to social and psychological factors in the causal processes leading to disease has received increasing attention. Underlying much of what constitutes medical practice is the **biomechanical/biomedical model**. This has its roots in the Cartesian revolution of the 17th century in which mind and body were seen as separate entities, the body being a physical entity activated by mental processes. According to this view, the body is akin to a machine, which can be corrected when things go wrong by procedures designed to repair damage or restore the functioning of its component parts. These procedures involve neutralizing the specific agents causing disease or modifying the pathological processes responsible for disease. Thus the model focuses on the causes and treatment of ill health and disease in terms of biological cause and effect. This approach largely ignores the part played by social, psychological, and economic factors in disease onset and recovery. Even in a speciality such as psychiatry, the biomedical model has prevailed in explaining abnormal behaviour. Genetic abnormalities and problems with the biochemistry or physical structure of the brain are some of the popular explanations for psychiatric disorders from the biomedical perspective.

The biomechanical/biomedical model is fully compatible with the **germ theory of disease**, which emerged at the end of the 19th century. Although the idea that disease was caused by a transmissible agent had existed since the 16th century, it was verified only during the latter half of the 19th century. The work of Pasteur and Koch showed that these agents were living organisms that enter the body via food, water, or air. From this theory emerged the doctrine of specific aetiology: the idea that each disease has a single and specific cause.

The germ theory suggests that the mere introduction of an organism into a community is sufficient to cause disease. This is clearly not the case; we are exposed to a wide variety of organisms yet rarely succumb to disease. Consequently, it is incorrect to designate an organism or other noxious agent as the sole cause of disease.

From an epidemiological point of view, such an agent is "necessary but not sufficient", since suitable conditions, with respect to the host and the environment, must be present for disease to develop (6). The epidemiological triangle portrays the interaction between agent, host, and environment (see figure below). The agent may be chemical (e.g., lead), biological (e.g., bacteria), or physical (e.g., violence); host factors may be genetic or acquired, and influence susceptibility to disease; environmental factors may be biological, social, or physical, and affect exposure and susceptibility. From this point of view, all diseases are multifactorial and can be prevented by procedures that modify either the host or the environment.

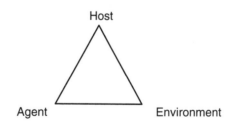

Often, in chronic degenerative disorders such as heart disease, no single agent can be identified. In order to explain disorders of this type, MacMahon and Pugh introduced the idea of a web of causation (7). Diseases such as heart disease develop through the interactions of many factors that form complex, interwoven chains. These factors may be biophysical, social, or psychological, and may promote or inhibit the development of the disease. For example, some of the factors implicated in heart disease are diet, smoking, physical inactivity, stress, Type A personality, obesity, cholesterol levels, hypertension, and diabetes. Some of these factors are also associated with the onset of other disorders such as cancer. More recently, the **theory of general susceptibility** has been developed to explain why some social groups are more vulnerable to disease in general. In this susceptibility theory, non-specific social and psychological factors are associated with a variety of health outcomes. For example, single, divorced, and widowed men have consistently higher mortality rates than married men. One explanation for these differences is that marital status is associated with a wide variety of psychological and lifestyle factors, some of which are related to the risk of disease and death. There is also an accumulating body of research that shows that a lack of social support or close social and emotional ties increases vulnerability to disease and death. This work is a direct challenge to the doctrine of specific aetiology.

2.   DETERMINANTS OF HEALTH

Traditionally, providers of health care working in hospitals, such as doctors and nurses, have been concerned primarily with diagnosing and treating existing disease in individuals (8). It has been widely believed that the quantity and quality of their services are the chief factors in determining the health of the population. Thus, the biomedical model has been pre-eminent. Furthermore, significant changes in health outcomes (such as decreasing morbidity and mortality rates) have been generally attributed to improvements in medical interventions. More recently, however, this view has been challenged and gradually replaced by more comprehensive concepts of health. The impetus for this broader view comes from two main sources.

First, a critical assessment of the history of disease reveals that major infectious diseases such as tuberculosis and cholera, which were the leading causes of death in western societies at the turn of this century, began to decline long before the introduction of effective therapy. Improvements in sanitation and general living conditions were much more important than medical intervention in reducing mortality due to these scourges. Second, the evaluation of the factors underlying today's major causes of death and disability has been illuminating. For example, motor vehicle accidents, which constitute the major cause of death and potential-years-of-life-lost in young adults, are largely the result of self-imposed risks and lifestyle habits. Mortality caused by accidents cannot be reduced by traditional forms of medical treatment, but rather by changes in behaviour, such as increased caution, sobriety, and use of seat belts. Therefore, a concept of health must include other factors in addition to traditional curative medicine.

A Canadian example of a more comprehensive view of the determinants of health is the health field concept put forward in 1974 by Marc Lalonde, Minister of Health, in *A New Perspective on the Health of Canadians* (9). Lalonde outlined four elements that interact to determine the health of Canadians: human biology, environment, lifestyle, and the health care organization. More recently, the fields have been modified to incorporate psychosocial factors such as gender and ethnicity. The fields are described on the following page.

2.1. HUMAN BIOLOGY

Human biology encompasses those aspects of health (both mental and physical) that are determined by the organic structure and physiological functioning of the human body. An individual's genetic make-up determines the likelihood of inherited disorders and predisposition to later acquired diseases. That person's constitution also determines susceptibility to risk factors that can arise from certain lifestyles and environments. Changes in the human body due to maturation and aging are important factors that can interact with the other three health field elements in determining the individual's state of health. Science has made great progress in understanding the complex processes of the human body and mind, but much remains to be elucidated.

2.2. THE ENVIRONMENT

The "physical" environment includes all factors external to the human body that may affect health. More recently, the concept of environment has expanded to include the "psychosocial" environment. Individuals often have little or no control over the presence of environmental risk factors but may be able to exercise some control over the degree of exposure.

2.2.1. The Physical Environment

Factors in the physical environment include the quality of air, water, and soil; the safety of food, drugs, and other products that humans consume or are exposed to; the physical handling and disposal of waste; and the control of excessive noise. The physical environment is both outdoors and indoors, and involves factors such as workplace ergonomics and indoor air quality (e.g., sick building syndrome). The physical environment can affect human health directly, for example by exposure to potentially hazardous agents such as chemicals or radiation, or indirectly, for example, by global warming, which is predicted to cause diminished food production. A major challenge is the development of economic production methods that sustain a healthy environment ("sustainable development") as a legacy for our children.

2.2.2. The Psychosocial Environment

The psychosocial environment also contributes to health and illness. Social and physical environments, the places where people live and work, education, and income and social supports, all have a major impact on health. To explore the role of social and psychological factors in disease, researchers have either adopted a historical perspective and investigated changes in the health of population over time, or have focused on specific factors that predispose an individual to illness. The best example of the former is provided by McKeown (10), who used careful historical analysis to show that the massive decline in mortality from infectious disease during the 18th and 19th centuries was not due to any specific medical interventions but was the product of social and environmental progress. In particular, improvements in agricultural production led to better nutrition and a population more resistant to infectious disease. Improvements in sanitation and clean water supplies reduced the exposure of the population to infectious organisms. By the time medicine had developed specific therapies for diseases such as tuberculosis, for example, 90% of the decline in mortality from that disease had already occurred.

Studies on contemporary population have looked at factors such as bereavement, social mobility, migration, cultural change, income, unemployment, and work hazards. Research on stressful life events and health applies a systematic approach to investigating social factors and illness, on the assumption that life changes, particularly those involving some form of loss, are stressful and render an individual vulnerable to health problems via a variety of mechanisms. Such events have been found to be related to the onset of psychiatric disorders such as depression and a range of physical illnesses (11). However, whether life stress leads to some form of illness depends on the presence of one or more mediating factors. Personality characteristics, coping styles, and the presence of social support are the main variables shown to influence the response to life stress. This is a complex area conceptually and methodologically, but current research indicates that an individual's social circumstances frequently exert a significant influence over health status.

The 1991 Ontario report of the Premier's Council on Health, Well-Being and Social Justice (12) on the determinants of health cites studies that conclude that both societal inequalities in income and powerlessness, or lack of perceived control, contribute to ill health in a community. Data from the Organization for Economic Cooperation and Development (OECD) indicate the lowest infant mortality and highest life expectancy occur where there are the least income inequalities. The study by Marmot et al. in the United Kingdom identified a strong association between the incidence of heart disease and the lack of decision-making latitude in the workplace (13). The Whitehall study demonstrated a clear relationship between place in the social hierarchy (as determined by position in the civil service in the United Kingdom) and mortality risk. Inequities may be horizontal, with unequal distribution of resources, or vertical, with those at a disadvantage without the resources to reduce differentials. Some social groups have markedly better health than others, with lower death rates and less illness and disability. It is for this reason that such inequities have recently been identified by the federal government and the government of Ontario as a major health policy issue. Socioeconomic status is the variable most commonly used in the analysis of inequities in health. All industrialized nations have some system for classifying their population into socioeconomic strata or groups. Such systems may be based on occupation, education or income, or some combination of all three. There are, of course, a number of other important variables related to health and mortality. Differences in health can also be connected to geographic location, gender, race, or ethnic origin, and employment status.

In Canada, until recently, relatively few data existed that documented the links between health and socioeconomic status. Data on provincial differences in health are more readily available. Nevertheless, the analysis of mortality data and data obtained from the Canada Health Survey provides evidence of the poorer health status of lower socioeconomic groups (14). In addition, Wilkins and Adams (15) used composite health indicators to show that overall life expectancy, years of life free of disability, and quality-adjusted life-years are directly related to income. Data from other countries have shown a clear inverse relationship between socioeconomic status and a wide range of health indicators, including acute and chronic illness rates, days of restricted activity, psychiatric symptoms, high blood pressure, height, obesity, low birth weight, prematurity, ability to conceive, and self-perceived health (16). Moreover, there is evidence to show that these differences have widened over the past four decades in spite of universal access to health care in many developed countries.

Explaining Socioeconomic Differences in Health

A number of explanations have been advanced to account for the association between socioeconomic status and health. The artefact explanation claims that such differences are not real but are a product of attempts to measure complex social entities such as socioeconomic status and health using inadequate instruments. However, the evidence concerning health inequities is overwhelming. Systematic gradients exist whether objective or subjective measures of health are used and whether socioeconomic status is measured by income, education, or occupation.

The theory of natural and social selection argues that inequities in health are created and maintained by a process of social mobility whereby healthy individuals move up the socioeconomic scale and less healthy individuals move down. Some studies confirm that conditions such as schizophrenia and chronic bronchitis often lead to a downward occupational drift, with the affected individual ending up in low-paid, unskilled, manual labour or unemployed. Other studies have shown that healthy women were more likely to be upwardly mobile at marriage, marrying men from a socioeconomic group higher than the one they were born in, while less healthy women tended to be downwardly mobile. Although these studies indicate that health can influence socioeconomic status, it is unlikely that this theory can fully account for the extent of the differences in health observed.

The materialist explanation suggests that inequities in health originate in material deprivation. That is, groups at the lower end of the socioeconomic scale lack adequate financial and other resources to maintain their physical and psychological well-being and to protect themselves from hazardous physical or social environments. Most of the evidence that supports this theory focuses on differences in income and wealth, working conditions, the quality of housing, and the nature of communities where people live. The lower socioeconomic groups are frequently disadvantaged in terms of all four of these factors. Evidence from numerous studies has demonstrated an inverse relationship between material deprivation and health. For example, differences in the health of children from different socioeconomic groups has been linked to poor quality housing and hazardous domestic environments. Overcrowding, damp conditions, and inadequate heating all affect health and are associated with increased rates of respiratory illness and deaths from accidents in the home. As well, people from lower socioeconomic groups often work in more hazardous environments and this is reflected in data on deaths from accidents at work, or deaths from occupationally related disease.

Cultural or behavioural theories seek explanations in reference to differences in knowledge, attitudes, and behaviours. Individuals in lower socioeconomic groups are considered less healthy because they consume health-damaging substances such as tobacco and alcohol at higher rates, have diets high in sugars and fats and low in fibre, are less likely to take exercise regularly, and make less use of preventive health services. This explanation is valid to the extent that lifestyles and consumption patterns are related to socioeconomic status and, in turn, are associated with the onset of conditions such as heart disease or cancer.

Clearly, the implications of the materialist and cultural explanations of inequities in health differ radically.

The materialist theory suggests that widespread social change is necessary to ensure that all individuals have equal opportunities for maintaining and improving their health. This involves a fundamental redistribution of resources in society in order to ensure that all have access to those goods and services necessary to produce health. The cultural theory is narrower in its implications and suggests that the remedy lies in health education to change health-damaging attitudes and behaviours. The problem with this approach is that it assumes such attitudes and behaviours are freely chosen, rather than environmentally induced, and it carries with it a tendency to blame the victim for situations over which they have relatively little control. As some have pointed out, cultural and behavioural patterns deleterious to health are rooted in the material conditions of life of people in the lowest socioeconomic groups. Efforts to change attitudes and behaviours are likely to fail if these material conditions are not addressed at the same time. This is embodied in the socioecological approach to health promotion, which regards social change as a prerequisite for changes at the individual level (17). Health-related behaviour does not occur independently of the influence of the surrounding physical and social environment.

A final factor that may contribute to differences in health status is inequality in access to and use of medical services. There is evidence from a number of Canadian jurisdictions that low-income groups use fewer family practitioner services in relation to need than their high-income counterparts. Differences in the quality of care have also been observed; patient-practitioner communication is one area in which the lower socioeconomic groups are particularly disadvantaged.

2.3. LIFESTYLE, BEHAVIOURS, AND RISK FACTORS

Lifestyle involves aspects of individuals' behaviour and surroundings that they control; although it takes into account that behaviour is influenced by the social and physical environment. A healthy lifestyle incorporates elements of social responsibility as well as individual responsibility and can be defined as comprising patterns of health-related behaviour, values, and attitudes adapted by groups of individuals in

Figure 1.1:   Risk Continuum

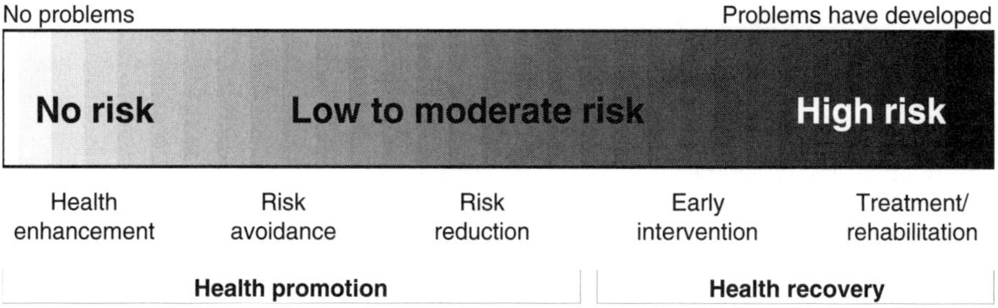

No problems   Problems have developed

No risk	Low to moderate risk	High risk

Health enhancement	Risk avoidance	Risk reduction	Early intervention	Treatment/ rehabilitation

Health promotion		Health recovery

Source: Ontario Ministry of Health: *A Framework for the Response to Alcohol and Drug Problems in Ontario*, 1988.

response to their social, cultural and economic environment" (18). The decisions that individuals make result in favourable or adverse consequences for health and play an important role in today's major health problems.

It is useful to consider the health effects of a lifestyle factor in terms of the degree of risk posed by a health-related behaviour. Figure 1.1 shows the risk continuum of alcohol consumption, an example of a substance abuse lifestyle factor (19). The level of risk indicates the most appropriate strategies, such as "health promotion" or "health recovery" programs. For individuals at minimal or no risk, further enhancement of health is appropriate, as is avoidance of risk. Consuming fewer than 14 drinks per week is generally defined as a low risk to health. For individuals at moderate levels of risk, reduction of risk is appropriate; they may be consuming more than 30 drinks per week and be experiencing problems such as impaired driving. Early (medical/social) intervention may be necessary. Higher levels of consumption are usually associated with significant health problems that require treatment and rehabilitation ("health recovery").

2.4. HEALTH CARE ORGANIZATION

The health care organization (HCO) is what is traditionally defined as the health care system. It includes medical and dental practice, nursing, hospitals, chronic care facilities, rehabilitation, drugs, public health services, and health services provided by allied health care professionals such as chiropractic, podiatric, and optometric services. The Canadian health care system is examined in detail in Chapters 12 to 17.

Although the health care system is primarily regarded as a means to alleviate or remediate the problems associated with ill health, it also contributes to morbidity and mortality. A New York hospital study found that 4% of patients had suffered an iatrogenic complication that prolonged hospital stay or resulted in measurable disability. Medication errors were common, occurring in 2 to 14% of patient stays, although not usually resulting in serious harm. Missed or incorrect diagnoses were also problematic (20). The extent of the problem in Canada has not been subject to systematic study.

2.4.1. Alternative Health Care

As the Canadian population becomes more cosmopolitan and heterogenous, many individuals seek to enhance their health by pursuing alternative health care modalities. A large number of traditions and practices are covered under this umbrella term. Homeopathy, naturopathy, acupuncture, ayurvedic medicine, herbology, and Aboriginal healing techniques are just a few examples. Epidemiologic studies have indicated that many Canadians seek alternative health care practices (21). Critics of alternative health care assert there is little or no evidence to support the efficacy of these modalities of care (22) and argue that they should not be funded by a public health care system. However, systematic analysis is ongoing, and scientific demonstration of benefit cannot be ruled out a priori for all practices.

2.5. EXPANDING THE DETERMINANTS OF HEALTH MODEL: POPULATION HEALTH

Population health is variously defined as the study of the determinants of health and disease, health status, and the degree to which health care affects the health of the community. The Canadian Institute of Advanced Research has instituted a population health program to extend the study of population health to incorporate the broad determinants of health. The conceptual framework for this approach is detailed in a book entitled *Why Are Some People Healthy and Others Not?* (23). This research framework seeks to explain how societal influences exert a profound influence on health and well-being throughout the life cycle. In particular, the integration of physical responses into social stimuli (psychoneuroimmunology) and the consequences of deprivation in early childhood development are currently being researched. The framework expands the Lalonde health field concept by synthesizing the vast empirical literature on diverse determinants and health outcomes. In broad terms, the population health model recognizes the following health determinants:

- Income and social status;
- Social support networks;
- Education;
- Employment and working conditions;
- Physical environment;
- Biology and genetic endowment;
- Personal health practices and coping skills;
- Healthy child development;
- Health services.

2.6. SPIRITUAL DIMENSIONS OF HEALTH

Spirituality encompasses the practices, beliefs, and values a person holds concerning his or her place in the cosmos. Spiritual people are often at peace with themselves or have what is called "inner peace" and feel connected with their fellow human beings and other creatures in a "meaningful and caring way" through their practice, beliefs, and values. Spirituality is related to, but not entirely synonymous with, religion, and its impact on health may be through a psychoneurohumoral mechanism that reduces stress and through social connectedness, which increases one's social network. The spiritual model incorporates a holistic approach in which healing plays a central role. Healing is different than treatment. Treatment focuses on discrete physical abnormalities with a view to mitigating them or curing the body. Healing applies to all dimensions of a person's existence: correcting a physical abnormality is but one aspect of a healing approach. How an illness affects the psychological and spiritual dimensions of the afflicted person's life must be considered. The use of sweat lodges in some Aboriginal healing practices illustrates this distinction. Prayers have been used in most cultures for healing; one randomized clinical trial indicated the power of intercessory prayer for the patients admitted to a coronary care unit (24).

2.6.1. Death and Dying

Technology has resulted in a range of techniques to prolong life. Such life-sustaining technologies have provoked concerns about their appropriate use, and more Canadians are reflecting upon the need to consider end-of-life care. Most provinces have introduced legislation regarding the use of advance directives, which permit individuals to document their preferences for the use of life-sustaining technologies while they are still competent. People may also nominate a proxy to make end-of-life decisions on their behalf. Related to this issue is the debate concerning euthanasia and physician-assisted suicide. The case of Susan Rodriguez, who had a chronic life-threatening and disabling condition and was assisted in terminating her life, brought the issue to the forefront of the Canadian consciousness in 1994 and stimulated vigorous debate that will no doubt continue for the foreseeable future.

3.   APPROACHES TO ACHIEVING HEALTH

Previous sections have described a shift in the concept of health from a predominantly biomedical view to a multidimensional concept. Interacting components of many aspects of life may affect health and are viewed as a resource for living. We now move on to a discussion of the implications for the prevention of disease and the attainment of health.

3.1. TRADITIONAL MODEL OF PREVENTION

Traditionally, there have been three approaches to disease prevention: primary, secondary, and tertiary. Primary prevention is aimed at preventing disease before it occurs, thereby reducing the incidence of disease. Examples include immunization programs, dietary recommendations, avoidance of initiating smoking, and the use of seat belts and other protective devices. Secondary prevention involves the early detection of disease and the treatment that may accompany screening. Tertiary prevention attempts to reduce death and disease by treatment and rehabilitation of diseased individuals, and is carried out by the existing health care system.

Many primary and secondary preventive measures for patients of medical practitioners are incorporated in the periodic health examination, which is fully described in Chapter 11. The remainder of this chapter concentrates on population health and emphasizes approaches that are more appropriate for the community.

3.2. HEALTH PROMOTION: EPP'S FRAMEWORK

The traditional model of prevention has commonly employed the modification of human biology (e.g., developing antibodies by vaccine), the environment (e.g., clean water supply), or the organization of health care services (e.g., mass screening for phenylketonuria). However, the paradigm shift in understanding the determinants of disease described in the Lalonde health field concept requires non-traditional approaches to prevention in order to have additional impact on the health of Canadians. The objective is to change unhealthy lifestyles and environments. These approaches are embodied in the concept of health promotion, which first gained legitimacy in the 1974 Lalonde document. A newly emergent concept is the use of different communication techniques to enhance health or to encourage the maintenance of an existing healthy lifestyle.

The Declaration of Alma Ata on Primary Health Care (25) in 1978 set the international stage for numerous initiatives in health promotion. Notable was *Targets for Health for All by 2000* (26) adopted by the European Region of the WHO. This document proposed improvements in health, specified the locus of action, and provided tools to monitor progress toward health goals. The United States began to develop health goals based on health promotion and disease prevention with the publication of *Healthy People*: *The Surgeon General's Report on Health Promotion and Disease Prevention* (27) published in 1979. This report was followed by the development of 226 specific objectives with target dates for achievement and, more recently, by a mid-course review.

Within Canada, the concepts of health promotion served as a basis for a reformulation of national and provincial health policies. At a national level, in 1986 the Honourable Jake Epp, Minister of National Health and Welfare, released *Achieving Health for All*: *A Framework for Health Promotion* (28). Subsequently, Health and Welfare Canada, the European Region of the WHO, and the Canadian Public Health Association endorsed the Ottawa Charter for Health Promotion (2), which provides a clear vision of current health promotion concepts and calls on all concerned to join forces to introduce strategies for health promotion that affect the moral and social values that support the Charter. In Ontario, three government reports strongly endorsed the principles of health promotion and made specific recommendations designed to incorporate these into government health policy (29-31). The Quebec government has undertaken a major health planning project called Objectif Santé (32), which incorporates principles of health promotion in selecting specific health improvement objectives.

Achieving Health for All outlined three major challenges that are not being addressed adequately by current health policies and practices. The first problem is that disadvantaged groups have significantly lower life expectancy, poorer health, and a higher prevalence of disability than the average Canadian (see Chapter 6); second, various forms of preventable diseases and injuries continue to undermine the health and quality of life of many Canadians; and third, many thousands of Canadians suffer from chronic disease, disability, or various forms of emotional stress, and lack adequate community support to help them cope and live meaningful, productive, and dignified lives. The Epp document calls for health promotion directed at these three problems and refers to the WHO's definition of health promotion: "the process of enabling people to increase control over, and to improve, their health". It outlines three mechanisms intrinsic to health promotion, namely self care (the decisions and actions that individuals take in the interest of their own health), mutual aid (the actions people take to help each other cope), and healthy environments (the creation of conditions and surroundings conducive to health). Implementation requires three strategies: fostering public participation, strengthening community health services, and coordinating healthy public policies. This approach integrates ideas from public health, health education, and public policy, and expands the term "health promotion" to complement and strengthen the existing system of health care. The differences between the concepts of disease prevention and health promotion are indicated in Table 1.1. The table also highlights the complementary nature of these approaches, which means they can be utilized in combination (33).

3.3. HEALTH PROMOTION STRATEGIES

A number of strategies have been developed or adapted for the promotion of health. Many of them are aimed at influencing healthy behaviours and the determinants of health that influence these behaviours. Methods that involve changes in lifestyle may include a number of approaches directed at the individual or community level. Health promotion approaches in general, as articulated in the Ottawa Charter, involve advocacy for health, the enabling of people to achieve the conditions necessary for reaching their full potential for health, and mediation by health care professionals between differing groups in society in the interests of health. Specific strategies include education, communication, legislation, fiscal measures, community organizational change, community development, and local community action (34). Legislation and fiscal

Table 1.1:   Disease Prevention versus Health Promotion Approach

Health promotion	Disease prevention
Health = positive and multidimensional concept	Health = absence of disease
Participatory model of health	Medical model
Aimed at the population in its total environment	Aimed mainly at high-risk groups in the population
Concerns a network of issues	Concerns a specific pathology
Diverse and complementary strategies	One-shot strategy
Facilitating and enabling approaches	Directive and persuasive strategies
Incentive measures offered to the population	Directive measures enforced in target groups
Changes in man's status and his environment sought by the program	Focused mostly on individuals and groups of subjects
Non-professional organizations, civic groups, local, municipal, regional and national governments necessary for achieving the goal of health promotion	Preventive programs considered the affairs of professional groups from health disciplines

Source: Stachenko, S., and Jenicek, M. *Conceptual Differences between Prevention and Health Promotion: Research Implications for Community Health Programs.* Canadian Journal of Public Health. 81:53-9, 1990. Reprinted with permission.

measures may affect policy that has not traditionally fallen under the purview of health, constituting a strategy called "healthy public policy". Communication and education, in conjunction with other approaches such as community organization, may be directed to whole population. This strategy is called community-based prevention. Finchman has provided an excellent Canadian review of the theory, strategies, and outcomes of community-based health promotion programs discussed below (35).

New Directions

The framework for population health has been combined with health promotion concepts in a document entitled *Population Health Promotion: An Integrated Model of Population Health and Health Promotion* (36). This document synthesizes the elements of the population health approach to the broad determinants of health with the strategies and techniques of health promotion as outlined in the Ottawa Charter and the Epp framework. Figure 1.2 shows the interrelationship of the elements of the population health promotion framework. Each element can be extracted so that health promotion strategies can be developed at the social, sectoral (e.g., the agricultural industry), local community, family, or individual level. The framework is also explicit in noting that the choice depends on values and assumptions about desirable health-related goals that must be mediated through evidence and evaluation. The model provides a synoptic view of the manner by which health promotion strategies can be conceived and implemented.

Figure 1.2:   Population Health Promotion Framework

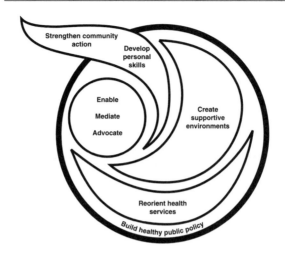

Source: Hamilton N. and Bhatti T. *Population Health Promotion.* Health Canada, 1996.

3.3.1. Health Education

Health education can be defined as any combination of learning experiences designed to facilitate voluntary actions conducive to health. The aim of health education is to encourage people to modify their lifestyles positively while also encouraging them to resist reverting to bad habits. People who have adopted unhealthy lifestyles often find it difficult to change their behaviour even if they want to. It is increasingly recognized that social influences affect behaviour. Without reinforcement from change in social norms, health education is less effective in producing a change in behaviour.

A number of theoretical views of behaviour change underlie the types of programs developed for health education. One unifying concept proposed by Green and Krenter (37) states that behaviour is a result of predisposing, reinforcing, and enabling factors. Predisposing factors comprise knowledge (for example, the health consequences of smoking), attitudes, beliefs, and values. Fishbein and Aizen (38) have found that the intention to change behaviour is also a strong predictor. Reinforcing factors (such as those provided by the social context of family, society, or health care professionals) involve reward or feedback for the discontinuation or adoption of behaviour. Enabling factors include skills such as behaviour modification techniques as well as the availability of relevant supports such as reasonably priced, low-fat foods that support dietary change.

Bandura (39) constructed an influential theory of social learning from a number of related concepts that must to be addressed in lifestyle education. There is a strong correlation between social learning principles and some health-related actions. The essential concept is of reciprocal determinism, which is recognition that social environment influences behaviour, which in turn affects environment. Behaviour is the result of personal and environmental factors. The importance of the social environment as the context for learning has been developed in the social influences model.

Apart from components of behavioural capability (the acquisition of skills and knowledge), reinforcements, and supportive social environments, there are other components of social learning theory. These are observation (such as with role models), expectations of positive results from behaviour change, expectancies (such as an improved appearance following weight loss, which may be a more potent motivator than the expected health benefits), perceptions of an individual's situation (e.g., what the consequences of pregnancy might be), and emotional factors that may pose barriers to behaviour change (such as anxiety associated with the anticipation of giving up a lifestyle habit).

Self-efficacy and self-control are components of behaviour change that are increasingly being incorporated into health education for sustained behaviour change. Self-efficacy refers to the cognitive state when one is confident that one can achieve a behaviour change. This may be reached by the achievement of short-term goals. Self-control relates to decision-making capacities for healthy choices and self-monitoring, such as those utilized in guided self-management programs for smoking cessation.

An important model, the health belief model (40) attempts to explain the factors influencing compliance (see Figure 1.3). This model suggests that behaviours undertaken by individuals in order to remain healthy, including the use of preventive services, are a function of a set of interacting beliefs. In order to be motivated to take action to avoid illness, an individual must be in a state of readiness to take action and must believe that the action will have positive consequences. In order to be ready to act, the individual needs to feel susceptible to the disease in question and to believe that it would have some significant impact on his or her life. Beliefs about the benefits of the action in question involve consideration of barriers to action such as time, cost, and inconvenience.

Current formulations of the model include the role of cues and modifying factors. Cues consist of specific events that act as a stimulus to preventive health behaviours. Modifying factors consist of sociodemographic variables such as age, sex, and race, sociopsychological variables such as personality and peer group pressure, and other variables such as knowledge of, and prior experience with, the disease. All of these factors influence the individual's perception of susceptibility to disease and seriousness, as well as perception of the benefits of health-related actions. This model has provided the foundation for many health education and awareness programs. One of the implications of this model is that these programs must be carefully targeted at specific social and cultural groups and must be based on a detailed understanding of their health beliefs.

More recently a stages-of-change model has provided a useful framework to understand how changes of lifestyle behaviour can be facilitated (see Figure 1.4) (41). In studies of cigarette smokers, four different stages were identified: stage 1 is a precontemplation stage where the individual was unaware of a behaviour-related health problem; stage 2 is a contemplation stage when change was considered; stage 3 is an action stage where initial attempts at change were made; and stage 4 is maintenance, or

Figure 1.3:   Health Belief Model

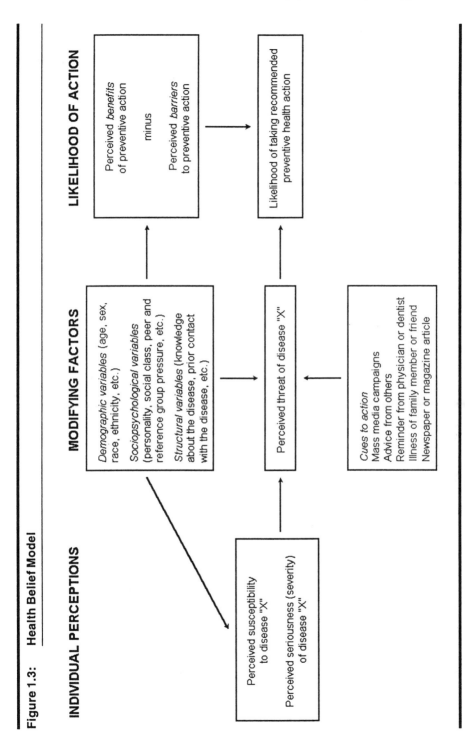

Source: Becker MH, Maiman LA.. *Sociobehavioral Determinants of Compliance with Health and Medical Care Recommendations. Medical Care* 13:1:12, 1975. Reproduced with permission.

long-term change. Individuals may not move through these stages in a linear fashion. There are barriers to change at each stage, as well as facilitative processes.

Evaluation of most health education programs has produced mixed results. Recent evidence indicates some effectiveness for skills training for young people to prevent smoking (in particular, peer-led learning) (42). There are indications that preventing alcohol abuse in drinking establishments by server-intervention education programs (which train servers to recognize and reduce client intoxication) has some effectiveness.

The models outlined above have also been applied to enhance compliance. A review of the literature by Butler et al. (43) indicates that the stages-of-change model can successfully aid the design of effective compliance strategies. Strategies that allow personal control over decision making also seem to be more successful in aiding behaviour change and increasing compliance.

3.3.2. Risk Reduction Strategies

An important concept that is emerging from the risk continuum is that of harm reduction (44, 45). Harm reduction holds that some behaviours cannot be eliminated by current knowledge and techniques. Consequently, harm reduction advocates tolerance of some degree of risk behaviour and seeks strategies designed to mitigate the adverse consequences associated with the behaviour. A good example of a harm reduction strategy is needle exchange. In a needle exchange program, the fact of intravenous drug use is acknowledged, but clean syringes are provided in order to lessen the risk of transmitting communicable diseases. Harm reduction strategies do not involve judgement of the unhealthy behaviour, although counselling may be offered if requested.

3.3.3. Communication/Behaviour Change

Information can be communicated effectively in a strategy to promote knowledge of health and its determinants. Mass media constitute an important tool for influencing awareness, knowledge, attitudes, and behaviour. The Stanford Five-City Study used mass media to affect behaviour in relation to cardiovascular risk factors on a community-wide basis (46). In the control city (which was comparable to the experimental community on a sociodemographic basis), prevalence of risk factors increased, while in the community in which given an intensive mass media approach was used there was a reduction in risk behaviours. A review of mass communication programs directed at alcohol abuse in Canada indicates that although attitudes and knowledge levels are affected, behaviour change frequently remains unchanged. There have been several studies that indicate that behaviour change was influenced (47). Mass media form one modality that assists in setting and framing the public agenda and is most effectively used in conjunction with other health promotion measures.

3.3.4. Social Marketing

Social marketing is another health promotion modality and applies the principles of commercial marketing to promote social change. It influences the acceptability of a

Figure 1.4:   The Stages of Change Model

The Five Stages of Change

Precontemplation: an individual is not seriously considering change (for all kinds of reasons) and isn't interested in any kind of intervention.

Contemplation: the individual begins to seriously consider making the change within the forseeable future (often defined as six months).

Preparation: the individual begins experimenting, making small changes. He or she resolves to make a serious attempt in the near future (usually defined as 30 days).

Action: the individual is actively involved in making the change, using different techniques.

Maintenance: the individual must learn to successfully cope with temptations to return to the previous behaviour pattern.

Adapted from: Prochaska JO, DiClemente CC, and Norcross JC, *In Search of How People Change. Applications to Addictive Behaviours.* Am Psychol 47(9):1102-1114, 1992.

social idea by a target group. Key concepts are the "marketing mix" of four variables: product, price, place, and promotion. The product may be "good health," for example (47). The price, a concept based on exchange theory, represents what consumers must give up if they accept the health promoter's offer. The place concerns the distribution channels used to reach the consumer, such as the distribution of leaflets on AIDS through clinics serving the population at risk for sexually transmitted diseases. Promotion is the way in which the product is promoted to the customer; examples are advertising or personal endorsements. Social marketing is a planned activity that involves target group analysis based on demographics and segmentation of the market for specific messages and channels. It is possible to increase the effectiveness of social marketing to reach non-responsive people by focusing the messages on the actual actions involved in a behaviour, the target of the action, or the context and time of the behaviour (48).

3.3.5. Healthy Public Policy

Healthy public policy is one of the major strategies for achieving health. For example, even though early models of cars had seat belts and the general public was somewhat aware of their benefit in case of an accident, few people used seat belts. Compliance improved when a fine was imposed by legislation if passengers were found not wearing seat belts. Rising health costs and the economic burden of motor vehicle accidents appeared to be a determining factor in the introduction of this legislation, especially since other countries had achieved positive results. Seat belt usage in Ontario increased to 71% with early and strict enforcement of the legislation in 1976, but adherence declined to 36% in 1978 as a result of less stringent enforcement by authorities (49), indicating that most people were unwilling to accept responsibility for their own health unless some authority ensured the behaviour occurred. With stricter enforcement of the law again, seat belt usage in Ontario climbed back to 91% in 1994.

Thus, despite people's awareness of certain risk-taking behaviour and its associated health hazards, many still resist change. Various adverse behaviour patterns appear more desirable and attractive by the use of sophisticated advertising techniques. The implementation of legal deterrents to individual behaviours such as seat belt legislation, anti-smoking bylaws, or legal drinking age is an approach to overcoming these barriers to change. Government control is also mediated by tax and pricing policies with the objective of reducing accessibility of certain "luxury" commodities (such as cigarettes and alcohol) to the public by raising prices. The effectiveness of these economic policies depends on the amount of the individual's disposable income. Programs based on personal motivation and behavioural change take much longer to effect change and involve a smaller percentage of the participating public. Yet such programs must not be ignored, because it is important for individuals to be responsible for their own health, in addition to the external imposition of rules and regulations.

The Epp document (28) differs from the Lalonde report (9), which mainly advocated healthy lifestyles and a safe environment. Epp's document better reflects current thinking at the international level, which has a broader perspective on health promotion and recommends healthy public policies for achieving good health for all. Healthy public policies espouse the concept that responsibility for improving health lies beyond traditional health policies, such as universal health insurance. Social policies favouring affordable housing, public transportation, and income maintenance have more impact on the health of the Canadian population than the infusion of additional resources in the health care sector. Due to the intersectoral and multisectoral nature of the determinants of health, healthy public policies must be part of the agenda of government departments and private agencies that would not normally consider health a priority.

3.3.6. Community Organization and Community Development

In the Epp document, enhanced public participation is a major strategy. The nature and extent of public participation can be conceptualized along a spectrum of increasing community capacity to respond to issues of community concern. Community efficacy represents the state of community confidence necessary to bring about desired social change (50). Mechanisms include lobbying, coalition-building, and political action. Community development refers to the process of community members identifying issues and problems affecting their community, and developing and acquiring, as necessary, the planning skills and capacity to bring about the implementation of change. Health care organizations, such as public health departments, may facilitate this community-initiated and directed process.

Community organization also involves the identification of problems within a community and the mobilizing of resources for change (51). However, the process is driven to some extent by the goals and strategies established by the health care sector, and assists the community to achieve the change. Three elements of community organization have been identified: social planning, which implies the rational solution of problems using the existing power structure, community locality development or the development of a community for an organized approach to a given problem, and social action, which implies a shift in power structures in the community. Organizing occurs when interest is focused on a concern by the development of leadership, commitment, bargaining, protest, education, and persuasion. This may result in changes within administrative structures themselves, or "inter-organizing" the development of joint structures for community problem solving.

These strategies can be integrated into a concept that views an entire community as the focus of health promotion. In the healthy cities framework, health-enhancing strategies are integrated into urban planning and community design (52). Elements of a healthy city include a clean and safe physical environment, a sustainable ecosystem, the meeting of basic human needs, and a strong and supportive community in which decision making is shared by all. The strategy involves including health promotion issues on the political agenda so that key decision makers and the community at large make prevention and health promotion highly visible and community supported. Over 300 cities are participating in a project sponsored by the WHO. Canadian involvement in the healthy cities movement is prominent, as the conception of the healthy cities movement originated by Trevor Hancock at the Beyond Health Care conference held in Toronto in 1984.

3.3.7. Community-Based Prevention

Recognition of the prevalence of multiple preventable factors in communities has resulted in the application of multiple health promotion modalities. The emergence of the community-based approach complements, or replaces, a high-risk approach that focuses on specific risk factors or special high-risk groups. For example, the Canadian Heart Health Initiative has pilot projects in many provinces that are population-based, multifactorial approaches that incorporate combinations of communication-behaviour change, community organization, and social marketing (53). Other programs such as the Heartbeat Wales Project, the Minnesota Heart Health Program, and the Pawtucket Program are using selections of the various approaches discussed above. Evidence supporting the effectiveness of community-wide prevention was initially provided by the North Karelia Project in Finland, which showed a reduction in cardiovascular mortality subsequent to the introduction of a community-wide prevention program, and the Stanford Five-City Project in which cardiovascular risk factors decreased after five years (46).

3.3.8. Innovation-Diffusion Theory

Complementary theories have developed to explain the process by which health promotion innovations spread in communities and to identify the most effective ways to encourage people to adopt a different behaviour. Roger's theory of diffusion conceptualizes a population as composed of innovators, early adapters, an early majority, a late majority, and those who resist most efforts for change. Community leaders tend to be early adapters and can be effective as project advisors. Other characteristics of an innovation affecting its adoption are whether it is simple, workable, reversible, flexible, advantageous, cost effective, low risk, and compatible with value systems. Elder has applied concepts of behaviour modification (i.e., positive and negative consequences) in a theory of behavioural community psychology.

4.   SUMMARY

This chapter outlines the concepts of health and disease, determinants of health, and approaches to achieving health.

Health has been defined in various ways. In this book, the definition set out by the WHO is used: *Health* is the ability to identify and to realize one's aspirations, to satisfy one's needs, and to change or cope with one's environment. Thus health is a daily resource rather than the objective of living, and emphasizes social and personal resources, and physical capacities.

Impairment is any loss or abnormality of psychosocial, physiological, or anatomical structure or function. *Disability* is any restriction or inability to perform an activity in a way considered normal, whereas *handicap* is the disadvantage experienced by someone with an impairment and disability that limits or prevents the fulfilment of a role that is normal for that person.

Illness behaviour can be any activity undertaken by someone who perceives a potential health problem for the purpose of defining his or her state of health and for undertaking an appropriate remedy. Illness behaviour depends on many factors, one of which is cultural background.

There are several theories of disease causation. One, the *biomechanical/biomedical model*, holds that the body is like a machine that can be corrected by procedures designed to repair damage or restore functioning. According to the *germ theory of disease*, a living organism enters the body via food, water, or air, and hence each disease has a single and specific cause. The most recent is the *theory of general susceptibility*, which holds that broad, non-specific social and psychological factors are associated with a variety of health outcomes.

The *determinants of health* include the individual's human biology (those aspects of both mental and physical health that arise out of the basic biology of humans or are due to the organic make up of the individual), the individual's physical and psychosocial environment (factors in the physical environment that include food, drugs, air and water quality, and waste disposal),   lifestyle, behaviour and modifiable risk factors (aspects of an individual's behaviour and surroundings over which he or she has some control), and health care organization.

Approaches to achieving health include prevention and health promotion strategies. There are three levels of *prevention*: primary, secondary, and tertiary. Primary prevention is aimed at preventing disease before it occurs. Secondary prevention involves early detection of disease and the treatment that may accompany screening. Tertiary prevention attempts to reduce complications by treatment and rehabilitation. *Health promotion* is defined as "the process of enabling people to increase control over, and to improve, their health". A number of *health promotion strategies* have been developed or adapted for the promotion of health and include education, communication-behaviour change, social marketing, healthy public policy (including fiscal measures and legislation), community development and organization, community-wide prevention, and diffusion of innovations.

5.   REFERENCES

1.   Culyer AJ. Health Indicators. Oxford: Martin Robertson, 1983.
2.   Canadian Public Health Association and WHO. Ottawa Charter for Health Promotion. Ottawa: Health and Welfare Canada, 1986.
3.   Wood P. The Language of Disablement: A Glossary Relating to Disease and its Consequences. International Journal of Rehabilitative Medicine 1980;2(2):86-92.
4.   Harper AC, Wood P, Chambers L, Cino PM, Singer J. An Epidemiological Description of Physical, Social and Psychological Problems in Multiple Sclerosis. Journal of Chronic Disease 1986;39(4):305-310.

5. Williams SJ, Bury MR. Impairment, Disability and Handicap in Chronic Respiratory Illness. Social Science and Medicine 1989;29(5):609-616.
6. Rothman KJ. Modern Epidemiology. Toronto: Little, Brown and Co., 1986.
7. MacMahon B, Pugh T. Epidemiological Principals and Methods. Boston: Little, Brown and Co., 1970.
8. Bunker JS, Frazier HS, Mosteller F. The Role of Medical Care in Determining Health: Creating an Inventory of Benefits. In Amick III BC, Levine S, Tarlov AR, Walsh D (Edso). Society and Health. New York: Oxford University Press, 1995.
9. Lalonde M. A New Perspective on the Health of Canadians. Ottawa: Ministry of Supply and Services, 1975.
10. McKeown T, Record RG and Turner RD. An Interpretation of Decline in Mortality in England and Wales During the Twentieth Century. Population Studies 1975;29(3):391-422.
11. Brown G, Harris T. The Social Origins of Depression. London: Tavistock, 1979.
12. Premier's Council on Health, Economics and Social Justice. Nurturing Health. A Framework for the Determinants of Health. Toronto: Healthy Public Policy Committee, 1991.
13. Marmot M. Socioeconomic Determinants of Coronary Heart Disease Mortality. International Journal of Epidemiology 1989; 18(suppl 1):196-202.
14. Manga P. Equality in Access and Inequalities in Health Status. In Coburn D, D'Arcy C, Torrance G, New P (Eds.). Health and Canadian Society. Markham: Fitzhenry and Whiteside, 1987.
15. Wilkins R, Adams O. Healthfulness of Life: A Unified View of Mortality, Institutionalization, and Non-Institutionalized Disability in Canada. Montreal: Institute for Research on Public Policy, 1983.
16. MacIntyre S. The Patterning of Health by Social Position in Contemporary Britain: Directions for Sociological Research. Social Science and Medicine 1986;23(4):393-415.
17. Community Health Information Section, Department of Public Health. Human Inequalities in the City of Toronto. Toronto: City of Toronto, 1991.
18. Conway J. With Gun and Camera in Darkest Ontario: Searching for Elusive Health Lifestyle Concept. Public Health and Epidemiology Reports Ontario 1992;3(16):268-269.
19. Ministry of Health. A Framework for the Response to Alcohol and Drug Problems in Ontario. Toronto: Government of Ontario, 1988.
20. Leape I. Error in Medicine. Journal of American Medical Association 1994; 272(23):1851-1857.
21. Verhoef M, Russel M, Love E. Alternative Medicine Use in Rural Alberta. Canadian Journal of Public Health 1994;85(5):308-309.
22. Brigden ML. Unproven Cancer Therapies: A Multi-Headed Hydra. Annals of Royal College of Physicians and Surgeons of Canada 1998;31(1):9-14.
23. Evans RG, Barer ML, Marmor TR. (Eds). Why Are Some People Healthy and Others Not? New York: Aldine de Gruyter, 1994.
24. Byrd R. Positive Therapeutic Effects of Intercessory Prayer in a Coronary Care Unit Population. Southern Medical Journal 1988;81(7):826-829.
25. World Health Organization. International Conference on Primary Health Care, Alma Ata, USSR, 1978. Geneva: WHO, 1978.
26. World Health Organization. Targets for Health for All by the Year 2000. Copenhagen: WHO Regional Office for Europe, 1984.
27. U.S. Department of Health Education and Welfare. Healthy People: The Surgeon General's Report on Health Promotion and Disease Prevention. Washington, DC: 1979.
28. Epp J. Achieving Health for All: A Framework for Health Promotion. Ottawa: Ministry of Supply and Services, 1986.

29. Report of the Ontario Health Review Panel, Evans J (Chair). Toward a Shared Direction for Health in Ontario. Toronto: Ministry of Health, Government of Ontario, 1987.

30. Ministry of Health, Spasoff RS (Chair). Health for All Ontario. Toronto: Government of Ontario, 1987.

31. Ministry of Health, Podborski S (Chair). Health Promotion Matters in Ontario: A Report of the Minister's Advisory Group on Health Promotion. Toronto: Government of Ontario, 1987.

32. Comité d'Étude sur la Promotion de la Santé. Objectif Santé. Quebéc: Direction Générale des Publications Gouvernementales, Gouvernement de Québec, 1984.

33. Stachenko S, Jenicek M. Conceptual Differences Between Prevention and Health Promotion: Research Implications for Community Health Programs. Canadian Journal of Public Health 1990;81(1):53-59.

34. Noack H, McQueen D. Health Promotion Indicators. Health Promotion 1988;3(1):1-125.

35. Finchman S. Community Health Promotion Programs. Social Science and Medicine 1992;35(3):239-249.

36. Hamilton N, Bhatti T. Population Health Promotion: An Integrated Model of Population Health and Health Promotion. Ottawa: Health Promotion Development Division, Health Canada, 1996.

37. Green LW, Kreuter MW. Health Promotion Planning; An Educational and Environmental Approach (2nd ed.) Toronto: Mayfield Publishing Company, 1991.

38. Fishbain M, Aizen I. Beliefs, Attitudes, Intentions and Behaviours: Introduction to Theory and Research. Massachusetts: Addison-Wesley Press, 1975.

39. Bandura A. Social Learning Theory. New York: General Learning Press, 1971.

40. Becker MH, Drachman RH, Kirscht JP. A New Approach to Explaining Sick-Role Behaviour in Low-Income Populations. American Journal of Public Health 1974;64(3):205-216.

41. DiClemente C, Prochaska JO, Fairhurst SK, et al. The Process of Smoking Cessation: An Analysis of Precontemplation, Contemplation, and Preparation Stages of Change. Journal of Consulting and Clinical Psychology 1991;59(2):295-304.

42. Shea S, Basch CA. Review of Five Major Community-Based Cardiovascular Disease Prevention Programs. Part 1: Rationale, Design and Theoretical Framework. American Journal of Health Promotion 1990;4(3):203-213.

43. Butler C, Rollnick S, Stott N. The Practitioner, the Patient and Resistance to Change: Recent Ideas on Compliance. Canadian Medical Association Journal 1996;154(9): 1357-1362.

44. Des Jarlais D. Harm Reduction: A Framework for Incorporating Science into Drug Policy. American Journal of Public Health 1995;85(1):10-11.

45. Canadian Centre on Substance Abuse National Working Group on Policy. Understanding Harm Reduction. The Journal 1997;26(4):8.

46. Shea S, Basch C. Review of Five Major Community-Based Disease Prevention Programs. Part 2: Intervention Strategies, Evaluation Methods, and Results. American Journal of Health Promotion 1990;4(4):279-287.

47. Hastings G, Haywood A. Social Marketing and Communication in Health Promotion. Health Promotion International 1991;6(2):135-145.

48. McDonald PA. Framework for Using Social Marketing with Non-Responsive High-Risk Populations. Public Health and Epidemiology Reports Ontario 1992;3(7):105-109.

49. Robertson LS. The Seat Belt Law in Ontario: Effects on Actual Use. Canadian Journal of Public Health 1978;69(2):154-157.

50. Wallerstein N. Powerlessness, Empowerment, and Health Implications for Health Promotion Programs. American Journal of Health Promotion 1992;6(3):199-205.

51. Bracht N, Tsouros A. Principles and Strategies of Effective Community Participation. Health Promotion International 1990;5(3):199-208.
52. Kickbusch I. Healthy Cities: A Working Project and Growing Movement. Health Promotion 1989;4(2):77-82.
53. The Canadian Heart Health Initiative, Health and Welfare Canada. Insert. Health Promotion 1992;30(4):2-19.

Chapter

2

Measurement and Investigation

As indicated in the previous chapter, concepts of health and disease are changing and are multidimensional. To measure health, both quantitative and qualitative data are used. The science of epidemiology has been widely used for quantitative approaches to studying the health of populations. This chapter provides an overview of the principles of epidemiology and some basics of statistics. The reader is referred to standard epidemiology texts for an in-depth treatment of this subject (1-4).

1. EPIDEMIOLOGICAL STUDIES

Epidemiology is "the study of the distribution and the determinants of health-related states and events (such as diseases) in specified populations, and the application of this study to the control of health problems" (5). The distribution of disease is studied in terms of person, place, and time. **Person** attributes include age, sex, race, and ethnicity. **Place** factors include location of residence, work, and school, and can involve comparisons between urban and rural, between north and south, and among different countries. **Time** factors describe the occurrence of health events per specified unit of time and trends over different periods of time. The determinants of diseases may be studied in terms of at-risk (demographic) groups, lifestyle factors (e.g., diet, smoking), occupation, and environment (physical, psychosocial, political, and economic).

In recent years the science of epidemiology has been well recognized for investigating epidemics and identifying new health problems in populations. Examples include "unusual" infectious diseases (e.g., AIDS, Lyme disease, Legionnaires' disease, toxic shock syndrome), exposure to environmental and occupational hazards (e.g., ozone pollution, pesticides, asbestos), and diseases for which no agent has yet been identified (e.g., Reye's syndrome, Kawasaki disease). Epidemiologists use certain methodologies to identify and evaluate the causal or contributing factors to disease, its distribution, and possible means of prevention.

1.1. DESCRIPTIVE STUDIES

An epidemiologic descriptive study describes the occurrence of disease or other phenomena in terms of person, place, and time. For example, a study of children in the care of child welfare agencies revealed that 400 per 1,000 such children were disabled. One cannot make any causal attribution from descriptive studies; those studies may, however, generate hypotheses that may be investigated by further study. In this example, one may hypothesize that children with disabilities are more likely to come into public wardship than those with no disabilities. This hypothesis may be tested in an analytic study.

1.2. ANALYTIC STUDIES

In analytic studies, a hypothesis is tested to discover if there is an association between a given disease, health state, or other dependent variable (outcome), and possible causative factors. Analytic studies are of two types: observational and experimental.

1.2.1. Observational Studies
There are four types of observational studies:

Ecological Studies
Ecological studies differ from other observational studies in that the method of analysis does not involve individuals, but analyses an aggregate. Commonly, geographic areas, such as countries or census tracts, are used as units of analysis, and differences between exposures and outcomes of interest are compared. The recent interest in dietary epidemiology stems from the comparison of disease rates among countries with varying diets.

Ecological studies generate hypotheses, so they cannot be used for the direct assessment of causal relationships because adequate control of all confounding variables cannot be achieved. Interpretation of ecological studies must avoid the ecological fallacy, whereby inferences about relationships between individuals are made inappropriately (6). Ecological data can provide accurate descriptions of the average exposure or the average risk of disease for populations, but nothing can be inferred about any particular individual in the population, because data were not collected on individuals.

Cross-sectional or Prevalence Study
In this type of study, the prevalence of diseases, disability, and risk factors are examined in a defined population at one particular time (5). The population is divided

into those with and without the disease, and then various characteristics of the two groups are examined. The total population can also be divided according to different variables such as age or sex. **Prevalence rates** are calculated by dividing the number of individuals who have an attribute or disease at a particular time by the population at risk of having that attribute or disease at the same point in time. Most data obtained in surveys, including census data, report prevalence rates.

Retrospective Study

Retrospective studies "test aetiological hypotheses in which inferences about exposure to the putative causal factor(s) are derived from data relating to characteristics of the persons under study or to events or experiences in their past" (5). "Retrospective" means looking back in time; hence, a retrospective study begins after the disease has already appeared. Usually it takes the form of a **case-control study**, in which persons with a rare disease of interest (cases) are compared to similar persons without the disease (controls) who have had similar opportunity for exposure to the presumed causal factor. Investigators collect data by examining medical and other relevant records, and by interviewing cases and controls. If the presumed factor (variable) is present in cases significantly more frequently than in controls, then an association exists between this variable and the disease. This association is expressed by the **odds ratio**, the ratio of the odds in favour of exposure among cases to the odds of exposure among non-cases.

Retrospective studies are less costly and time consuming than prospective studies, but they may suffer from recall bias; people with a disease may be more prone to recalling, or believing, that they were exposed to a possible causal factor, compared to those who are free of disease. Retrospective studies may also show a spurious association between a factor and a health outcome because of unrecognized **confounding**. Confounding occurs when a variable is related to both the exposure and the outcome but is either not measured or is unequally distributed in the comparison groups. For example, a study that sought to investigate the relationship between coffee drinking and heart disease found a strong relationship between increased coffee consumption and heart disease but did not measure cigarette smoking. In this case it is likely that the association between coffee drinking and heart disease is confounded by cigarette smoking, if in fact more smokers are found among those with heart disease in a subsequent study.

An example of a retrospective study is an investigation by Denson et al. (7) into the relationship between smoking mothers and hyperactive children. The cases were the mothers of 20 hyperkinetic children. The mothers of 20 children with dyslexia (reading disabilities) and the mothers of 20 children brought to the emergency room as a result of minor accidents comprised two control groups. Controls were matched to cases by age, sex, and socioeconomic status, so that there was no significant difference between the three groups on these variables. The use of matched controls permits a study to attain significance with relatively few subjects. Study results indicated that the mothers of hyperkinetic children smoked significantly more (23 cigarettes per day on average) than the mothers of children in the two control groups, who smoked on average six and eight cigarettes a day respectively. This does not prove that maternal

Table 2.1:   Comparison of Cohort and Case-Control Studies

	Cohort study	Case-control study
Advantages	Provides incidence rates, relative risk, and attributable risk Less bias Can get natural history of disease Can study many diseases	Small number of subjects Quick to do Suitable for rare diseases Inexpensive Can study many factors
Disadvantages	Large number of subjects Long follow-up Attrition Costly Changes over time Locked into factor under investigation	Recall bias Provides only odds ratio (an estimate of relative risk) Problems in control group selection Does not yield incidence rate Incomplete recall Locked into disease

smoking causes the hyperkinetic syndrome, but the association in this study and others should stimulate more research into a possible mechanism.

Prospective or Cohort Study

This type of study may be considered an organized observation of a natural experiment. A **cohort** is a group of people with a common characteristic (e.g., year of birth, residence, occupation, or exposure to a suspected cause of disease) that may be followed over time by investigators. Hence cohort studies are also called **prospective** (looking forward in time). (Some cohort studies are called "retrospective" if the whole period of observation is historical, but the cohort's outcomes are still analysed from the beginning to the end of the period, that is, forward in direction.). From a defined population free of the disease under study, a cohort who becomes exposed to the hypothesized causal factor is chosen, along with a "control cohort" who ideally has the same characteristics except that it is not exposed to this factor. Both groups are followed for a certain period of time (e.g., 5, 10, or 20 years) and the observed occurrence of disease or other outcomes in the two cohorts are compared.

Prospective studies provide an estimate of the **incidence rate**, the rate at which new disease or other events in a defined population occur over a given time period. The numerator consists of the number of new events (e.g., new cases of a disease diagnosed or reported) over a given time period, and its denominator is the number of people in the population in whom the cases occurred. Prospective studies can also provide an estimate of **attributable risk**, the rate of a health outcome attributable to the risk factor for this outcome. In addition, prospective studies can furnish an estimate of **relative risk**, the ratio of the incidence of a health outcome (disease or death) among the exposed to that among the unexposed.

Incidence density can also be calculated from prospective studies and is defined as the number of new cases that occur per unit of population-time (for example, person-years at risk). At times, it is difficult to follow a cohort who is exposed to an agent for an extended period. In such cases, the total length of time each person is exposed becomes the denominator for the calculation of incidence density (i.e., the number of new cases divided by the person-years at risk). An example is expressing the incidence rate of lung cancer in terms of 1,000 person-years exposed to smoking.

Prospective studies have the great advantage that possible risk factors are identified before the disease appears, thus reducing the possibility of many sources of **bias** (systematic error in making inferences and making and recording observations). However, these studies are expensive and not useful for studying rare diseases, and it takes many years before results can be analysed. Uncontrolled confounding factors may also lead to a spurious association between the exposure factor and the health outcomes under study. Table 2.1 summarizes the advantages and disadvantages of case-control and cohort studies.

A classical cohort study is one carried out in Framingham, Massachusetts, used here to show the different concepts outlined above (8). Of the total 10,000 men and women in Framingham, 5,209 randomly selected individuals were recruited into the study and followed for several years. Health habit history, physical examination, and appropriate laboratory investigations were recorded initially and at two-year intervals. The investigator was interested in studying the effect of high-density lipoprotein (HDL) cholesterol levels on coronary heart disease (CHD). (High levels of HDL cholesterol are known to have a protective effect for CHD.) He found that the incidence of CHD in men was 176.5/1,000 when HDL cholesterol levels were less than 25 mg/mL, whereas it was 25/1,000 when HDL cholesterol levels were between 65 and 74 mg/mL. From these data, one can conclude that the *attributable risk* of low levels of HDL cholesterol compared to high levels is 151.5/1,000 (176.5/1,000-25/1,000). The *relative risk* for developing CHD with lower HDL cholesterol levels compared to higher levels is 7.1 (176.5/1,000 divided by 25/1,000).

1.2.2. Experimental Studies

Experimental studies are those in which conditions are under the direct control of the investigator, and they are conducted like laboratory experiments. In a **therapeutic trial (randomized clinical trial)**, a group of people with a disease is randomized into two or more groups. It is expected that randomization will ensure equal distribution of all major demographic characteristics, such as age, sex, and socioeconomic status. One group is subjected to the intervention being evaluated, usually a treatment, while all other groups (**controls**) are given either an inactive treatment (**placebo**) or current standard treatment. When subjects are blinded to their treatment status, this procedure is called a **single-blind** trial. The effectiveness of the treatment can only be evaluated when there is a comparison group, because the health status of individuals or groups changes constantly. Outcomes for both groups ideally are assessed by an individual who does not know to which group each person belongs, thus reducing the possibility of bias in the observer. Trials where neither participant nor observer knows the group assignment are called **double-blind** clinical trials. If the health outcomes in the treatment group are statistically significantly better than those in the control group, then the treatment is considered to have been effective in this trial.

Although many clinical trials evaluate new drugs or operations, alternative forms of health care delivery can also be studied in this way. For example, Shah et al. (9) examined the attitudes of parents whose children were sent home rather than kept in hospital after minor surgery. Children scheduled to have surgery were randomly assigned to two groups: the experimental group, whose members were discharged by eight hours after surgery and were provided with home care; and the control group, whose members were kept in hospital for the usual one to three days. The groups were similar in age, sex, socioeconomic status, and type of surgery. After the children had recovered from surgery, the parents were asked about their child's symptoms and their satisfaction with the treatment. Parents were also asked about their preference for care (i.e., whether they would prefer their children to be hospitalized for minor surgery or prefer them to be at home on the same day as surgery). There were 116 children in each group. Most parents of the control children (66.4%) preferred hospitalization, but the parents of experimental subjects favoured home care (78.4%). Thus, it appears that such home care is well accepted by those who have experienced it.

Although trials can yield reliable and valid results, there are many situations in which trials cannot be carried out on humans. If a treatment is known to be superior, it would not be ethical to deprive people in the control group of the treatment. If a factor is thought to cause or predispose a person toward a disease, ethical considerations forbid deliberately exposing humans. Furthermore, recent experience with trials for new treatments for AIDS has shown that personal desire to have the new treatment can result in unblinding and contamination of the trial. This has led to innovative new strategies such as **open-arm** trials where some of the participants can choose the therapy they wish to receive. This poses new challenges for the statistical interpretation of the trial, but enables participants to exert more control over their fate.

With regard to studying the effect of removing an environmental factor thought to cause disease (for example, some kinds of air pollutant), a comparison study of two communities that already have different levels of the pollutant would be much cheaper and faster than a trial in which the pollutant levels were lowered and levels of disease tracked over time. **Community trials** of preventive health interventions are delivered to whole populations. One community is given an intervention (mass regimen) while another serves as a control. This methodology, for example, was used to evaluate the effects of naturally fluoridated water supplies on the prevalence of dental caries. There are intrinsic reasons why community trials are likely to produce more equivocal results than randomized clinical trials. Community trials are quasi-experimental, since allocation of the intervention is not randomized among individuals in the communities. It is particularly difficult to control for contamination, which occurs when the comparison communities also receive some of the intervention, and **confounding** is also a concern. Frequently, the outcomes observed are risk behaviour changes in the population, which are intermediate rather than "final" health outcome data.

Recently, a new type of research technique has appeared in the literature, termed **meta-analysis** (10). Meta-analyses are "studies of studies", synthesizing the results of many studies. Initially, a thorough search for all relevant studies, published and unpublished, is required; the studies are critically reviewed and their results combined statistically. Usually meta-analysis is applied to clinical trial data, but it may be applied to other analytic studies as well. By pooling the data from many sources, meta-analysis can reduce the alpha and beta errors described later in this chapter. Its purposes include increasing statistical power for outcome assessment and subgroup evaluation, resolving uncertainty, improving estimates of effect by increasing sample size, and providing answers to questions not posed by the original trials. In recent years, the number of clinical trials has multiplied, and several trials of the same treatment may be published serially, often over a span of ten years or more. At what point should one stop doing more trials? Lau and his colleagues (11) have described a method of using meta-analysis in which the results of clinical trials are accumulated as they are published. This procedure is called cumulative meta-analysis, which could be used to identify a significant difference between an existing treatment and an experimental one as information from such trials accrues. Such ongoing analyses may help investigators to decide whether continued study of a problem is needed.

There is an international effort to collect and collate all randomized trials relevant to clinical medicine. The **Cochrane Collaboration** is an international collaboration of health care researchers to create a central and accessible database of all evidence related to the delivery of health care. In Canada, the Cochrane Collaborative Centre is located at McMaster University in Hamilton. The database can be accessed through the web site which is listed at the end of book.

1.2.3. Clinical Epidemiology

An important source of information on the natural history, prognosis, and outcome of disease states comes from the observations and actions of practising physicians. Clinical epidemiology represents the application, modification, and refinement of epidemiologic techniques to individual patient care. The purpose of clinical epidemiology is to collect systematic information from the practice of medicine in order to increase the accuracy, reliability, validity, and effectiveness of clinical care. An important facet of this is the development of clinically relevant disease and outcome taxonomies. This field is known as **clinimetrics** (12).

Clinical epidemiology is concerned with the accuracy of diagnostic strategies and uses a variety of statistical techniques such as **decision analysis** and **Bayesian analysis** to study the most efficient use of diagnostic technology. Statistical techniques are also used to study the natural history and prognosis of diseases, with a particular emphasis on the extent to which medical intervention improves outcomes.

Closely related to clinical epidemiology is the technique of **critical appraisal**. Critical appraisal has been defined by Sackett et al. (3) as the "application of certain rules of evidence to clinical (symptoms and signs), paraclinical (laboratory and other diagnostic tests), and published data (advocating specific treatment manoeuvres or purporting to establish the aetiology or prognosis of disease) in order to determine their validity (closeness to the truth) and applicability (usefulness in one's own clinical practice)". A series of articles outlining the principles of critical appraisal has been published (13) and is available over the web sites listed in Appendix B. The application of the techniques of clinical epidemiology and critical appraisal constitute **evidence-based medicine**.

1.2.4. Causal Associations

The types of studies outlined in the previous sections are undertaken, frequently in a step-wise fashion, with the overall objective of identifying and establishing associations between exposure to factor(s) and disease. Each type of study has its strengths and limitations. *Descriptive studies* generate hypotheses about potential risk factors. *Prevalence studies* can identify potential risk factors in a specific population, which can be further investigated by *case-control studies*. By comparing rates of exposure in cases of disease with those free of the disease, case-control studies indirectly give an estimate of relative risk. *Cohort studies* take more resources and time as subjects are followed over a long period; however, the relative risk of disease following exposure to a putative risk factor, as well as absolute risk, can be accurately determined. Randomized *experimental (clinical) trials* give the highest calibre information on the effect of a factor or intervention on individuals. Community intervention studies, although only quasi-experimental, provide this information for communities. Before a conclusion can be drawn about whether an exposure causes a chronic disease (i.e., a **causal association**), the following questions established by Hill (14) should be considered:

- **Experimental evidence:** Is there experimental or quasi-experimental evidence that removal of the putative causative factor results in reduction of disease incidence?
- **Consistency of the association:** Do the findings of studies of the same and different design in different populations demonstrate the same association?
- **Strength of the association:** How large is the relative risk of the outcome in relation to exposure?
- **Dose-response:** Does the severity of the likelihood of the outcome increase as the amount, intensity, or duration of the exposure increases?
- **Temporal relationship:** Did the exposure occur before the onset of the disease?
- **Plausibility:** Is the association plausible, given the existing basic science and clinical knowledge about the disease?
- **Coherence:** Does the association make sense in terms of the theory and knowledge about the disease process?
- **Specificity:** Is the association specific for a particular disease or group of diseases? (In practice, however, this often is not satisfied.)
- **Analogy:** Do other established associations provide a model for this type of relationship?

1.2.5. Qualitative Research

Many important issues in public health cannot be adequately addressed by quantitative methods. Issues relating to the attitudes and beliefs of community members or health care practitioners may be best explored using qualitative research techniques. Qualitative research uses interpretive and naturalistic approaches to study research questions. Studies are carried out in natural non-experimental situations. Unlike the quantitative approach, which places a high value on reliable, accurate measurement and the generalizability of results, qualitative research focuses on explaining and understanding the particular process. Narrative accounts replace statistical summaries (15).

A variety of qualitative research techniques, developed in the social sciences, have found applications in the health care field. **Focus groups** use group interviews to generate data for thematic analysis. In-depth interviews, such as **key informant** interviews, seek to garner information from individuals with special insight into health issues. Consensus methods such as **Delphi and nominal groups** seek to establish the extent of agreement, often among experts, in cases of unclear evidence.

2. INVESTIGATION OF DISEASE IN POPULATIONS

The above section provided an overview of different epidemiological methods in studying health and disease in the population. The following describes several situations in which these methods are applied to investigate non-communicable disease in populations.

2.1. CLUSTERS OF DISEASE

One of the most frequent problems faced by local health units or a provincial department of health is the concern of local residents and practising physicians about apparently excessive numbers of health problems or diseases in their community. For example, residents may express concern about an apparent excess number of cancer deaths or birth defects in their community. The excess number of cases is often referred to as a cluster. Caldwell (16) defines a **cluster** as "a number of like or similar things occurring together in time and space". This definition includes the notion of disease aggregation and its aetiology. In common usage in epidemiology, "cluster" is used for noninfectious diseases, while "epidemic" and "outbreak" refer to infectious disease.

The first step in investigation is to identify the type of disease cluster: clustering of possibly related diseases within the same person, clustering within families or other interpersonal networks, clustering in time (i.e., cases of the same disease within a short period), clustering in space (i.e., within close geographic proximity), or clustering in both time and space.

Next, the population at risk of exposure to the putative causal agent of the disease (e.g., a suspected environmental carcinogen) must be determined. A similar but non-exposed group is defined as a reference population (control group) for comparison. A "case" definition is formulated and cases, both new and existing, are actively ascertained in both the exposed and the reference populations within a standard time frame for observation. By means of statistical tests, the observed number of cases in the population at risk can be compared to the "expected" number in the reference population.

If a statistically significant excess of cases (a "true cluster") is found, then appropriate epidemiological studies are needed to assess the degree of exposure to the suspected causal factor (e.g., a chemical or physical agent) and to test the hypothesis that this agent is indeed a cause of, or significant risk factor for, the disease in question. The Centre for Disease Control has published a comprehensive guide to the analysis of clusters in populations (17).

2.3. ASYMPTOMATIC DISEASE

Prior to the development of symptoms, or physical signs noticeable to health care professionals, diseases may be present in affected people without their knowledge (asymptomatic disease). Diabetes, hypertension, and cancer (such as breast cancer or cancer of the uterine cervix) fall into this category. The commonly used method for detecting asymptomatic disease in a population is screening. **Screening** is defined as "the presumptive identification of unrecognized disease or defect by the application of tests, examinations or other procedures which can be applied rapidly" (18). Thus, the goal of a screening program is early detection — identifying which asymptomatic people in the community probably have the disease and which probably do not. Examples of screening procedures are mammography for breast cancer and Papanicolaou tests for cervical cancer.

2.3.1. Types of Screening
There are three types of screening that can be applied to a community.

For example **mass screening** for tuberculosis by chest x-ray is done in many developing countries where the disease is still highly prevalent. It is not widely performed in developed countries where the prevalence is low.

Selective screening is performed on selected subgroups of a population at increased risk of developing certain diseases. Tay-Sachs disease (transmitted by a recessive gene, resulting in mental retardation and premature death) is quite common among French Canadians in some parts of Quebec. Thus, screening for carriers coupled with genetic counselling may be worthwhile in this population.

Multiphasic screening programs include a medical history, physical examination, and various measurements and investigations. The objective is to detect as many diseases as possible with one screening intervention. Screening of this nature is done by large organizations, especially U.S. organizations (such as Kaiser Permanente and the Health Insurance Plan of New York) that operate prepaid group health plans.

2.3.2. Characteristics of Screening
People with positive screening tests do not always have the disease (see Figure 2.1). Screening tests are not diagnostic tests. People with positive or questionable results must be referred for diagnostic evaluation. For screening to fulfil its intended

Figure 2.1:   Mass Screening

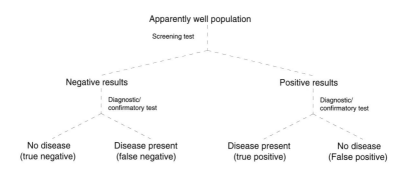

$$Sensitivity = \frac{true\ positives\,(TP)}{true\ positives\,(TP) + false\ negatives\,(FN)} \times 100\%$$

$$Specificity = \frac{true\ negatives\,(TN)}{true\ negatives\,(TN) + false\ positives\,(FP)} \times 100\%$$

purpose, there should be adequate, effective, and accessible methods of diagnosis and early treatment for diseased individuals.

Screening tests are evaluated in terms of their validity, reliability, and yield. The **validity** of a screening test is measured by the frequency with which the result of the test is confirmed by an accurate diagnostic method and is often expressed in terms of its sensitivity and specificity. **Sensitivity** is the proportion (percentage) of truly diseased persons identified as diseased by a screening test. **Specificity** is the proportion (percentage) of truly non-diseased persons who are so identified by the test (see Figure 2.1). Both sensitivity and specificity are characteristics of a given test, and do not change when applied to populations with varying prevalence of disease.

Tests with low sensitivity and specificity (i.e., low percentages of correctly identifying those who have and do not have the disease respectively) are poor screening tests. To have high sensitivity, screening tests must produce few false negative results; for high specificity, few false positive results should arise. A screening test is never 100% sensitive and specific. High sensitivity is gained at the expense of specificity and vice versa. Raising test sensitivity will result in loss of specificity and the investigation of false positives.

Table 2.2:   Result of a Hypothetical Screening Test

		Disease present	
		YES	**NO**
Result of test	**POSITIVE**	True positive	False positive
	NEGATIVE	False negative	True negative

$$\text{Positive Predictive Value} = \frac{\text{true positives (TP)}}{\text{true positives (TP) + false positives (FP)}} \times 100\%$$

$$\text{Negative Predictive Value} = \frac{\text{true negatives (TN)}}{\text{true negatives (TN) + false negatives (FN)}} \times 100\ \%$$

Positive predictive value is measured as the proportion of true positives in all test positives (i.e., the proportion of cases who truly have the disease among those with positive tests) (see Table 2.2). The predictive value of a positive test tends to be higher when the disease is more prevalent (see Table 2.3). The **negative predictive value** is the test's ability to identify all those who truly do not have the disease among all those who tested negative. The predictive value of a negative test decreases with increasing disease prevalence.

The **reliability** of a screening test refers to its ability to produce consistent results when applied to different populations or repeatedly to the same individual. The **yield** from a screening test is the amount of previously unrecognized disease detected in the population; it depends on the sensitivity of the screening test as well as the prevalence of unrecognized disease in a population. For example, the yield from the Papanicolaou test is very low among women who have never had sexual intercourse but is much higher among sexually active females.

2.3.3. Criteria for the Population-Based Screening Program

As new tests or procedures emerge for screening for a disease, there are pressures on health care professionals and the health care system to adopt and institutionalize them. However, screening can only be justified if the following criteria are met (19):

- Diseases for which screening is used should be important health problems. When there is an extremely low incidence of a disease in a population, the cost and effort

Table 2.3:   Predictive Values of a Positive Test with 99% Sensitivity and 95% Specificity at Three Levels of Prevalence

Item	Level of prevalence		
	1 percent	10 percent	20 percent
a) Number in population	1,000	1,000	1,000
b) Diseased	10	100	200
c) Not diseased	990	900	800
d) True positive [b x 0.99]	10	99	198
e) False positive [c x (1 - 0.95)]	50	45	40
f) Total positive [d + e]	60	144	238
g) Predictive value of a positive test [d/f]	17%	69%	83%

of mass screening may be prohibitive. Epidemiological studies to determine the incidence and prevalence of various diseases in a community may be necessary before embarking on any large-scale screening operations.

- Facilities for diagnosis and treatment should be available, because lack of follow-up negates any possible benefit of the screening test.
- Effective non-controversial treatment for people with confirmed disease should be available.
- Screening tests should have high sensitivity and specificity; screening must be safe, rapidly applied, and acceptable to the screened population (for example, while chest radiographs or a blood test may not bother most individuals, the discomfort produced by sigmoidoscopy may be unacceptable).
- The natural history of the disease (i.e., the precursor, asymptomatic, and symptomatic stages) should be thoroughly understood. If controlled studies have demonstrated that the natural history of the disease is not favourably altered by earlier detection and treatment, then screening for that particular disease should not be instituted. For example, periodic screening by chest x-rays for lung cancer does not improve the prognosis of the disease. Primary prevention methods such as cessation or prevention of smoking are more effective than chest x-ray screening in controlling lung cancer.
- Prior agreement or policy must stipulate what action will be taken for borderline results in order to avoid the problem of over-diagnosis of disease.
- Comparing the costs and efficiency of various screening methods for a disease is essential for achieving maximum benefit for minimum cost.
- Control and screened groups should be compared at regular intervals to establish whether the screening procedure and subsequent investigations have any greater effect than regular observation of the control groups. In one study, it was demonstrated that systematic, regular examination of a control group of individuals

appeared to exert a similar effect on blood pressure, glucose tolerance, and cholesterol level compared to the screened group.
- Compliance with screening recommendations is essential. There may be no benefit in screening unless diagnosed individuals comply with effective treatment.
- Screening programs should be a continuing process rather than being done "one time only."

Beyond these accepted criteria, there are issues that must be considered before instituting a provincial or national program (20):
- Are the screening program requirements for time, money, and costs appropriate for the community?
- Are other equally worthy procedures and efforts being given equal consideration or are existing resources being redirected unnecessarily?
- Does the procedure create new medical risks, and how are these assessed in relation to the procedure?
- Does the procedure place additional strain on health care resources in a disproportionate manner to the magnitude of the health problem being studied?
- What are the limitations of using screening assessments as a widespread diagnostic tool in relation to other diagnostic approaches?
- Are there specific ethical or moral issues raised by the program?
- How will the objectives of the screening program be communicated to the various target populations at risk?

The introduction of various forms of screening can be effective in secondarily preventing illness and improving the health of populations. A consideration of possible harms must be addressed before instituting a screening program, as summarized by Marshall in a recent series of articles (21-23).

3. RELEVANT STATISTICAL CONCEPTS

Statistics are frequently used in studying the health and disease of populations. Statistics deal with the collection, classification, description, analysis, interpretation, and presentation of data and are the backbone of all epidemiologic research. A brief summary is provided here; more detailed discussion is available in standard statistical textbooks (24, 25).

In general, statistics can be either descriptive or inferential. **Descriptive statistics** are counts of events or other characteristics of interest and give information about the nature of a group. For example, census data can provide a description of the population by age or region. **Inferential statistics** are used to compare and look for differences between groups and regions.

A population can consist of individuals, events, observations, or any other grouping. Data can be derived from an entire population or from a sample. In epidemiology, data are usually available only on a sample of the population. Sampling may involve random selection, systematic selection, stratified selection, or cluster selection, or may be non-random (convenience) in nature. The sampling strategy influences the amount of bias likely to be encountered in making inferences from the data.

Data collected can be either grouped or ungrouped, qualitative or quantitative. In quantitative epidemiology, data are collected on **variables**. A variable is a category of measurement that can take on a variety of values. Data can be either continuous or discrete. A **continuous variable** is one that has an infinite number of evenly spaced potential values between any two values. Age is an example of a continuous variable. **Discrete variables** can be ordinal or nominal. An **ordinal variable** is one where values are chosen from a limited number of possible values, but there is no possibility of a value between the other values. In cancer staging, stage 1 is regarded as less severe than stage 4, but the distance between stage 1 and stage 2 cannot be measured. The data can therefore be ordered. Similarly, the number of children in a family is ordinal, in that the difference between the first and second child is one of order, and it is not possible to have more than one but less than two children. **Nominal variables** are also categorical, but not ordered. There are a finite number of values that the variable can take, but the data cannot be ordered. Ethnic status is an example of nominal data.

Health data consist of sets of numerical information about anything related to health. They are the basic scientific tools with which health and disease are studied, but, like any tools, they must be of suitable quality to do the job expected. First, data must be **reliable** — when the same group of people is measured more than once, similar values must be obtained. Second, data must be **valid** — it must relate to the problem studied. For example, we expect hospital admissions to provide a valid assessment of the incidence of third-degree (very severe) burns, but not to measure the incidence of diabetes, since most people with early diabetes are not hospitalized. **Validity** reflects the degree to which a measurement measures what it purports to measure. Also, data in the health field must have sufficient resolution to give the answers being sought; like a microscopist, the epidemiologist may need to see one part of the problem in great detail. For example, a report of a slight increase in the national incidence of tuberculosis would not indicate where the cases were or in what groups of people they occurred. No action could be taken until these details were determined by using epidemiologic and statistical techniques. Third, data must be **precise** — the measuring instrument defines how "sharply" it can provide a value. For example, a measurement of four decimal places is more precise than two decimal places. Unfortunately, very precise data may be neither valid nor reliable.

Data can be analysed to determine its distributional characteristics. Common methods of examining data are **bar graphs** for discrete data and **histograms** for continuous data. The frequency with which values occur is referred to as **distribution.** The most common and well-known distribution is the **normal** or **Gaussian** distribution, which resembles a bell (see Figure 2.2). Distributions can often be succinctly summarized mathematically by numeric values called **parameters**. For the normal distribution, a **measure of the central tendency** (the mean) and a **measure of the variation of the data** in the distribution (the standard deviation) are all that is required to summarize the distribution. The **mean** is calculated by summing all the observations and dividing by the number of observations. It is expressed mathematically as follows:

$$\bar{x} = \sum \frac{x_i}{n}$$

Related to the mean are the variance and the standard deviation. The **variance** expresses the amount of dispersion in the data and is calculated by taking the sum of the squares of the deviations from the mean value and dividing by the sample size subtracting one observation. It is represented mathematically as follows:

$$s^2 = \frac{\sum (x - \bar{x})^2}{n - 1}$$

The **standard deviation** is merely the square root of the variance:

$$s = \sqrt{\frac{\sum (x - \bar{x})^2}{n - 1}}$$

Other important aspects of distributions are the **median**, which describes the value above and below which 50% of the values lie. The **mode** describes the data value that is observed most frequently. Another measure of the variability of data is the range, which reflects the difference between the highest and lowest values in the distribution.

Statistical techniques are used to test hypotheses and determine the degree to which an effect or difference exists between two or more comparison groups. Tests of statistical significance are chosen on the basis of the type of data being analysed. Statistical tests also differ on the type of distribution the data is thought to approximate.

Statistical testing requires the statement of a null and alternative hypothesis. The **null hypothesis** states that there is, in fact, no real difference between the groups being compared, and that the differences seen are due to chance. Thus, a p-value of 0.05 or less allows one to reject the null hypothesis and select the alternative hypothesis (i.e., that there is, in fact, a difference between the groups being compared). It must be pointed out that at a p-value less than 0.05 there is still a small chance (1 in 20) that random variation may be responsible for the observed difference.

Table 2.4 indicates the type of errors that can occur in the interpretation of data. The truth, or gold standard, is whether the intervention confers benefit or not. A **Type I** or **alpha error** is the incorrect rejection of a null hypothesis or asserting that there is a difference between treatments when in fact there is not. Thus, in a situation of p=0.05, there is a 5% chance, or 1 out of 20 chance, of rejecting a null hypothesis that should not be rejected.

A **Type II** or **beta error** occurs when the null hypothesis is not rejected when it should be or when there is a failure to recognize a difference in the result of an intervention when it is actually present.

Figure 2.2:   Distribution Curves

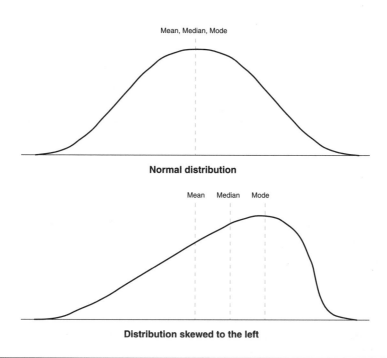

Normal distribution

Distribution skewed to the left

The chance of a Type II error occurring is used to determine the **power** of a study, which is 1 minus beta. The power of a study is the probability that a difference will be detected when there is indeed a difference. Power is a function of the sample size of the study. A small study may fail to reject the null hypothesis because the numbers were too small to detect a significant difference. Therefore, it is crucial to consult a statistician before commencing a study to ensure that the sample size is adequate.

Study results are usually reported by either a p-value or confidence interval. A **p-value** is used to determine whether to reject the null hypothesis. If the level of significance is set at 0.05, then if a significance test yields a probability less than 0.05, the null hypothesis is rejected. A p-value is not the probability that the null hypothesis is true. Rather, it is the probability of the observed result or more extreme results that might have been observed under the assumption that the null hypothesis is true. It is easiest to think of a p-value as a decision rule. If the observed value is less than the preset alpha (which is a conventional decision), then the null hypothesis can be rejected.

Table 2.4:   Type I and Type II Error Probabilities

		Truth	
		Treatment benefits (H_1)	**No benefit (H_0)**
Result from the study	**POSITIVE**	**True positive** Correctly reject H_0 $p = 1 - \beta$	**False positive** Type I error Incorrectly reject H_0 $p = \alpha$
	NEGATIVE	**False negative** Type II error Incorrectly do not reject H_0 $p = \beta$	**True negative** Correctly do not reject H_0 $p = 1 - \alpha$

A **confidence interval** is a summary of the data in the original units of measure. A confidence interval can give information on the variability of the data, the sample size, and the magnitude of the effect size demonstrated in the study. A 95% confidence interval includes a point estimate, which is the best estimate of the value of the population parameter given the data from the sample. The range of values around the point estimate calculated from the study population indicate the possible values that may be found as the true population estimate. It is likely that in 100 repetitions of a study, the true population estimate would be contained in the interval 95 times. For example, if a study reports a p-value of 0.01, one can conclude that it is statistically significant, but cannot infer the magnitude of effect or the precision of the estimate. If the same study yields a relative risk of 1.6 with 95% confidence levels of 1.2 to 1.8, one can infer that the sample size was large enough to give a precise estimate, and that the effect though significant was consistent with a 20% to 80% increase in risk. A wide confidence interval indicates a small sample size and is an imprecise quantification of effect indicating uncertainty about the estimate. Most medical journals require both p-values and confidence intervals (26).

Statistical significance is distinct from clinical relevance or importance. As p-values are a function of sample size, a large study can report statistically significant results that are trivial. Similarly, a small study could neglect to show a difference when one existed. Any uncertainty about the interpretation of a study in the literature should prompt the reader to consult a knowledgeable statistician or epidemiologist in the same manner one would consult a specialist over a puzzling clinical case.

A wide variety of statistical techniques exists in the literature. With the advent of powerful computers, **multivariate analysis** has become increasingly common. Whereas **univariate analysis** is used to examine the relationship between two variables, a multivariate model allows for a number of relevant variables to be related to an outcome of interest. The most common form of multivariate analysis is **regression** analysis. Multiple regression can take a number of forms. Linear, logistic, and proportional hazards are some examples of different types of regression techniques. Commonly, an outcome such as mortality is related to a set of potential risk factors such as smoking status, age, gender, blood pressure, and blood cholesterol level to give an estimate of the contribution each factor makes when the potential confounding effects of the other variables are controlled.

3.1. RATIOS, PROPORTIONS, AND RATES

Usually, health data take into account the population where the events have occurred. Hence, in most situations, one needs a numerator, that is, the occurrence of an event under observation, and a denominator, that is, size of population where the event occurred. As disease is relatively rare, rates are expressed in terms of per 100, 1,000, 10,000, or 100,000 population. For example, the smoking prevalence for a given population may be expressed as 40% whereas death rates are expressed as 7 deaths per 1,000 people per year. For example, lung cancer in males, which is rare, is expressed as 55 per 100,000 population per year. Similarly, use of hospital days is expressed as days per 1,000 population.

The commonly used means of data expression are ratio, proportion, and rate. A **ratio** is an expression of the relationship between two items that are usually independent of each other. If there are 6 males and 12 females, then the ratio of males to females is 1:2.

A **proportion** is the relationship of a part to its whole expressed as a percentage. If there are 25 ill persons out of 100 persons, then the proportion of ill persons is 25%.

A **rate** is an expression of the probability of an occurrence of an event in a defined population at risk during a specific time period.

3.1.1. Odds Ratio and Relative Risk

The risk of disease for individuals may be measured by either relative risk or odds ratio. To calculate these risk measures, data on the number of persons who have the disease or do not have it and those who were exposed to the suspected causal or risk factor or not exposed are arranged in a two-by-two table in the following manner:

		Disease (cases)	No disease (control)
Exposure	POSITIVE	a	b
	NEGATIVE	c	d

The **relative risk** (RR) of those exposed having the disease, compared to the unexposed is:

$$\left(\frac{a}{a+b}\right) \div \left(\frac{c}{c+d}\right)$$

The **odds ratio** (OR) of a case having been exposed, compared to a control, is (a x d)/(b x c). One can see that for rare diseases, for example, where the values of a and c are small, the formula for RR approximates (a/b)/(c/d), which equals (a x d)/(b x c). In such a scenario, the OR (derived from a case-control study) is a suitable estimate of the RR (derived from the more costly cohort study).

3.1.2. Attributable Fraction/Population Attributable Risk

Attributable fraction or **population attributable risk (PAR)** is a measure of the amount of disease associated with an exposure within a population. This can be derived by subtracting the incidence rate in the unexposed groups from the incidence rate in the total population and dividing by the incidence rate in the total population. This indicator provides an estimate of the proportion of cases that may be ascribed to the factor in question. PAR can also be calculated directly from the relative risk and the prevalence of exposure to the risk factor in the population.

3.2. OTHER MEASURES OF EFFECT ON SIZE: ABSOLUTE AND RELATIVE RISK REDUCTION AND NUMBER NEEDED TO TREAT

Clinical trials are traditionally reported in terms of the reduction of the outcome measure associated with the intervention in comparison to a placebo or alternative treatment. There are three equivalent statistical measures of trial data: the relative risk reduction, the absolute risk reduction, and the number needed to treat. It is important to note that framing results in these different but mathematically equivalent ways influences practitioners and planners in their willingness to employ an intervention (21, 27).

These concepts can be illustrated with the following example. A randomized trial shows a rate of 34% in the placebo group and a rate of 28% in the treatment group. This is equivalent to a relative risk reduction of 21% and an absolute risk reduction of 6%. The number needed to treat shows how many individuals would need to comply fully with the intervention to prevent one outcome (28). It is the reciprocal of the absolute risk reduction, in this case 1/0.06, or 17 individuals. Practitioners' willingness either to accept or recommend a therapy can be influenced by the way these numbers can be presented.

3.2.1. Rate Standardization

The comparison of rates for important health outcomes between different geographical regions is a common way of analysing health data. However, it is important that such comparisons be legitimate. Epidemiologists rely on techniques of rate standardization to ensure that comparisons are unbiased.

For example, as risk of dying varies widely by age (i.e., older people are at a greater risk of dying than younger ones), the annual frequency of deaths in a population depends on its age composition. Simply comparing the crude death rates of two populations may give a false impression. The crude death rate in the Aboriginal population of Canada is 5.5/1,000, compared with 7.2/1,000 for the entire Canadian population. However, 38% of the Aboriginal population is under 15 years of age, compared with only 23% for the Canadian population. The basic principle of **standardization** is to introduce a standard population with a fixed age and sex structure. For example, an age-standardized mortality rate is the overall death rate that a population would have if it had the standard age structure. Age-standardized rates are sometimes called age-adjusted rates because the standardization is an actuarial way of adjusting the crude rate to remove the effect of any difference between actual age structure in the population and the standard age structure. The two approaches to standardization are the direct method and the indirect method.

Direct Method

When age-specific mortality rates are available for the study population, the age-standardized mortality rate (SRATE) is obtained by calculating the weighted average of these age-specific rates, using the number of persons in the respective age groups in the standard population as the weights. It is expressed in notation as:

$$\text{SRATE} = \frac{Pi \times mi}{Pi}$$

where SRATE is the age-standardized mortality rate, mi is the age-specific mortality rate in the study population for persons in age group i, and Pi is the number of persons in the age group in the standard population. Comparisons of different standardized rates are valid only if they are based on the same standard population. However, there is no single standard population acceptable for all purposes. The most commonly used standard populations for international comparison are the world standard population (a hypothetical model). For Canada, the 1971 population of Canada is used as the standard. This is done to permit comparisons to national statistics compiled by Statistics Canada, since that is their choice of standard population. For the above example, Aboriginal age-sex specific death rates are applied to the reference population (the 1971 Canadian population) and the death rate is recalculated to obtain the standardized rate. In this instance, it is 10.5 per 1,000 population, which is much higher than the earlier crude death rates obtained for the Aboriginal or Canadian populations. Thus, age-standardized rates are the annual number of deaths per 1,000 population that would be observed in the population if it had the same age composition as a reference (or standard) population. This is referred to as the direct method of standardization.

Indirect Method

Indirect standardization is a comparison of observed deaths in a study population and the number of deaths that would be expected if the population had the same mortality rate as the standard population; it is therefore a ratio rather than a standardized rate. The most commonly used ratio is the standardized mortality ratio (SMR):

$$SMR = \frac{mi \times pi}{Mi \times pi}$$

SMR is the standardized mortality ratio, mi is the age-specific mortality rate in the study population for people in age group i, pi is the number of people in age group i in the study population, and Mi is the age-specific mortality rate in the standard population. When comparing the mortality or morbidity of a region with that of another, SRATE is preferable to SMR because the former is calculated by applying the age-specific mortality rates of each region to only one standard population distribution. However, if the comparison is made between a region and the province, then the use of SMR is preferred because the denominators of SMRs (i.e., the expected number of deaths in regions) are all based on one set of age-specific mortality rates, i.e., the provincial experience. Hence the standardized mortality ratio (SMR) is the ratio of observed deaths to expected deaths per 100 population. This ratio is frequently used in occupational health studies and the expected number of deaths is obtained from the comparison population (usually a larger population such as the national one). For example, if the mortality rate in industry X is 200 per 1,000 persons and the national mortality rate is 150 per 1,000 persons, then the SMR is 133.

4.   SUMMARY

This chapter examined the data quality, epidemiologic studies, investigation of diseases in populations, and some relevant statistical concepts. Health data consist of sets of numerical information about anything related to health and are compiled from many sources. These data must meet three criteria: they must be reliable, valid, and have sufficient resolution.

Epidemiologic studies are a commonly used method for data collection and analysis. *Epidemiology* is the study of the distribution (which is studied in terms of person, place, and time) and the determinants of disease, health-related states, and events in populations. Epidemiology can be applied to control health problems. The two types of epidemiological studies are descriptive and analytical.

A *descriptive study* investigates the occurrence of a phenomenon in relation to person, time, and place. Causal associations should not be drawn from the results of a descriptive study; however, the results may lend themselves to an hypothesis for investigation of a causal association or relationship.

In *analytic studies*, a hypothesis is tested to find out if there is an association between a given disease, health state, or other dependent variable, and possible causative factors. There are two types of analytic studies: observational and experimental.

Observational studies include ecologic studies, which can compare aggregated variables between different geographical areas, and cross-sectional or prevalence studies, which examine the relationship between diseases and other variables of interest as they exist in a defined population at one particular time. The population is divided into those with and without the disease and then various characteristics of the two groups are examined. This type of study reveals the prevalence of disease, disability, and risk factors in a given population at one point in time. A third type of observational study is the retrospective study, used to test aetiological hypotheses in which inferences about exposure to the putative causal factor or factors are derived from data relating to characteristics of the people under study or to events or experiences in their past; this study takes the form of a case-control study in which people (cases) with the disease are compared with similar people without the disease (controls) who have also had the opportunity for exposure. Hence, a retrospective study begins after the disease has appeared. In prospective studies or cohort studies, a cohort (a group of people with common characteristics) is identified, and the initial characteristics and health status are compared to those of a control cohort (chosen on the same basis as the original cohort, except for exposure to the suspected cause of disease); both groups are followed for a certain time period to observe for evidence of disease or other outcomes, yielding incidence rates, attributable risk, relative risk, and incidence density.

Experimental studies are those in which conditions are under the direct control of the investigation, and are conducted like laboratory experiments. These studies include randomized clinical trials or therapeutic trials and community trials. In a therapeutic trial, subjects with a disease are randomized into two or more groups. One group is subjected to the intervention being evaluated, usually a treatment, while the control group is given either an inactive treatment (placebo) or current standard treatment. Subjects are usually unaware of their treatment status, in a procedure called a single-blind trial. Trials where neither the participant nor observer knows the group assignment are called double-blind clinical trials. If the final outcomes show a statistically significant difference between the study group and the controls, then the results obtained are usually attributed to the treatment. The community trial is used when a comparison study of two communities is desired in order to see what effects a variable has on the health of a community. One community is given an intervention while the other serves as a control.

Clinical epidemiology represents the application, modification, and refinement of epidemiologic techniques to individual patient care. The purpose of clinical epidemiology is to collect systematic information from the practice of medicine in order to increase the accuracy, reliability, validity, and effectiveness of clinical care. An important facet of this is the development of clinically relevant disease and outcome taxonomies. This field is known as clinimetrics.

For a *causal association* (i.e., to establish causality), there must be sufficient experimental evidence, consistency of association, strength of association, dose-response, correct temporal relationship, plausibility, coherence, specificity, and analogy.

Critical appraisal has been defined as the "application of certain rules of evidence to clinical (symptoms and signs), paraclinical (laboratory and other diagnostic tests), and published data (advocating specific treatment manoeuvres or purporting to establish the aetiology or prognosis of disease) in order to determine their validity (closeness to the truth) and applicability (usefulness in one's own clinical practice)" (3). The application of the techniques of clinical epidemiology and critical appraisal constitute evidence-based medicine.

Qualitative research uses interpretive and naturalistic approaches to study research questions. Studies are carried out in natural non-experimental situations. Narrative accounts replace statistical summaries. A variety of qualitative research techniques, developed in the social sciences, have found applications in the health care field.

The method commonly used for detecting asymptomatic disease is *screening*. In order to screen for a disease, a number of criteria must be met. There are various types of screening that can be carried out within a community, such as mass screening and selective screening. Screening tests are evaluated in terms of their validity, reliability, and yield. The validity of a screening test is measured by the frequency with which the result of the test is confirmed by an accurate diagnostic method, and is often expressed in terms of its sensitivity and specificity. The sensitivity of a test is the proportion of truly diseased who are identified as diseased by a test. Specificity is the proportion of truly non-diseased persons who are so identified by the test. Tests with low sensitivity and low specificity are poor screening tests. However, no screening test is 100% sensitive or specific, and high sensitivity is gained at the expense of specificity and vice versa. The reliability of a screening test refers to its ability to produce consistent results when applied to various screened populations or even repeatedly on the same individual. The yield from a screening test is the amount of unrecognized disease that is detected in the population, and thus depends on the sensitivity of the screening test as well as the prevalence of unrecognized disease in a population.

Statistics deal with the collection, classification, description, analysis, interpretation, and presentation of data, and form the backbone of all epidemiological research.

5.   REFERENCES

1.   Beaglehole R, Bonita R, Kjellstromm T. Basic Epidemiology (1st ed.). Geneva: World Health Organization, 1993.
2.   Fletcher RH, Fletcher SW, Wagner EH. Clinical Epidemiology. (3rd ed.) Philadelphia: Williams and Wilkins, 1996.

3. Sackett D, Haynes R, Tugwell P. Clinical Epidemiology: A Basic Science for Clinical Medicine (2nd ed.). Toronto: Little, Brown and Co., 1991.
4. Coggon D, Rose G, Barker DJP. Epidemiology for the Uninitiated (http://www.bmj.com/epidem/epid.html), May 1997.
5. Last JM. A Dictionary of Epidemiology. (3rd ed.) New York: Oxford University Press, 1995.
6. Kelsey J, Thompson W, Evans A. Methods in Observational Epidemiology. New York: Oxford University Press, 1986.
7. Denson R, Nanson J, McWatters M. Hyperkinesis and Maternal Smoking. Canadian Psychological Association Journal 1975;20(3):183-187.
8. Castel W. Epidemiology of Coronary Heart Disease: The Framingham Study. American Journal of Medicine 1984; 76(2A):11-12.
9. Shah C, Robinson G, Kinnis C, Davenport H. Day Care Surgery for Children: A Controlled Study of Medical Complications and Parental Attitudes. Medical Care 1972;10(5):437-450.
10. Spitzer W. The Challenge of Meta-Analysis. Journal of Clinical Epidemiology 1995;48(1):1-4.
11. Lau J, Antman E, Jimenez-Silva J, Kupelnick B, Mosteller F, Chalmers T. Cumulative Meta-Analysis of Therapeutic Trials for Myocardial Infection. New England Journal of Medicine 1992;327(2):241-247.
12. Feinstein A. Clinimetrics. New Haven: Yale University Press, 1987.
13. Jaeschke R, Guyatt G, Sackett D, et al. User's Guide to the Medical Literature. III How to Use an Article About a Diagnostic Test. A. Are the Results of the Study Valid? Journal of American Medical Association 1994;271(5):389-391.
14. Hill AB. The Environment and Disease: Association or Causation? Proceedings of Royal Society of Medicine 1965;58(295-300).
15. Pope C, Mays N. Reaching the Parts Other Methods Cannot Reach: An Introduction to Qualitative Methods in Health and Health Services Research. British Medical Journal 1995;311:42-45.
16. Caldwell G. Time-Space Clusters. Health Environment Digest 1989;3(5):4-5.
17. Guidelines for Investigating of Health Effects. Morbidity and Mortality Weekly Report 1990; 39(RR-11):1-23.
18. Whitby L. Screening For Disease: Definitions and Criteria. Lancet 1974;2(3):819-821.
19. Glausnov I, Dowd J, Jaksic E, et al. Repetitive Health Examination as an Intervention Measure. Bulletin. World Health Organization 1973;49(4):423-432.
20. Task Force on the Use and Provision of Medical Services. 1989-1990 Annual Report. Toronto: Government of Ontario and Ontario Medical Association, 1990.
21. Marshall K. Prevention. How Much Harm? How Much Benefit? 1. The Influence of Reporting Methods on Perception of Benefits. Canadian Medical Association Journal 1996;154(10):1493-1499.
22. Marshall K. Prevention. How Much Harm? How Much Benefit? 3. Physical, Psychological and Social Harm. Canadian Medical Association Journal 1996;155(2):169-176.
23. Marshall K. Prevention. How Much Harm? How Much Benefit? 4. The Ethics of Informed Consent for Preventive Screening Programs. Canadian Medical Association Journal 1996;155(4):377-383.
24. Glantz S. Primer of Biostatistics (2nd ed.). New York: McGraw-Hill Inc., 1987.
25. Leaverton P. A Review of Biostatistics. A Program for Self-Instruction (4th ed.). Boston: Little, Brown and Co., 1986.

26. Walter S. Methods of Reporting Statistical Results from Medical Research Studies. American Journal of Epidemiology 1995;141:896-906.

27. Naylor CD, Chen E, Strauss B. Measured Enthusiasm: Does the Method of Reporting Trial Results Alter Perceptions of Therapeutic Effectiveness? Archives of Internal Medicine 1992;117:916-921.

28. Laupacis A, Sackett D, Roberts R. An Assessment of Clinically Useful Measures of the Consequences of Treatment. New England Journal of Medicine 1988;318:1728-1733.

Part Two

Health of Canadians

3

Health Indicators and Data Sources

The rational planning and evaluation of services to meet the health care needs of a population must be based on data on the health status of that population and how it is evolving. As government involvement in the provision of health care has increased, interest in the measurement of health and demand for data on the health of the population for which governments are responsible have increased. Many contemporary trends reinforce and consolidate that interest, particularly demographical changes, patterns of disease and illness, and medical practice, as well as changes in technology, the need for meaningful outcome measures, and the increasing costs of health care.

The measurement of health dates from the 17th century, when governments first began to collect information on death and its causes. Mortality statistics continue to be a major source of information about health, and are useful primarily in developing countries where death rates remain high. In industrialized countries where death rates are much lower, mortality statistics and associated measures such as life expectancy are no longer adequate indicators of health; they do not take into consideration illness that does not result in death or the often profound disability and distress that may accompany such illness. Following contemporary concerns about the quality of life, this broader definition of health has made its measurement more complex. It is now necessary to take into account the physical, psychological, and social status of the individual.

Chapter Two outlined the various ways in which data, once collected, can be summarized and analysed by various statistical techniques. This chapter describes the variety of data sources used for the health status of Canadians. Examples of the indicators and descriptive statistics derived from these sources will be given.

1. HEALTH INDICATORS

Health indicators are qualitative and quantitative statistical summaries that describe the health of a population. An **indicator** is a statistic that gives a meaningful indirect depiction of the health of a community. For example, mortality rates are an endpoint indicator of the burden of illness in a population. Comparing rates between communities can give an indication of underlying differences between these communities. Mortality rates alone do not suffice to describe the health of a community, because they address only one dimension. An **index** is the weighted average of related indicators designed to describe a phenomenon. A well-known example of this is the Consumer Price Index, used by economists as a measure of important economic events such as inflation and consumer demand. Indicators and indices are useful for depicting trends over time and giving capsule summaries of various aspects of community health. Ideally, indicators are derived from data that are reliable and valid, collected on a frequent basis, and sensitive to changes in the community so that planning and intervention strategies can be promptly implemented when warranted by changes in the indicator.

A useful hierarchy of community health indicators, which addresses health in its broad sense and is used in the Canada and Quebec Health Surveys, considers health on three main levels: determinants, health status, and consequences. Each of these levels incorporates biological, psychological, and social elements. Determinants of health are the prepathological components that can be associated with the development of health problems. Health status deals with pathological states; there may be health problems, morbid states or illnesses, diagnosed by health care professionals or through self-assessment, or even by a third party, with seriousness ranging from the most benign to the most severe (1). Consequences are the effects of health problems on the individual, such as a disability, on the health care system, such as hospitalization, and on society in general, including the economic burden.

The following section provides specific definitions and methodologies for deriving some representative common health indicators. A comprehensive description of health indicators for Canada is presented in Chapters Four and Five. It is important to note that there is no ideal taxonomy of indicators. This framework is only a guide to categorizing information on many aspects of health. Additionally, there are few indicators for some aspects that are considered important and for which further research is needed. Health promotion activities are a case in point, although some progress has been made in this direction. Ease of access to health services is another health indicator, which may in itself only be an indirect, proxy measure for the underlying concept.

The abundance of data on different types of indicators relevant to the spectrum of the determinants of health has led to the development of reports of community health status. The Canadian Institute for Health Information has published a list of 60 indicators that are useful for the production of community health status reports (1). Different health districts within Quebec currently use these indicators. Local health authorities, planning bodies, and community groups have found these indicators of immense value in understanding the challenges to be faced in providing comprehensive health care and social services to their populations.

1.1.   DETERMINANTS

1.1.1. Environment

As discussed in Chapter One, the environment encompasses both the physical and psychosocial milieu to which the population is exposed.

Physical Environment

These indicators are an integral component of monitoring progress toward a safe and clean physical environment. An example of an environmental health indicator is the Air Quality Index (AQI) that is measured continuously and summarized daily. The AQI is a composite of six commonly measured air pollutants that have evidence of adverse human health effects, namely carbon monoxide, total suspended particulate, ozone, sulphur, nitrogen dioxide, and total reduced sulphur compounds. When the AQI exceeds certain thresholds, health warnings can be issued so that people in vulnerable groups can avoid inhaling outdoor air.

Other indicators of environmental health include water quality measurements of drinking water and recreational water. The number of days that beaches are closed to swimmers because of elevated bacterial counts can also serve as an indicator of recreational water quality.

Psychosocial Environment

Indicators of the psychosocial environment incorporate demographic indicators, such as the age and gender of the population, and population growth rate, which are discussed in the next chapter. Definitions of natality and fertility rates and life expectancy, which are demographic indicators, are given below:

Crude Birth Rate: The annual number of live births per 1,000 population.

General Fertility Rate: The annual number of live births per 1,000 women between ages 15 and 49. This is a more refined measure of fertility, as it includes only those likely to give birth.

Total Fertility Rate: The average number of children who would be born alive to a woman during her lifetime if she were to pass through all her childbearing years conforming to the age-specific fertility rates of a given year.

Life Expectancy at Birth: The average number of years a newborn is expected to live if current mortality trends continue. It is a crude indication of the intrinsic health of a population, or the integrated result for basics of the interaction of many determinants of health and disease.

Indicators of the social environment also include demographic indicators that have more influence on the social context. These include ethnicity, language, family size, proportion of single-parent families, proportion of low birth weight infants (births of infants weighing less than 2,500 grams), and proportion of elderly persons (the health of the elderly is discussed in Chapter Six). Socioeconomic indicators include educational levels, literacy, unemployment rates, and income distribution.

1.1.2. Lifestyle, Behaviours, and Risk Factors

Survey data can supply a rich source of lifestyle, behaviour, and risk-factor indicators, which are discussed in detail in the next two chapters. Indicators such as the proportion of high-risk drinkers, the proportion of smokers by age and sex, the proportion of sexually active individuals who regularly use condoms, and estimates of the use of recreational and prescription drugs all give valuable insight into the patterns of health in the community.

1.1.3. Indicators of Human Biology

These determinants of health include age and gender. Women, men, children, and the elderly have different potential for health and disease. Due to the interaction with social and economic conditions, age and gender have been incorporated in social environment determinants. Genetic inheritance is currently the best example of this human biology indicator. The Human Genome Project offers the potential for complete knowledge of the human gene and the identification of an individual's genetic make-up. Mass screening programs for phenylketonuria (PKU) are well established, and genetic screening occurs for Tay-Sachs disease and the sickle cell trait and is anticipated for cystic fibrosis. Ethical issues are raised by genetic screening for diseases, as it may stigmatize the individuals (2). The implications of mass genetic screening will likely emerge as a public health concern.

1.1.4. Indicators of Health Services

Analysis of administrative data collected by the health care system provides information about people seeking formal health care. Examples include the numbers of health care providers such as physicians, nurses, or dentists per 1,000 Canadians. The number of beds per 1,000 population is also of interest.

1.2. HEALTH STATUS

Health status indicators include **subjective assessments**, such as the perception of one's own health or the proportion of people reporting one or more health problems in surveys. **Objective indicators** of health status include mortality, hospital morbidity, and non-hospital morbidity and are collected from records of consultation. Morbidity is generally measured in terms of disease incidence and prevalence rates, and also in terms of hospital use. The latter is made up of the number of individuals who are discharged from hospital or who have died divided by the number of people in the population. Some objective indicators of community health status are indicated on page 62, and their derivations are summarized in Table 3.1.

Table 3.1:   Derivations of Commonly Used Health Status Indicators

$$\text{Incidence rate} = \frac{\#\text{ of new cases of disease in a time interval}}{\text{population at risk}} \times 1{,}000$$

$$\text{Prevalence rate} = \frac{\#\text{ of existing cases of disease at a point}}{\text{total population}} \times 1{,}000$$

$$\text{Hospital morbidity rate} = \frac{\text{total }\#\text{ of hospital separations in a year}}{\text{total population at midyear}} \times 1{,}000$$

$$\text{Perinatal mortality rate} = \frac{\text{annual }\#\text{ of stillbirths} + \text{live births dying under 7 days}}{\text{total births (still and live)}} \times 1{,}000$$

$$\text{Neonatal mortality rate} = \frac{\text{annual }\#\text{ of deaths of children under 28 days}}{\text{annual live births}} \times 1{,}000$$

$$\text{Maternal mortality rate} = \frac{\text{annual }\#\text{ of deaths from puerperal causes per year}}{\text{annual live births}} \times 1{,}000$$

$$\text{Infant mortality rate} = \frac{\text{annual }\#\text{ of deaths under one year of age}}{\text{annual live births}} \times 1{,}000$$

$$\text{Crude death rate} = \frac{\text{annual }\#\text{ of deaths}}{\text{total population}} \times 1{,}000$$

$$\text{Age and/or sex specific death rate} = \frac{\text{annual }\#\text{ of deaths in a specific subgroup}}{\text{total population in that subgroup}} \times 1{,}000$$

$$\text{Standardized mortality ratio (SMR)} = \frac{\text{total observed deaths}}{\text{expected deaths}} \times 100$$

$$\text{Proportionate mortality ratio (PMR)} = \frac{\text{deaths from a specific cause}}{\text{total deaths}} \times 100$$

$$\text{Case fatality rate} = \frac{\#\text{ of deaths from a specific disease}}{\text{total }\#\text{ of cases of that disease}} \times 100$$

Infant Mortality Rate: The annual number of deaths in babies less than one year of age per 1,000 live births in the same year. The infant mortality rate is commonly used for comparing health among different countries.

Crude Death Rate: The annual number of deaths per 1,000 population.

Perinatal Mortality Rate: The annual number of stillbirths (gestation of 20 weeks or more) and early neonatal deaths (within the first seven days of life) per 1,000 stillbirths and live births. Perinatal mortality usually reflects standards of perinatal care, maternal nutrition, and obstetric and paediatric care.

Neonatal Mortality Rate: The annual number of deaths in a year of children under 28 days of age per 1,000 live births in the same year.

Maternal Mortality Rate: The annual number of maternal deaths from puerperal causes within 42 days of delivery per 100,000 live births in the same year.

Age and/or Sex Specific Death Rate: The annual number of deaths in a particular age and gender group per 1,000 population in that sub-group.

Potential Years of Life Lost (PYLL): The total years of life lost before age 75 years for people who become deceased between birth and the 75th year of life. It shows the burden of premature deaths by different causes and the cost in terms of person-years lost to society.

Proportionate Mortality Ratio (PMR): The ratio of deaths from a specific cause to the total number of deaths in a given period.

Case-Fatality Rate: The number of deaths from a specific disease per total number of cases of that disease in a given time period.

1.3. CONSEQUENCES

Indicators of the consequences of health problems include the economic burden (the direct and indirect costs of disease), indicators of the economic evaluation of health programs relating effectiveness to costs, rate of hospitalization, disability, and prescription drug use.

Economic Burden of Disease

Economics relates to the utilization of society's resources. Resources utilized for one purpose are unavailable for another, a concept known as opportunity cost. The economic burden of disease has become increasingly prominent in recent years. This section describes the meaning and precision of measurement of this concept.

The costs of disease are measured in terms of direct and indirect costs. Estimates of direct costs measure the expenditure for prevention and treatment of disease. They include: personal health care, which consists of institutional costs, non-hospital medical care costs, and other costs, such as dental care, prescribed drugs; publicly funded health care costs; education; and research.

Estimates of indirect costs measure the loss of productive services due to morbidity and mortality. They include financial loss due to premature death or loss of workdays due to temporary or permanent disability. For example, the number of person-years of productive work lost because of automobile accidents is an indirect cost, or indirect burden, of disease. Usually, data limitations and conceptual problems limit the scope and accuracy of these estimates.

Gross National Product

The proportion of the gross national product (GNP) or the gross domestic product (GDP) spent on health expenditure and the per capita expenditure (the average amount spent per person) on health by government are both indicators of the burden of disease. GNP measures all the goods and services produced by a country in a given year and is a measure of productivity. GDP includes all resources available to the country, irrespective of whether earned by local production or foreign investment in the country. It is useful for international comparisons. The per capita measure is limited according to what costs are included and the scope of adjustment for demographic characteristics of the population.

Economic Evaluation of Health Programs

Health programs may be evaluated in terms of their effects on morbidity and mortality (health outcomes), in terms of changes in behaviour (impact), and from an economic perspective (i.e., utilization of resources). Economic indicators, which may be factors in choosing between competing programs, are derived from different types of economic analysis.

Community Effectiveness

For these analyses, direct and indirect costs are measured as described above and expressed in dollars, related to the effectiveness of programs. The differences in the analyses lie in how the effects of a program are conceptualized and measured. Whether desired outcomes are achieved by an intervention in ideal conditions, such as in a randomized control trial, is called its efficacy. However, the efficacy of an intervention is only one component of its usefulness as applied in the community. Community effectiveness also depends on coverage and compliance. Coverage is the proportion of the target or at-risk population reached by the program: Is it directed to, accessible to and available to those who would maximally benefit? Compliance deals with provider and consumer compliance. Provider compliance indicates the degree to which health care providers cooperate with providing the program and all its elements. Consumer compliance indicates the degree to which those who need the intervention use it. This can be expressed in the following relationship:

$$\frac{\text{Community}}{\text{Effectiveness}} = \text{efficacy} \times \text{coverage} \times \frac{\text{provider}}{\text{compliance}} \times \frac{\text{consumer}}{\text{compliance}}$$

Quality of Life

The concept of quality of life has been used increasingly in the health care sector in the assessment of the benefit of a procedure, drug, or service provided, as the major objective is to improve the quality of life and not merely to increase longevity by these interventions. Torrance et al. (3) describe the health-related quality of life, which measures a broad array of physical, social, and emotional functions accrued by the intervention. Examples are sensory function (speech, sight, hearing), mobility and physical function, emotional function, cognitive function, self-care function related to activities of daily living, and the level of pain and discomfort.

In quantitative terms, one approach to measuring quality of life is the **quality-adjusted life year (QALY)**. A QALY is the modification of the actual anticipated duration of survival by the expected level of functioning and quality of life for that period as measured by health care providers.

An important economic concept is that of efficiency. A program is efficient if it achieves desired results with a minimum of inputs. Inputs, or resources utilized, are usually calculated in dollars, and effectiveness is quantified in the same manner. There are three approaches to evaluating the relative efficiency of health programs. These are described below:

Cost-Effectiveness Analysis. Cost-effectiveness analysis can be used when the outcomes of procedures or programs vary, but the outcomes can be expressed by a common natural unit such as life years gained (4). The effectiveness of the interventions can then be compared and expressed in dollar figures per natural unit of that outcome. For example, one could calculate the cost of an intervention per year of life gained, or per millimetre of mercury of blood pressure reduction.

Cost-Benefit Analysis. The effects of programs are expressed in health-related terms and then converted to dollar terms. For example, years of life gained are translated to dollars that could be earned during this period for a person of working age. The ratio of the benefits to costs are compared for different programs.

Cost-Utility Analysis. Cost-utility analysis refers to the subjective level of well-being experienced by people in differing states of health. It can be measured using a variety of techniques such as time trade-offs and the standard gamble. Cost-utility analysis seeks to incorporate the utility of quantity and quality of life in a summary measure such as QALY. Interventions can then be compared in terms of the QALYs gained or lost. Readers are referred to the article by Laupacis et al. for further details (5).

Hospital Separation Rate. The number of hospital separations (discharges and deaths) recorded in the year per 1,000 population. It reflects the frequency at which hospital care is sought, and is influenced by a number of factors such as the availability of care.

Hospital Days of Care. The total number of days of care for all hospitals per 1,000 population in a year. This rate may also be expressed for certain diseases to allow comparisons.

Disability Days. Days spent in bed, days during which the individual has to abandon principal activities, or days when activities are restricted for health reasons are considered disability days. These are quantified as the annual rate of disability days per 1,000 population.

2.   SOURCES OF HEALTH DATA

There is a large volume of Canadian health data available for interpretation. However, these data are scattered and often hidden in governmental and non-governmental publications. The following are some common data sources in Canada. The abundance of health-related data, from a variety of disparate sources, poses problems for comparability. As well, the need to share information across a variety of jurisdictions creates challenges for the development of compatible information systems. The challenges are not merely technical. The advent of powerful computers and algorithms for linking databases also cause significant ethical and social problems.

2.1.   CENSUS DATA

Statistics Canada conducts a national census every five years in June. All citizens are required by law to participate and complete the short census form (form 2A); a sample of 20% complete a more detailed form (form 2B; the long form). The census is the major source of information on population and demographic information, and is the chief source of numerator information for the calculation of rates. It also serves as the denominator for the calculation of certain rates. Census undercounting is usually about 3%. Data are collected on many variables, including age, sex, language spoken at home, place of birth, education, and economic status, and are aggregated on a geographic basis according to census tracts. This permits the analysis of census data on a geographic basis.

2.2. SURVEYS

A health survey is a cross-sectional study usually conducted by interview and/or examination of a sample of the population. It can also be conducted with a self-administered questionnaire, by telephone, mail, or personal interview. It can be done regularly and repeatedly (to analyse trends), or as needed to investigate a special problem (e.g., blood lead levels of children living near lead smelters in Toronto). Health surveys directed at a selected or representative sample of the population do not follow individuals over time, or produce retrospective or prospective studies for testing associations (e.g., cause and disease, treatment and result). However, they are useful for surveillance of levels of illness, impairment, disability, and many related social factors in people who do not necessarily contact the health care system.

Although simple in theory, surveys pose many methodological problems. Respondents have been shown to forget even major events. If the questionnaire is neither designed properly nor presented conscientiously, it may give ambiguous or misleading results. If interviewers are not adequately trained, they can easily influence the quality of responses. There is also a problem with missing data.

The federal government established the National Health Information Council (NHIC) to formulate plans on the need for data for the health sector (6). In 1991, the NHIC recommended that an ongoing national survey of population health be conducted. This recommendation was based on the knowledge of the economic and fiscal pressures on the health care system and on the requirement for information to improve the quality of health in Canada as well as the effectiveness and efficiency of health care services. The survey was first done by Statistics Canada in 1994 and is repeated every two years; the second phase was completed in 1996. The objectives of this National Population Health Survey (NPHS) (7) are to:

- aid in the development of public policies by providing measures of the health status of the population;
- provide data that assist in understanding the determinants of health;
- collect data on the economic, social, demographic, occupational, and environmental correlates of health;
- increase the understanding of the relationship between health status and the use of health care resources, including alternative as well as traditional services;
- follow a selected group of people over time to provide information on the dynamic process of health and illness;
- provide the provinces and territories and other clients with a template for a health survey that they can modify to supplement content and/or sample;
- allow the possibility of linking survey data to routinely collected administrative data such as vital statistics, environmental measures, community variables, and health care service utilization.

A number of national and provincial surveys of importance have been conducted in the last five decades (8). General health-related surveys in the past two decades include:

- Canada Health Survey (1978);
- General Social Surveys (1985, 1991);
- Health Promotion Surveys (1985, 1990);
- Ontario Health Surveys (1990, 1997);
- Quebec Health Surveys (1987, 1993).

Medically related surveys include:

- Blood Pressure (1985);
- Heart Health (1985-90).

Surveys devoted to health determinants, special populations, and lifestyles include:

- Canada Alcohol and Other Drugs Survey (1994);
- Surveys of smoking in Canada;
- Youth Smoking Survey (1994);
- Violence Against Women Survey (1993);
- Aboriginal Peoples Survey (1991);
- National Longitudinal Survey of Children (1994);
- Labour force surveys.

In 1991 and 1997, Statistics Canada and the Laboratory Centre for Disease Control produced an overview of the major population based surveys in Canada (8, 9). Recently, the Canadian Institute for Health Information (CIHI) also published a resource guide for data sharing that contains an appendix with an excellent description of the major health-related surveys ongoing or proposed in Canada (10).

2.3. ADMINISTRATIVE DATA

Perhaps the most uniformly recorded and reliable health data are administrative (e.g., rates of hospital admission, treatments, and discharge diagnoses). Administrative and professional bodies demand this information for use in the planning and evaluation of medical care. Administrative data for hospitalization in most provinces are summarized yearly and entered into a central provincial file, such as the one operated by the CIHI. At present, the main function of the CIHI is to prepare easily audited reports for hospitals to use in quality control and planning, but the data may also be used for research. Data are also gathered by all provincial health insurance plans, workers' compensation boards, drug utilization plans, and dental health plans. Usually, administrative data are more useful in studying health care rather than the distribution and causes of disease.

The broad utility of administrative data for an understanding of health services has been shown by research institutions in Manitoba and Ontario. The Manitoba Centre for Health Policy and Evaluation and the Institute for Clinical Evaluative Sciences in Ontario (ICES) make extensive use of administrative data to document variations in the delivery of health care services and examples of excellence. Two editions of an atlas of health care services have been published by ICES and are indispensable tools for understanding the role of the health care system in the broader determinants of health (11,12). Similarly, the Manitoba Centre for Health Policy and Evaluation produces regular reports on health services utilization.

2.4. REGISTRIES

Disease registries for chronic diseases, especially cancer, are another important source of data, particularly if they are population based. In all provinces, cancer reports are sent by private practitioners, clinics, and pathology departments, and each patient's name and clinical information are entered in a central registry. The completeness of the registry is checked by searching for notations of cancer on death certificates. If the registry is complete, the name of any person who died of cancer should already be entered in the registry records, as cancer is usually detected before death. A 95% agreement between death certificates and registry is the goal in most provinces. If registries are well kept, they can provide incidence and prevalence data.

There are other registries, including one for disabled children in British Columbia and the Canadian National Institute for the Blind. Currently, the following disease registries operate nationally:

- Canadian Cancer Registry;
- Canadian Organ Replacement Register;
- Canadian Tuberculosis Reporting System;
- Notifiable Disease Reporting System;
- Therapeutic Abortion Database.

It is anticipated that more registries will be developed in the future. Chronic Diseases in Canada, a report published by Health Canada, has analyses on disease registries in Canada (13, 14).

2.5. REPORTS

Reports are another source of health data. There are five types:

- Medical officers of health, physicians, and other health care professionals report unusual occurrences or apparent increases in disease rates to provincial or federal agencies responsible for surveillance.
- Many infectious diseases (e.g., measles, chicken pox) and sexually transmitted diseases are reportable — that is, the law requires that they be reported to the local health authority. This provides the data for incidence rates of infectious diseases. The list of reportable diseases in a province is available from the provincial health department or ministry. In Ontario, there are over 50 reportable diseases. These include diseases ranging from AIDS to yersiniosis. As of 1990, the Ontario Ministry of Health required municipal public health departments to record all reportable diseases of which they were notified on a central computer system. The system, which is called the Reportable Disease Information System, provides an up-to-date, province-wide reportable disease database. An example of reportable diseases is given in Table 3.2, which lists those that must be reported in Ontario.

Cancer is also reportable by law in a number of provinces. It must be stressed that under-reporting is the norm and so official figures are always lower than the actual incidence of disease.

- Case studies and clinical surveys of a specific disease appear frequently in medical journals. Selected case reports and notifiable disease data are published every two weeks by Health Canada in the *Canadian Communicable Disease Report*. Such data may be useful in following trends and spotting new epidemics; however, it may be difficult to calculate incidence and prevalence rates from these reports, because the precise number of cases and the population base from which they come are unknown. *Chronic Diseases in Canada* provides information on trends in chronic diseases.

- Another source of reports is the provincial workers' compensation board. In each province, notification of industrial accidents and diseases is required to facilitate claim processing and preventive activities. These data can provide incidence information on industrial accidents and diseases.

- *Health Reports* is a quarterly publication of the CIHI and Statistics Canada, and was started in 1989. This serial gives readers convenient access to essential health data and the general and disease-specific trends in risk factors, morbidity, mortality, and disabilities. Canadian hospital statistics are also listed in every issue, as are other available data. This serial is an excellent source of current health statistics.

2.6. VITAL STATISTICS

The record of the basic events of the human life cycle — birth, marriage and death — is appropriately called vital statistics. Throughout history, governments have kept some kind of register of their citizens. As early as 1608, an "Ordinance" in Quebec required the clergy to register births, marriages, and deaths in each parish. By 1667, this registration was required in duplicate, and one copy was forwarded to the "Judge Royal". In late 17th century England, John Graunt systematized record-keeping, and since then, vital statistics have been the most reliable and consistently recorded data source in the health field.

2.6.1. Birth Certificate

Figure 3.1 is an abridged facsimile of a Statement of Live Birth in Ontario. In Canada, the parents are responsible for filing the certificate with the municipal clerk. Note the relatively limited health information on the birth certificate. There is no medical history of the mother, or description of the birth itself. Another form, the Notice of Live Birth or Stillbirth, must be filled out by the attending physician and filed with the provincial registrar. This form provides no information about the father, and records the length of the gestation period and the presence of congenital deformities obvious at birth.

Table 3.2   List of Reportable Diseases in Ontario, 1991

Acquired Immunodeficiency Syndrome
Amebiasis
Anthrax
Botulism
Brucellosis
Campylobacter enteritis
Chancroid
Chickenpox (Varicella)
Chlamydia trachomatis infections
Cholera
Cytomegalovirus infection, congenital
Diphtheria
Encephalitis, including:
    Primary, viral
    Post-infectious
    Vaccine-related
    Subacute sclerosing panencephalitis
    Unspecified
Food poisoning, all causes
Gastroenteritis, institutional outbreaks
Giardiasis, except asymptomatic cases
Gonorrhoea
Haemophilus influenzae b disease, invasive
Hemorrhagic fevers, including:
    Ebola virus disease
    Marburg virus disease
    Other viral causes
Hepatitis, viral
    Hepatitis A
    Hepatitis B
    Hepatitis C
    Hepatitis D (Delta hepatitis)
Herpes, neonatal infection
Influenza
Lassa Fever

Legionellosis
Leprosy
Listeriosis
Lyme Disease
Malaria
Measles
Meningitis, acute
    i. bacterial
    ii. viral
    iii. other
Meningococcal disease, invasive
Mumps
Ophthalmia neonatorum
Pratyphoid Fever
Pertussis (Whooping Cough)
Plague
Poliomyelitis, acute
Psittacosis/Ornithosis
Q Fever
Rabies
Rubella
Rubella, congential syndrome
Salmonellosis
Shigellosis
Syphilis
Tetanus
Toxic Shock-like Syndrome
Trichinosis
Tuberculosis
Tularemia
Typhoid Fever
Verotoxin-producing E. coli
Yellow Fever
Yersiniosis

2.6.2. Death Certificate

A death certificate must be signed by a licensed physician and includes cause of death, person's name, birth date, sex, and place of residence and death. Figure 3.2 illustrates the part that lists the causes of death. As can be seen, there are three distinct sections for the cause of death. The immediate cause of death is recorded on the first line; for example, a certificate for an elderly person dying of pneumonia with no other fatal health conditions has pneumonia recorded there. The second entity is called "antecedent causes", which means that there may be a condition or disease that gave rise to the immediate cause of death. For example, an immediate cause of death in a woman could be metastatic or secondary cancer of the lung; if the condition led to this was cancer of the breast, then cancer of the breast would appear on the second line. The

Figure 3.1:   Birth Certificate, Province of Ontario

Province of Ontario (Canada)   Office of the Registrar-General   *(Abridged)*

CHILD	1.	2. Sex of child
Last name		
Given names		

Date of birth	3. Month (by name) day year of birth	4. Please state if mother is: Married, widowed, divorced or single (the term "common law" or "separated" not to be used)

Place of birth	5. Name of hospital (If not in hospital give exact location where birth occurred)	
	Borough, city, town, village, township (by name)	Regional municipality, county or district

PARENTS	FATHER	MOTHER
Name	6. Surname of child's father	10. Name before marriage
	All given names	All given names
Birthplace	7. City, town, or other place of birth (by name)	11. City, town, or other place of birth (by name)
	Province (or country if outside Canada)	Province (or country if outside Canada)
Birth date	8. Month (by name), day, year of birth — Age (at time of this birth)	12. Month (by name), day, year of birth — Age (at time of this birth)
Usual residence of mother	14. Complete street address; if rural, give exact location and post office or rural route address	
	Borough, city, town, village, township (by name); regional municipality, county or district; province (or country)	
Mailing address of mother	15. Complete mailing address (if different from 14). If rural give post office or rural route address	

OTHER	16. Duration of pregnancy (in completed weeks)	17. Number of children ever born to this mother (including this birth)	Number live born	Number stillborn (after 20 weeks pregnancy)

BIRTH PARTICULARS	18. Weight of child at birth ____ ____ or ____ lbs. oz. grams	19. Kind of birth (single, twin, or triplet)	20. If twin or triplet, whether this child was born 1st, 2nd, or 3rd.

ATTENDANT	21. Name of attending physician (or other attendant)	☐ Physician
	Complete mailing address	☐ Nurse
		☐ Other

Figure 3.2   Death Certificate

CAUSE OF DEATH

Part One

Immediate cause of death	(a) _____
	due to, or as a consequence of
Antecedent causes, if any, giving rise to the immediate cause (a) above, stating the *underlying cause last*	(b) _____
	due to, or as a consequence of
	(c) _____

Part Two

Other significant conditions contributing to the death but not causally related to the immediate cause (a) above	_____
	_____

third section is "any other significant conditions" that contributed to the death but did not directly cause it. For example, on the death certificate of a person who has chronic bronchitis and dies of uraemia as a result of chronic nephritis, uraemia would be listed as the immediate cause of death (line a), chronic nephritis would be listed as the antecedent cause of death (line b), and chronic bronchitis would be listed in the second part as another significant condition. When both the immediate cause of death and the antecedent cause are recorded on the death certificate, then the antecedent cause is the one used for data analysis for cause-specific mortality. Other significant conditions may also be recorded separately.

The current system for recording cause of death information has been described as unreliable. Problems exist in the ambiguity of the instructions and disease definitions set out by the World Health Organization for use by the physician or coroner when filling out a death certificate. A recent critique suggests the need for greater validity in recording cause of death data (15).

Some causes of death require notification of death to the coroner (or medical examiner). In such cases, a physician must not sign the death certificate. These include situations where there is reason to suspect that the person died by violent means or undue negligence or in an unexplained manner, death in a correctional institution, in police custody, in maternally related situations (e.g., abortion), after anaesthesia, in seniors' homes and in work places, and associated with involuntary residence in an institution. Each province has its own statute governing the causes to be notified to the coroner.

Birth and death data usually provide the fertility rate, infant mortality rate, crude death rate, life expectancy at birth, potential years of life lost, and all other mortality rates described earlier.

2.7. CONSUMPTION DATA

Various production and consumption data can be related to health. The most obvious of these is food. The figures for tonnage of food produced or imported each year are adjusted according to current levels of supplies to produce a "disappearance" figure: the amount of foodstuffs that need to be replaced each year. In general, it is possible to determine the proportion of various foodstuffs actually eaten by humans, so the average per capita consumption of meat, for example, can be calculated for any year. Although this information is useful for following long-term historical trends (compared with dietary inventories of the type collected in surveys carried out by Nutrition Canada), such data are not very reliable, as they tell us little about the habits of any individual. In the same way, annual production of cigarettes or litres of alcohol can be related to long-term trends in health. More indirectly, data on industrial processes involving hazardous substances, such as asbestos or substances emitting pollutants (e.g., sulphur dioxide from the pulp and paper industry), may be related to levels of health.

3.   RECORD LINKAGE

A wide variety of health data (vital statistics, registries, surveys and reports) is collected about each individual and recorded in many places. Many people feel that if these data were collected in one place, a very useful profile of social, biological, and personal data could be constructed. Relationships between possible causes of disease (industrial exposure, levels of pollution, social conditions, family history) and the individual's history of disease would yield much more precise information than the other sources of data already described. Furthermore, the Canadian system of "geocoding" social and demographic information according to the postal code, and the existence of a centralized agency (Statistics Canada, the ultimate collector and publisher of a great volume and variety of data) set the stage for this record linkage. The 1991 Task Force on Health Information advised that the capacity for linkage of different data elements was critical to fulfilling the potential of the development of systems for health data (6).

Approaches to record linkage include integrating health records at the level of the individual patient from different sources and over time. Record linkage can be achieved by the allocation of personal identifiers, possibly on a lifetime basis, a strategy that has been considered at the provincial level. However, these are not likely to be portable between provinces. Linkage can also be achieved, with varying degrees of accuracy, by matching based on probabilities of linking personal identifying data in two or more data banks. These include the surname, surname at birth (if applicable), first name, date of birth, place of birth, and any other identifiers such as the social insurance number. A record is strongly matched when a high percentage of similarities is obtained. If matched, records for individuals in the two data banks may be merged; however, these data must be of good quality and be sufficiently detailed for the information to be useful.

Record linkage can be employed for both the purposes of administration and research. Health records contain sensitive information about individuals. Linkage and data sharing must be carried out under conditions of strict confidentiality. Confidentiality requirements and consent procedures differ in research and administrative contexts. Data used for administrative purposes can have a direct impact on an individual, whereas research data rarely target individuals, but deal with unlinked aggregate data. In general, it is customary for data collected for administrative purposes to be used for research; the converse is never the case unless explicit consent for such use has been obtained.

Several provinces and the federal government have legislation that protects personal health information. The legislation usually outlines sanctions and punishments that can be brought to bear for violations of confidentiality. Other safeguards for data confidentiality include:

- a mechanism to obtain consent if administrative data are intended for research purposes;
- a means of informing data subjects on the possible uses of their information;
- a means of scrambling personal identifiers so that individuals are not identifiable;
- adequate legal and physical security controls so that data is secure and access granted only to those with justified access (10).

4.   INTERNET AND INFORMATICS

The development of the Internet has made possible both rapid access to databases and the global transfer of information. Most of the data sources listed above, as well as most major scientific journals, are now accessible electronically and can be easily found through search engines. These databases may contain their own powerful search engines that facilitate ease of access. They also contain extensive links to other related sites. Useful sites are listed at the end of the book in an appendix.

Informatics is the discipline that studies the application of computer technology to the retrieval and analysis of health information. Informatics is likely to become a critical knowledge skill for health care workers, and linked computer databases and the Internet will likely become a central and indispensable part of the provision of health care in the 21st century.

5.   SUMMARY

This chapter dealt with health indicators and sources of health data. *Health indicators* are qualitative and quantitative measures that indicate the health of a population, and are examined on three dimensions, namely determinants, health status and consequences. Each level has biological, psychological, and social elements.

Determinants are factors that are not actual health problems but are believed to be related to the development of disease. The determinants of health include the environment, lifestyle factors, behaviour and risk factors, human biology and the health care system.

The environment encompasses both the physical aspects and the psychosocial milieu experienced by the population.

With respect to the physical environment, Canadians may be exposed to toxic substances or other environmental hazards from a variety of sources, including food, water, air, soil, and consumer products. Indicators of the psychosocial environment incorporate demographic indicators, such as the age and sex of the population and population growth rate. Indicators of the social environment also include sociodemographic variables (such as ethnicity, language, and family size) and socioeconomic variables (which include education level, literacy, unemployment rates, and income distribution). Lifestyle factors, behaviours, and risk factors are measured in many ways, for example by the proportion of the population who are smokers, who are obese, or who wear seat belts.

The determinants of human biology include age and sex. Men, women, children, and the elderly have different potential for health and ill health. Another indicator is genetic inheritance.

Health status is viewed in terms of health problems that are concrete, medical conditions of individuals or groups, or pathology. Health status indicators include subjective assessments (such as the inclusion of questions concerning the perception of one's own health) and objective indicators (such as mortality, hospital morbidity, and non-hospital morbidity).

Consequences are the effects of health problems on the individual (such as disability), on the health care system (such as hospitalization), and on society in general, including economic burden. Indicators of the consequences of health problems include economic burden (incorporating direct and indirect costs of ill health), the economic evaluation of health programs relating effectiveness to costs, rate of hospitalization, disability, and prescription drug use.

There are several *data sources* in Canada. These consist of surveys, administrative data, registries, reports, vital statistics, consumption data, and record linkage. Surveys usually provide prevalence rates for risk factors, disease, disability, and utilization of health services, and can also be used to explore relationships among these factors. Recent surveys of interest include the Canada Health Survey, Canada Fitness Survey, Canada Student Health Survey, General Social Survey, National Alcohol and Other Drugs Surveys, and the Canadian Heart Health Survey. The most uniformly recorded and reliable health data are administrative. Administrative and professional bodies demand this information for use in planning and evaluation of medical care, and it is more useful in studying health care rather than the distribution and cause of disease. Disease registries for certain chronic diseases also provide incidence and prevalence data. Reports that provide health data include *Health Reports*, workers' compensation boards publications, and the *Canadian Communicable Diseases Report*. The events of the human life cycle — birth, marriage, death — are called vital statistics, and data usually provide the fertility rate, infant mortality rate, crude death rate, life expectancy at birth, and all other mortality rates.

6. REFERENCES

1.   Community Health Information Systems Working Group, Chevalier S. Community Health Indicators: Definitions and Interpretations. Ottawa: Canadian Institute for Health Information, 1995.
2.   Markel H. The Stigma of Disease: Implications of Genetic Screening. American Journal of Medicine 1992;93(2):209-215.
3.   Torrance G et al. Risk-Benefit and Quality-of-Life Analyses of Prescription Drugs. Ottawa: Health and Welfare Canada, 1990.
4.   Robinson R. Economic Evaluation and Health Care: What Does it Mean? British Medical Journal 1993;1993(307):670-673.
5.   Laupacis A, Feeny D, Detsky AS, Tugwell PX. How Attractive Does a New Technology Have to be to Warrant Adoption and Utilization? Tentative Guidelines for Using Clinical and Economic Evaluations. Canadian Medical Association Journal 1992;146(4):473-481.
6.   National Health Information Council. Health Information for Canada 1991, Report of the Task Force on Health Information. Ottawa: Health and Welfare Canada, 1991.
7.   Tambay J, Catlin G. Sample Design of the National Population Health Survey. Health Reports 1995;7(1):29-39.
8.   Kendall O, Lipskie T, MacEachern S. Canadian Health Surveys, 1950-1997. Chronic Diseases in Canada 1997;18(2):70-90.
9.   Adams O, Ramsay T, Millar W. Overview of Selected Health Surveys in Canada, 1985 to 1991. Health Reports 1992;4(1):25-52.
10.   Canadian Institute for Health Information. Health Data Sharing in Canada: A Resource Guide. Ottawa: Canadian Institute for Health Information, 1995.
11.   Naylor CD, Anderson G, Goel V. Patterns of Health Care in Ontario: The ICES Practice Atlas (1st ed.). Ottawa: Canadian Medical Association, 1994.
12.   Goel V, Williams J, Anderson G. Patterns of Health Care in Ontario: The ICES Practice Atlas, vol. 2. Ottawa: Canadian Medical Association, 1996.
13.   Health and Welfare Canada. Special Diseases Registries Issue, Part B. Chronic Disease in Canada 1988;9(4):66-76.
14.   Health and Welfare Canada. Special Diseases Registries Issue, Part A. Chronic Disease in Canada 1988; 9(3): 50-63.
15.   Lindahl BI, Glattre E, Lahti R, et al. The WHO Principles for Registering Causes of Death: Suggestions for Improvement. Journal of Clinical Epidemiology 1990;43(5):467-474.

Determinants of Health and Disease

Chapter Four describes health determinants in the Canadian population, using the health field concept explained in Chapter One and the health indicators outlined in Chapter Three. Many statistics are listed here for two reasons: to compile data in a single source and to illustrate how each of these determinants affects on health and the health care delivery system in Canada. The next chapter describes the measurable outcomes of the interaction of these determinants of health. Health care organization, which contributes significantly to health, is also discussed in Part III of the book.

1. HUMAN BIOLOGY

The genetic potential of the individual has an impact on a person's health in many complex ways, many of which are poorly understood. There are, however, a few well-explained situations. Mutant genes lead to congenital malformations and genetic disorders within the population. For example, in Canadian (Old Colony) Mennonites, who are descended from a small number of founding families and whose conservative members practise endogamy, due to familial aggregations of autosomal recessive and dominant conditions, some diseases of multifactorial origin and other inherited conditions occur frequently (1). Those diseases include insulin-dependent diabetes melitis, auto-immune diseases, and Tourette's syndrome, which were described initially in Mennonites living in a sub-district of Alberta. Clusters of malformations, inborn errors of metabolism, and other inherited disorders were found in Mennonite families in rural areas of three other western provinces and southern Ontario. In Quebec, there is a high prevalence of the gene for Tay-Sachs disease among the French Canadian population and the incidence of sickle cell haemoglobinopathy (HbS) is estimated at 9 cases per 100,000, occurring mainly in the Black population and those of Central American ancestry (2). Nova Scotia has an indigenous Black population that is genetically predisposed to carriage or expression of the gene for sickle cell anaemia.

Age and sex are important determinants of health; due to their interaction with social and economic factors, they are discussed in the next section on demography, sociodemography, and socioeconomic indicators.

2.   THE ENVIRONMENT

2.1.   THE PSYCHOSOCIAL ENVIRONMENT

Demography is the study of populations, especially with reference to size, density, fertility, mortality, growth, age distribution, migration, and vital statistics. Sociodemographic and socioeconomic indicators represent the interaction of these factors with social and economic conditions. Most of the data in this section come from the 1996 Census of Canada (3-8) for age, sex, marital status, household composition, language, ethnic origin, education, and visible minority, and from the User's Guide to *Community Health Indicators* (9), the latter being a valuable source of references for definitions and data on determinants of health for Canada. The framework for categorizing community health indicators in the User's Guide provided the basis, with some exceptions, for the organization of this chapter as well as Chapter Five, Health Status and Consequences. Data obtained from sources apart from the two indicated are specifically referenced.

2.1.1. Demography
On May 14, 1996, Canada's population was 29,963,631, of whom 49.5% were male. Of the total population, 20.0%, 67.8%, and 12.2% were in the age groups 0-14 years, 15-64 years, and 65 years and over, respectively. Among those aged 65 and over, 57.8% of the population was female. In 2001, the Canadian population is projected to be 31.9 million people; 49.5% will be male. It is estimated that in 2001, the population of people aged 65 and older will constitute 12.7% of the total population (10). Marital status of people aged 15 and over revealed that 32.2% were single, and 51.2%, 3.0%, 7.2%, and 6.4% were married, separated, divorced, and widowed respectively. In 1996, there were total of 7.8 million families living in private households with or without children at home; almost three quarters (73.7%) were married couples, 1 in 10 (11.8%) were common-law families, and 14.5% were lone-parent families.

Population distributions by age and sex between 1901 and 2001 indicate that the population has more than doubled since 1941 (see Figure 4.1). The ratio of males to females has remained roughly constant, but there has been a definite change in the age distribution. In 1901, there were proportionately more children under age 14 compared with 1996, because of early age at marriage and large family size, as is the case in most developing countries. These factors are reflected in the total fertility rate (TFR) expressed as number of children a woman can expect to have in her lifetime based on the age-specific fertility rates of a given year. In 1941, compared with earlier years, there

Figure 4.1:   Populations Pyramids, 1901-2001, Canada

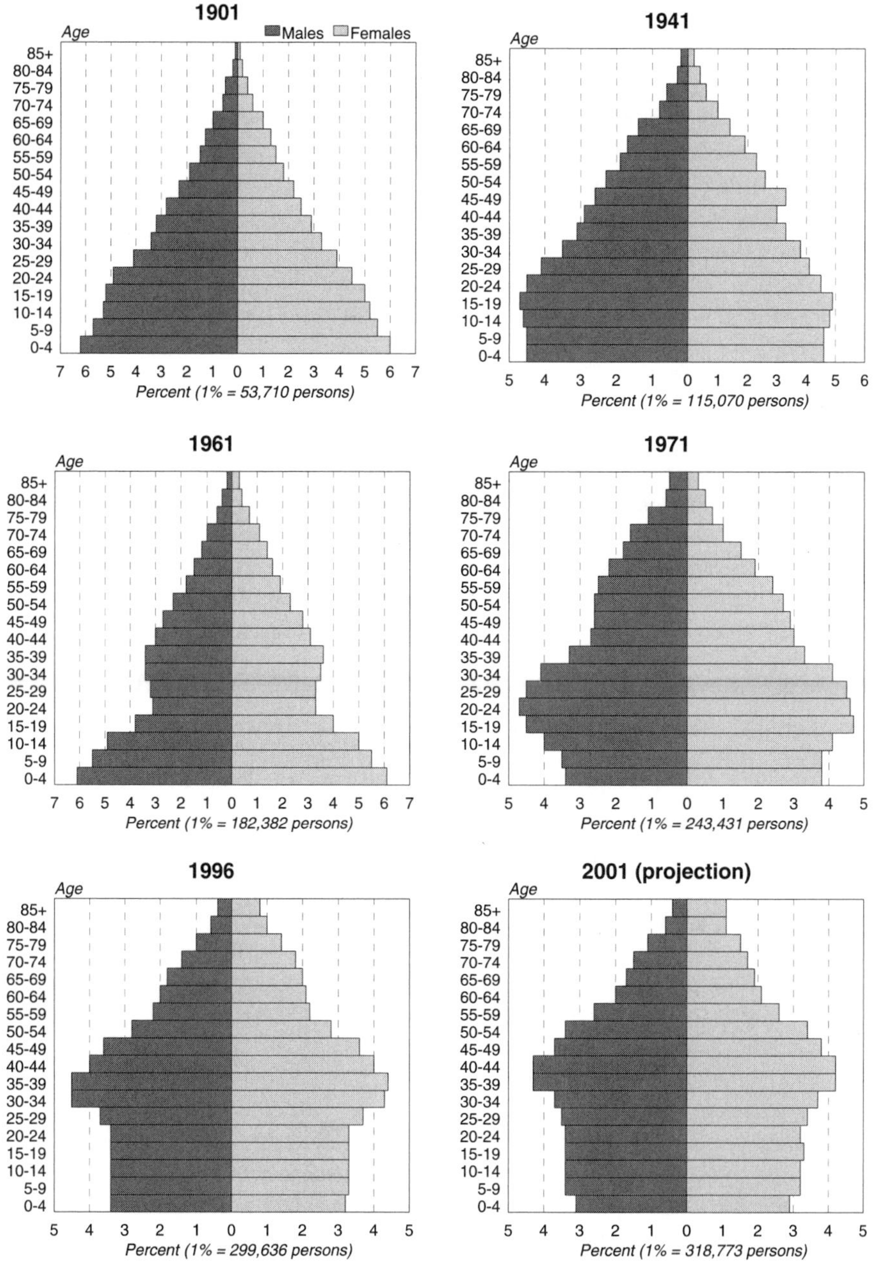

1901

Age — Males ▣ Females

Percent (1% = 53,710 persons)

1941

Age

Percent (1% = 115,070 persons)

1961

Age

Percent (1% = 182,382 persons)

1971

Age

Percent (1% = 243,431 persons)

1996

Age

Percent (1% = 299,636 persons)

2001 (projection)

Age

Percent (1% = 318,773 persons)

Source: Statistics Canada.

were proportionately fewer children under age 14. This was largely due to postponed childbirth during the Great Depression and World War II, which is reflected in low fertility rates during this period. In the late 1940s, the number of births increased during what is popularly described as the postwar "baby boom", and by 1961, there were proportionately more children under age 14. Generally, birth and fertility rates have been declining since the baby boom, and the effect on the population's age distribution may be traced in Figure 4.1. Since 1974, the TFR has remained below the level of 2.1, which is the replacement level needed for maintenance of the population at a steady state (11). Total fertility rate for the year 1994 was 1.66 per woman. Due to increased industrialization, level of education, and availability of contraception, family size fell gradually during the later part of the century.

With the availability of better contraception, more liberal abortion laws, and more women participating in the labour force, the proportion of children under aged 14 decreased in 1971, and the number between ages 15 and 29 increased. The decrease in the proportion of young children in the population is reflected in the decreased demand for paediatricians and paediatric units in general hospitals. A temporary increase in this proportion was predicted to occur when the baby boomers grew up and produced families, but has not happened. In 1996, the baby boomers contributed to the increase in the group aged 39 to 49. The population over age 65, particularly the number of females in this group, shows a remarkable increase from the previous years.

Population growth is the sum of natural increase and net migration. Natural increase is the difference between the number of births and number of deaths. For example, for the period of 1991 to 1996, there was a total of 1,945,000 births and 1,030,000 deaths. Thus, the natural increase was 915,000 persons. Net migration is the difference between immigration and emigration. Immigration has always been an important source of population growth in Canada. Between 1991 and 1996, the number of immigrants coming to the country was 1,156,000, whereas 228,000 people emigrated from Canada. Thus, the net migration was 928,000 persons. In essence, Canada's population increased by 1.84 million people between 1991 and 1996: natural increase contributed 49.6% and net migration 50.4%. Average annual growth rate of the population was 1.28% between 1992 and 1996.

Geographic distribution also affects the health status of a population. Approximately three quarters of the Canadian population live within 320 kilometers of the border between Canada and the United States, and the remaining population is spread over a vast land mass. Historically, providing health care services to a widely dispersed population in northern Canada has been a challenge.

Life Expectancy

Life expectancy has traditionally been the index of health most commonly used for international comparisons, as relevant data are readily available. Life expectancy at birth in Canada increased significantly between 1941 and 1996 from 63.0 to 75.7 years for males, and from 66.3 to 81.3 years for females; in 1996 overall life expectancy for both sexes combined was 78.6 years. The chief reason is the significant decline in infant mortality, from 61 deaths per 1,000 live births in 1941 to 6.1 in 1995. Life expectancy has increased significantly more for females than for males, such that the gap has broadened from 3.3 years in 1941 to 5.7 years in 1996. This is due to a decline in death rates among women at all ages over a longer period than for males. This increasing difference between the sexes appears to be levelling off (12). By contrast, Japan had the highest life expectancy at birth in 1995 — 82.8 for females and 76.4 for males. Life expectancies in other developed countries are listed in Chapter 12.

The sex differential in death rates may be partly attributed to differences in lifestyle, such as smoking, drinking, and occupation. Males have traditionally experienced higher mortality from ischemic heart disease, respiratory diseases, and lung cancer, as well as motor vehicle and other accidents, all of which are related to lifestyle. The influence of biological factors seems to be important, since infant males have higher mortality rates as well.

2.1.2. Sociodemographic Indicators
Aging

One important demographic change with far-reaching implications is the rise in the proportion of the population over age 65, largely due to increased longevity and a decreased proportion of children in the population. The number of seniors has more than doubled in the past 25 years; even since 1991, the percentage increase (11.4%) is double the increase (+5.7%) recorded for the population as a whole. The level rose in every province and territory. The significance of this change for health care lies in the fact that in 1991, seniors, who comprise 11% of the population, accounted for 40% of all patient days in general hospitals, allied special hospitals, and mental hospitals. The highest median age ever was recorded in Canada in 1996: 34.5 years for males and 36.1 for females. Both medians were almost two years higher than in 1991. Aging is discussed in more detail in Chapter Six.

Immigrant Population

The composition of the Canadian population is changing in relation to ethnicity, and is expected to continue to change as more immigrants are allowed into Canada in order to offset the decreasing Canadian fertility rate. The 1996 census showed that Canada was home to about five million immigrants, including the more than one million who had arrived between 1991 and 1996. The total number of immigrants represented 17.4% of the population in 1996, the largest share in more than 50 years. This share had remained at around 15% to 16% between 1951 and 1991.

Sources of immigration to Canada have also changed greatly. In 1996, the European-born continued to account for the largest proportion (47%) of all immigrants living in Canada but this figure has declined steadily since 1965. Asia and the Middle East (31%) were the second and the remainder (22%) were from other parts of the world. Seven of the ten most frequently reported countries of birth for recent immigrants were the Asian countries of Hong Kong, China, India, the Philippines, Sri Lanka, and Taiwan.

The impact of recent immigration is most clearly seen in big cities. In 1996, Toronto had the largest immigrant population of all the 25 census metropolitan areas, with 42% of its population being immigrants, followed by Vancouver (35%) and Montreal (18%).

Ethnicity

In 1996, 18.3 million people (64%) reported one ethnic origin, and 10.2 million (36%) reported more than one. Approximately 5.3 million people (19%) reported their ethnic origin as Canadian and an additional 3.5 million (12%) listed Canadian plus an-other origin. Most people listed as Canadian were born in Canada and had English or French as their first language. This suggests that many of these respondents come from families that have been in Canada for several generations. About 4.9 million people, or 17% of the population, listed their ancestry as British, and about 2.7 million, or 9%, reported French-only ancestry (French Canadian or Acadian). About 2.9 million (10%) people reported a combination of British, French, or Canadian origins. A further 4.6 million (16%) people reported an ancestry of either British, French, or Canadian origin, in combination with some other origin, many being mixed European and British ancestry. About 8.1 million (28%) people reported origins other than the British Isles, France, or Canada, and 3.7 million reported a single European origin. Most frequent ethnic origins other than Canadian, English, and French were Scottish (4.3 million), Irish (2.8 million), Italian (1.2 million), Ukrainian (1 million), Dutch (916,000), Polish (787,000), Jewish (353,000), and Norwegian (346,000). Aboriginal, Chinese, and South Asian origins were also among the top 15 ethnic origins (see next section). About 1.1 million reported Aboriginal ancestry.

Visible Minorities

In the 1996 census, the definition of a visible minority was taken from the *Employment Equity Act:* "persons, other than Aboriginal peoples, who are non-Caucasian in race or non-white in colour." The regulations of the Act specify the following groups as visible minorities: Chinese, South Asians, Blacks, Arabs, West Asians, Filipinos, Southeast Asians, Latin Americans, Japanese, Koreans, and Pacific Islanders.

In 1996, Canada was home to 3.2 million people who identified themselves as members of a visible minority. They represented 11.2% of the total population in Canada. About three in every ten were born in Canada, and the rest were immigrants. In British Columbia, 18% of the population were a visible minority; in Ontario, the figure was 16%. Seven out every ten visible minority persons lived in metropolitan Toronto, Vancouver, or Montreal. Toronto was home to 42% of the total visible minority population in Canada, and 18% lived in Vancouver and 13% in Montreal. A total of 860,000 or 3% of total population, identified themselves as Chinese in the 1996 census, constituting the largest visible minority population. The next largest groups were 671,000 (2.4%) South Asians and 574,000 (2%) Blacks. Together, Chinese, South Asians, and Blacks represented two thirds of the visible minority population in Canada.

Language

Given the ethnic diversity described above, it is not surprising that in 1996, 4.7 million people reported a first language other than French or English. This is defined as the first language learned at home in childhood and still understood by the individual at the time of the census. The most common first languages listed were English (67.6%), French (22.6%), and Aboriginal languages (0.5%); the remainder (9.3%) spoke non-official languages (that is, neither French nor English). The non-official languages most frequently listed as a first language were Chinese, Italian, Punjabi, Spanish, Portuguese, Polish, and German. Approximately half a million (473,475) Canadians do not speak either official language.

Religion

In 1991, the majority of Canadians were Christians (Catholic, 45.7%, and Protestant, 36.3%) followed by Eastern Orthodox (1.4%), Jewish (1.2%), Islam (0.9%), Hindu (0.6%), and Sikh (0.5%); 12.5% listed no religious affiliation. The remainder belonged to other religious faiths.

Family Environments

Over the past 20 years, it has been recognized that family abuse and violence affect the health of individual family members. There are three principal types of family violence: wife battering or spousal abuse, child abuse, and elder abuse. Abuse is threatening or intolerable behaviour that may involve physical violence and threats. Wife battering constitutes 76% of reported family violence; however, there is significant under-reporting. The Violence Against Women Survey (13) was conducted by Statistics Canada in 1993 and reported that 10% of women age 18 and over had experienced violence in the 12 months preceding the survey; 51% of Canadian women have experienced at least one incident of physical or sexual violence since the age of 16. In the 12 months prior to the survey, their partners had assaulted 3%. Nearly one half (45%) of wife assault cases were violent enough to cause physical injury to the woman, necessitating medical attention in 40%. Almost one third (29%) of those who had ever been married or lived common law reported being assaulted by their partner. Thus, 2.6 million Canadian women have been the victims of wife assault. The methods of assault include pushing, grabbing, or shoving (25%); threatening (19%); slapping (15%); throwing objects (11%); kicking, biting, or hitting (11%); battery (9%); sexual assault (8%); choking (7%); striking with an object (6%); and using a gun or knife (5%). Violence was reported more or less evenly across every socioeconomic group. In 1988, 15% of all homicide victims in Canada were women murdered by their male partners. A 1994-95 survey of transition homes reported a total of 85,259 admissions of women and dependent children to shelters in the preceding year. These women and children logged a total of over one million resident days in the shelters during the year (14) (see also Chapter Seven).

Child abuse consists of neglect, physical, emotional, or sexual abuse. The data available from a random sample (n=9,953) of general population over age 15 as a supplement to Ontario Health Survey done in 1990 provides the most comprehensive picture in this area (15). One in three boys (31.2%) and one in five girls (21.1%) suffers physical abuse during childhood; one in eight (12.8%) girls and one in 23 (4.3%) boys suffer sexual abuse. These rates are much higher than those reported earlier. Contrary to the common belief that parents and step-parents are the chief perpetrators of sexual abuse, the survey found that adults who were unrelated either by blood or marriage were most often identified as the abuser. In Canada between 1985 and 1990, the presumed child-abuse mortality for infants under one year of age was 2.7 per 100,000 live births.

Elder abuse includes emotional, financial, physical neglect, and maltreatment, including questionable institutionalization (see Chapter Six for the details on elder abuse). It is estimated that approximately 4% of elderly Canadians (approximately 1 in 25 over age 65) may be abused annually (16).

2.1.3. Socioeconomic Indicators

The composition of the population in terms of educational, income, and employment characteristics influences health status. The proportion of live births to mothers who have fewer than 11 years of schooling to total live births is one indicator of socioeconomic status that identifies a high rate of premature birth, low birth weight, and perinatal and infant mortality rate, because mothers in this group tend to be poor. In Quebec, in 1990, 15.3% of all live births reported were to mothers with fewer than 11 years of education. The figures for the rest of Canada are not available. In 1996, 34.8% of the population had less than high school education (7).

The mother's age at the time of the birth of an infant influences the number of low birth-weight infants, prematurity, and perinatal morbidity. In 1993, 6.1% of Canadian births were to mothers under age 20 and 10.7% were born to mothers age 35 and over. There is an increased risk for infants in both age groups (17).

In 1994, the Adult Literacy Survey reported that 16.6% of the adult population has literacy limitations, and can only read at a level 1 prose level (18). Prose is defined as printed material from texts, editorials, news stories, poems, and fiction. Most tasks at level 1 require the reader to locate one piece of information in the text that is identical or synonymous to information given in a directive. These limitations may affect health directly in terms of the inappropriate use of medication, inability to communicate effectively with health care workers, or difficulty in following instructions (including safety instructions at work). As already mentioned, unhealthy lifestyles due to limited access to health information also affect health status. This latter concept has been termed health literacy.

Income is another major socioeconomic indicator. Statistics Canada has determined low-income cut-off points based on a survey of family expenditures; these are adjusted annually in line with the Consumer Price Index and are used to determine poverty levels. A family that spends more than 56.2% of income on the basic needs of accommodation, food, and clothing falls below the cut-off. These levels are adjusted for family size and location.

In 1985, 15.9% of Canadian families were living in poverty, whereas in 1996, 17.9% of the families lived below the poverty line. This figure excludes the residents of the Yukon Territory, Northwest Territories, and First Nations communities.

The average family income in Canada in 1996 was $56,629. Unemployment rates in Canada are high, having increased from 7.4% in 1981 to over 11.0% in early 1990s, to just under 9.0% in 1998.

The lone-parent status of families, particularly families headed by females, often denotes disadvantage to children as many of these families live below the poverty line. In 1996, there were 14.5% lone-parent families whereas in 1991 there were 13.0%. Of the 1.1 million lone-parent families, the majority (83.0%) were headed by a female, and nearly one quarter (24.0%) of all female lone parents were single. Almost one in every five children — just under 1.8 million children — in Canada lived with a lone parent in 1996. The effects of poverty on the health of children is described in Chapter Six.

The proportion of welfare recipients indicates those who cannot adequately meet their own needs or those of their dependants because of their inability to find work, or because of the loss of a spouse who is the main support of the family, or because of illness, disability, or other reasons. Welfare payments fall below the previously described low-income cut-off points set by Statistics Canada. For Canada as a whole, 14.4% of the population received welfare support in March 1993, compared to 6% in March 1990.

Living alone may be associated with social isolation and possibly with lower socioeconomic status and a higher incidence of suicide. In 1996 in Canada, about 2.6 million individuals (11.7% of the population aged 15 and over) lived alone, and the number of people over age 65 constituted just over one third (35.6%) of people living alone. The extended survival of senior women and the breakdown of families are major contributing causes.

Although homeless men and women do not have illnesses that differ from the general population, homelessness is associated with increased health risks. Many homeless persons are ex-patients of mental health institutions, runaway teenagers, women and children escaping from domestic violence, seniors, alcoholics, and Aboriginal peoples. The estimates for number of homeless varies because it is difficult to count them; however, the various estimates put the number in the range of 130,000 to 250,000 (19).

The social environment includes the working environment. The significance of safety in the work environment is illustrated by the fact that in Canada there were 703 work-related fatalities in 1996 (20). The number and characteristics of work-related health problems are changing as working environments change. Since World War II, a gradual shift of the labour force has occurred from goods-producing jobs in manufacturing, construction, and primary industries to less hazardous service-producing jobs, for example in finance, amusement, and business services. The increased participation of women in the workforce, generally in the service sector, has led to new concerns about the safety of the working environment for the pregnant mother and fetus. In 1991, one fifth to one third of the workforce, depending on the hazard, reported that they were exposed to unpleasant and potentially unhealthy working conditions. The most exposures were to dust (34%) and computer screens (31%), followed by loud noise (26%), poor air quality (23%), and dangerous chemicals (19%) (21). The effect of working environment on health is described in Chapter Ten.

It is apparent from the preceding discussion that both demographic and socioeconomic determinants strongly affect the overall health status of a population, particularly health problems concentrated in certain gender, age, ethnic, or income subgroups. It follows then that demographic and socioeconomic determinants are essential considerations for the effective planning of health care.

2.1.4. The Physical Environment

The environment has been widely discussed in the media in the past two decades, usually in regard to the pollution of air and water from industrial and domestic sources. A federal report that gives a good overview of environment and health in Canada (22) indicated that in 1990, 97% of Canadians surveyed were concerned about the effect of environmental pollution. Environmental health problems range from acute poisoning or chronic irritation to cancer or genetic damage (23). Although the negative impact of the environment on health has been publicized, the positive effect of the naturally occuring substances in the environment must not be forgotten; it can have a directly beneficial effect on health, such as the protection against dental caries enjoyed by the 37% of Canadians whose local water supply is "naturally" fluoridated.

Specific information on many of the environmental indicators defined as determinants of health in Chapter Three is presented in Chapter Nine, which deals with environmental health.

Agricultural Risks

At least two million Canadians are involved in activities related to agriculture or livestock on family farms. There are concerns about health and safety issues in modern, competitive agriculture, which is largely dependent on mechanization and the use of pesticides, herbicides, fertilizers, fungicides, and efficient feeding techniques (24). Grain workers and swine and poultry producers are at significant risk for respiratory disorders, the latter as a result of intensive feeding techniques and confinement of poultry. Disabling injuries from accidents are underestimated as they are poorly studied in Canada. Occupational exposure to chemicals such as solvents and fungicides have been linked with neuro-degenerative disease, respiratory disease, and cancer in case reports (25).

Outdoor Air Quality

Over the past 20 years Canada has made significant gains in improving air quality. There has been a decline in the concentration of hazardous air pollutants such as sulphur dioxide, nitrogen dioxide, lead, dust, and smoke. Ground-level ozone, which creates smog, is one of the most serious air pollution problems in Canadian cities (26). Generally, ozone levels hover around 80% of maximum acceptable levels. In 1994, Toronto and Vancouver had the highest number of days that were rated fair to poor (71%) in terms of air quality; Halifax had the lowest (6%).

3.   LIFESTYLE AND BEHAVIOURAL RISK FACTORS

The Lalonde report placed great emphasis on lifestyle elements and the personal behaviour of Canadians as a major factor in determining their health. The following discussion shows that this emphasis was not misplaced. Much of our knowledge about Canadian behaviour comes from Canada's Health Promotion Survey in 1990 (27), the National Population Health Survey of 1994, and the Technical Appendix of the *Report on the Health of Canadians*, which provides data from various current sources about lifestyle and behavioural risk factors (21). The more recent information on cardiovascular risk factors on a national basis comes from the Canadian Heart Health Survey (28) and, with regard to tobacco, from the Addiction Research Foundation's *Facts on Tobacco* (29).

3.1. STRESS

Chronic stress has a significant impact on the health of Canadians. In the 1994/95 Population Health Survey, one in four (26%) Canadians reported as experiencing high chronic stress, and the remaining equally divided between moderate stress (38%) and low stress (36%). Women are more likely than men to report high stress (29% versus 23% respectively). This is true for all ages except the youngest (age 18-19). The least educated group is more than twice as likely as university graduates to report high stress (31% versus 14% respectively). Men and women between the ages of 35 and 44 reported the highest rates of stress. It is also worth noting that stress is particularly predominant among working parents (75%) and that as stress increases, so too does the rate of family dysfunction (30).

Smoking is related to stress: in 1994, 46% of men who reported high levels of chronic stress smoked, compared to 27% of men who experienced low levels of stress. The association is even more pronounced in women, ranging from 45% for those with high stress levels to 21% among women with low stress levels.

3.2. SUBSTANCE ABUSE

Substance abuse refers to the problems associated with the use of alcohol and tobacco, overuse of tranquillizers and sedatives, and use of illicit drugs such as cannabis, cocaine, heroin, and LSD. The most commonly used substances are alcohol and tobacco. The risk-continuum framework for assessing the health risks of substance abuse is described in Chapter One.

3.2.1. Tobacco

Large decreases in tobacco consumption in Canada have been recorded recently. For the period of 1980 to 1990, Statistics Canada reported a 35% decline in tobacco consumption as measured by cigarettes smoked by people age 15 and over. In 1989 alone, overall tobacco consumption fell by 6.8%, mainly as a result of decreased cigarette consumption (31, 32). Between 1990 and 1994, no differences were reported, although it is likely that the prevalence of cigarette smoking continued to decline from 1991 to 1993, reversed itself in 1993, and then increased between 1993 and 1994 due to reduced tobacco taxes in 1994 (29). The increase in the tobacco tax that was announced in the federal budget of February 1998 is expected to reverse the smoking trends. According to Statistics Canada, over the last four years the proportion of Canadians who smoke has increased from 26% of the population age 15 and over in 1990 to 31% in 1994 (about 5.4 million people). However, the smoking rates of males and females have converged, as more women have taken up smoking while male smokers have declined. The 1994 National Population Health Survey reported that approximately 33% of males and 29% of females age 15 and older are current smokers. Thirteen per cent of males and 7% of females smoke more than 25 cigarettes per day. For the age group 15-19, 20% of males are daily smokers, as are 12% of females. Men in the 25-44 age group are more likely to smoke regularly (37%) than women (34%), although this gap has narrowed over time. Sex differences in smoking behaviour are not apparent among those over age 45. Among people aged 15 to 64, 30% of men and 29% of women smoke regularly; among those over age 65, 18% of men and 15% of women smoke regularly (see Chapter Seven).

A 1993 survey of Ontario students reported that 25.2% of females and 22.5% of males smoked (33). This was an upward trend from 1991 (21.5% and 21.9% respectively). In 1993, 15.0% of females and 9% of males between age 13 and 14 were considered beginning smokers (i.e., fewer than 100 cigarettes smoked in the last 30 days) (29), and 9.4% of grade seven students smoked. High school students are not representative, however, of all youth. It is reported that 92% of street youth smoke daily (34).

Smoking is much more common among the Canadian-born population than among immigrants. Recent non-European immigrants (residing in Canada 10 years or less) were significantly more likely to have never smoked than their Canadian-born counterparts (75% versus 34%), and 56% of recent European immigrants have never smoked. Low smoking rates among female immigrants from non-European countries are reflected in the high rates of people who have never smoked among them (88%), compared to female immigrants from Europe (69%) and Canadian-born women (38%) (35). For the health impact of smoking and prevention, see Chapter Seven.

3.2.2. Alcohol

The 1994 National Population Health Survey reported that 79% of Canadians over age 15 years are drinkers (i.e., consumed alcoholic beverages at least once in the 12 months prior to the survey). Another 12% of the population reported they are former drinkers, having consumed alcohol at some time earlier in their lives, while 10% reported that they have never consumed an alcoholic beverage. A drink in this survey was defined as one bottle of beer, one glass of draft beer, one glass of wine, one wine cooler, or one straight or mixed drink with 44 millilitres (1.5 ounces) of hard liquor. The number of drinks consumed by current drinkers aged 15 and over in the week preceding the survey was as follows: fewer than one drink for 29% of current drinkers, 1-6 drinks for 42%, 7-13 drinks for 16%, 14 or more drinks for 11%, and no drinks for 2%. The trend indicates that more adults are drinking: 58% of the population surveyed reporting that they were current drinkers in 1994 (consumed alcohol at least once a month) compared to 55% in the 1991 Social Survey. Males consume disproportionately more alcohol than females at all ages (see Chapter Seven).

After age 24, there is an inverse relationship between age and the prevalence of alcohol consumption. Drinking is more likely to occur among those in the workforce, those with higher incomes and those with higher education. According to a CAGE questionnaire (see Chapter Seven), it was estimated 4.1% of Canadians had an alcohol dependence in 1994 (36).

The per capita consumption of alcohol for Canadian adults increased steadily from 7.1 litres (of absolute alcohol) in 1958 to around 11.0 litres during a plateau from 1975 to 1981 (37). Since 1981, per capita consumption has declined to approximately 7.9 litres of absolute alcohol per year in 1991 (half of this is consumed as beer) (38). Per capita sales of the alcoholic beverages in 1994/95 for wine was 10.0 litres, for spirit 5.4, and for beer 86.5 litres.

Alcohol remains an important factor in health problems such as cirrhosis, motor vehicle accidents, family violence, and violent deaths (see Chapter Seven for details on health impact of alcohol). There has, however, been a decline in the number of people charged with impaired driving offences in Canada since 1984.

Repeated surveys of Ontario students in different grades between 1983 and 1993 have shown a significant reduction of alcohol use in both sexes from 71.7% to 56.2% with a steady decline occurring during these years (39). Similar rates have been found in students in Nova Scotia (40). There does, however, appear to be a concentration of problem drinking in those who report heavy use (particularly for males).

3.2.3. Drugs

The General Social Survey of 1993 (41) indicated that as many as one in five adult Canadians, or 4,200,000 people, have used an illegal substance at least once over their lifetime. The most widely used illicit drug was cannabis (marijuana and hashish) used by 20% of Canadians over their lifetime, whereas 4% reported its use in 12 months prior to the survey. In general, the use of illegal drugs by Canadians has declined. The decline in cannabis use is most evident among adults; however, use among those between ages 15 and 19 increased from 9% in 1990 to 10.3% in 1993. Use of cannabis was more than twice as common among men (5.9%) as for women (2.5%) in 1993. The highest rate of current use was among respondents between ages 20 and 24 (9.7%).

Only about 3% of all Canadians over age 15 have ever tried cocaine or crack at some time in their lives. The highest rate of current users for cocaine was among respondents 18-19 years of age. A significant decline in the use of cocaine was observed between 1989 and 1993 (from 1.4% to 0.3%) in all age groups. The proportion of Canadians who have used LSD, speed, or heroin over the past year has been relatively stable between 1989 and 1993 (approximately 0.3%); 0.4% of Canadians reported using these substances during the year preceding the survey. A very small proportion of Canadians (1.3%) had injected themselves with drugs using needles shared with someone else. This implies that approximately 235,000 Canadians shared a needle on at least one occasion.

A less widely perceived problem is the overuse and the inappropriate use of over-the-counter and prescribed medications. The Canada Health Survey (42) found that 48% of Canadians take some type of medication in any given 48-hour period, but only 60% do so on the advice of a physician. The General Social Survey indicated the proportion of Canadians using prescription drugs 30 days prior to the survey were as follows: 69.8% used aspirin, 3.8% used tranquillizers, 4.2% used sleeping pills, 8.2% used codeine or meperidine (Demerol), 2.5% used antidepressants, and 0.6% used diet pills. Generally, usage rates were higher among women than men. Seniors are highly medicated, taking on average 15 prescriptions per year per person in Canada, with those in Nova Scotia taking an average of over 24 prescriptions per year per person (38).

3.3. PROBLEM GAMBLING

Problem gambling is predicted to become a prominent social problem that will have an impact on health and the health care system in the near future. Gamblers can be placed along a continuum that ranges from no problems at one end to "pathological" at the other, as described in the risk continuum discussed in Chapter One. Problem gambling is a catch-all term used to cover all patterns of gambling behaviour that "compromise, disrupt, or damage personal, family, or vocational pursuits" (43). Rates of current problem gamblers are as follows: British Columbia 3.5%, Alberta 5.4%, Saskatchewan 2.7%, Manitoba 4.3%, New Brunswick 4.5%, and Nova Scotia 3.9%. There are no distinctions by wealth, class, age, race, or gender. It has also been observed that 30% of the average male problem gamblers have cross-addictions to alcohol, drugs, or sex.

Problem gambling carries with it a number of negative social impacts including lowered productivity, family problems, and criminal activities leading to prosecution and incarceration. Ontario's Addiction Research Foundation also reported that 20% of all problem gamblers attempt suicide at least once. Over the past few years, gambling has become a norm in society, but must now be recognized for the serious negative personal and societal consequences that result from problem gambling, which is a form of addiction.

3.4. NUTRITION

Food Consumption

Good nutrition is fundamental to maintaining good health and preventing disease and reducing its severity. According to 1996 figures on the Canadian food supply, Canadians have increased their consumption of vegetables by almost a quarter over the past two decades (44). In 1996, each individual ate almost 180 kilograms of vegetables, up 22% from 147 kilograms 20 years ago. Fresh varieties were most popular, accounting for more than three quarters of all vegetables consumed. Potatoes, the traditional favourite, led the way as consumption reached almost 70 kilograms per person in 1996. Lettuce, carrots, onions, tomatoes, and cabbage also remained popular consumer choices. Total fruit consumption reached just over 120 kilograms per person in 1996, up over 17% from the mid 1970s. Again, fresh varieties were by far the clear preference among consumers. Bananas topped the list at over 13 kilograms per person, followed by apples, at 11 kilograms. Canadians were also including more fish and shellfish products in their diet, although red meat and poultry remained the most popular choices for many consumers. In 1996, total fish consumption reached almost 9 kilograms per person, up by more than 2 kilograms from the 1991 level (44). The growing preference for fresh and frozen shellfish was responsible for most of this increase.

Although the best information available on nutritional intake and physical health for all Canada was gathered by Nutrition Canada in 1973, it is now outdated. A number of provinces such as Ontario and Manitoba have initiated or completed dietary surveys to assess the nutritional status of their population.

A recent survey from Quebec provides much needed information on nutrient intake of various age groups (45). It found that the average calorie intakes for males and females between ages 18 and 34 were 2,916 kilocalories and 1,866 kilocalories respectively; for males and females between ages 35 and 49, it was 2,606 kilocalories and 1,726 kilocalories; for males and females between ages 50 and 64, it was 2,248 kilocalories and 1,612 kilocalories; and males and females between ages 65 and 74, it was 2,136 kilocalories and 1,528 kilocalories. Except for males age 18 to 34, all other age and sex groups had lower total calorie intake compared with the recommended levels for persons during light activity. When intake of different nutrients were compared with the recommended level for most micronutrients such as magnesium, phosphate, zinc, thiamin, riboflavin, proteins, and vitamins A, C, B6, and B12, Quebecers were found to be taking adequate amounts. However, fat content, particularly saturated fat, was higher than recommended for all age and sex groups; iron intake was lower for females aged 18 to 49, as was folate for females aged 65 to 74. Compared with the previous results from Quebec in the 1971 Nutrition Canada Survey, Quebecers were consuming fewer calories, less fat including saturated fats, less cholesterol, and fewer carbohydrates. However, they were consuming more protein, polyunsaturated fats, and fibre, which reflects the nationwide trends (see Chapter Seven).

Body Mass Index

The National Population Health Survey (1994) determined the proportion of overweight and underweight adults by measuring the Body Mass Index (BMI). The BMI is calculated as weight in kilograms divided by the square of height in metres. This survey found that 43% of the Canadians age 20 to 64 had a BMI in the range of 20 to 25 (acceptable weight), 9% had a BMI lower than 20 (underweight), 16% had a BMI of 25-27 (possibly overweight), and 23% had a BMI higher than 27 (overweight). Young women in particular were more likely to be underweight (25% of women aged 20 to 24). Men, particularly middle-aged men (aged 45 to 54), were more likely to be overweight (33%). Over 50% of Canadians want to change their weight, primarily through weight loss. About 68% of women at an acceptable weight want to lose weight, as do 22% of women in the underweight category. Losing weight in the future is seen by 10% of Canadians as the most important action to improve health.

A particular concern that is relevant to nutrition for immigrants to Canada is the cultural lack of familiarity with the types of food available in Canada and a lack of domestic skill in preparing a varied diet using available foods. Although single male Ethiopian refugees were found to have generally adequate nutrient intakes, their diets in Canada (46) were found to be lacking in variety and in fruits and vegetables other than large quantities of orange juice. Refugees more skilled in preparing available food felt more satisfied with their eating habits, and had higher BMI (although overall BMIs and arm circumference measures for the group were lower than Canadian and American standards).

3.4.1. Plasma Lipids and Lipoproteins

It is well known that high blood cholesterol levels and other lipoprotein disorders are associated with increased risk for cardiovascular disease. Among those aged 18 to 74, 48% of male and 43% of female participants in the Canada Heart Health Survey had total plasma cholesterol levels greater than 5.2 millimoles per litre (mmol/L). Lower levels have been advised by a number of authorities. Eighteen per cent of males and 16% of females had levels of total cholesterol in the high-risk category of greater than 6.2 mmol/L. Serum cholesterol levels in males rose with age up to the age of 45 to 64, whereas levels were stable in younger females and increased dramatically among those aged 45 to 54. Eight per cent (of both sexes) had high-density lipoprotein levels (HDL) in the high-risk category below 0.9 mmol/L. Fifteen per cent (of both sexes) had levels of low-density lipoprotein (LDL) above the high-risk level of 2.3 mmol/L and the same percentage had high-risk triglyceride levels above 1.3 mmol/L (see Chapter Seven).

3.5. USE OF PROTECTIVE DEVICES

Seat Belts

Motor vehicle accidents are a leading cause of death and injury in Canada, especially in young adults. The established role of seat belts in reducing fatalities has been well publicized. In 1994, seat belt use by drivers in Canada was 92%, by vehicle occupants 87%, and by children under age five 70% (26). The prevalence of correct use of restraints for children under age five was only 30% of those wearing them.

There are interprovincial variations: Quebec has the highest rates of 94% and Manitoba has 86%. Territories have the lowest rate of just under 80% (47). Furthermore, there are regional variations within provinces. A 1991 survey in Ontario indicated an overall usage rate for those over age 16 of 80.9% , which had increased significantly from 69.6% in 1984; however, a rate of only 73.5% was reported for Northern Ontario (48). The lowest rates of seat belt use occur among impaired drivers and young drivers, the two groups who have the highest accident rates. These low percentages also clearly suggest the need for further safety education about correct usage of child restraints; the most common misuse of child seats was not securing the strap (see Chapter Seven).

Bicycle Helmets

Estimates from the 1994/95 survey indicate that there were approximately 6.4 million Canadian cyclists of whom only one in five (19%) always wear a helmet when riding. If those who wear a helmet most of the time are included, this figure rises slightly to fewer than one in four (23%). Overall use of helmets is similar between males and females, although it does vary substantially within the age groups. Among those aged 12 to 14 and those over age 44, males are more likely to wear helmets, in contrast to cyclists in their teens or early 20s (see Chapter Seven).

3.6. PHYSICAL ACTIVITY AND FITNESS

The National Population Health Survey reported the frequency of exercise by Canadians over the age of 15 in three categories. Energy expenditure (EE) was estimated for each activity in which respondents engaged during their leisure time, in order to derive their level of physical activity. Average daily EE was calculated by multiplying the number of times the respondent engaged in an activity over a 12-month period by the average duration in hours, then by the energy cost of the activity, and then dividing by 365. Respondents with an estimated EE of 3.0 or more kilocalories per kilograms per day (kcal/kg/day) are considered physically active. A value between 1.5 and 2.9 kcal/kg/day indicates moderate physical activity, while respondents with an estimated EE less than 1.5 kcal/kg/day are considered inactive.

In 1994, over half the population (56%) reported that they were inactive, 27% were moderately active, and 17% were physically active. Daily physical activity decreases with age to middle adulthood and then increases after age 44 for men. Canadians most likely to engage in daily exercise in their leisure time are men and women age 15 to 19. Active use of leisure time becomes more common as education, income, and occupational status increase in all age groups and in both sexes. Too much leisure time is still claimed by watching television, reading, listening to radio, and other activities of a sometimes educational but sedentary nature. In 1995, Canadians spent an average of 23.2 hours a week watching television, with Quebec viewers watching the most in viewing time (26.2 hours) and British Columbians watching the least of all Canadians (21.2 hours) (49). Canadians age 18 to 24 watched a mere 15.1 hours per week in viewing time. However, there is some evidence that more leisure time is being devoted to exercise (see Chapter Seven).

3.7. SEXUAL PRACTICES

While there are no large-scale studies on human sexuality in Canada, the AIDS epidemic has generated much interest in this field. The recent reports *AIDS in Canada: Knowledge, Behaviour and Attitudes of Adults* (50) and the *Canada Youth and AIDS Study* (51) have provided the necessary information about sexuality. Many of today's adolescents begin their sexual experiences by age 14. Nearly one half of the grade 11 respondents had sexual intercourse. Although fewer younger students had sexual intercourse, the percentages are still high: 26% of grade nine respondents (more males than females), and at least 12% of males and 8% of females in grade seven. Approximately 75% of college and university students and about 85% of early school-leavers reported having had sexual intercourse at least once in their lifetime. Eighty-six per cent of adult Canadians have had sexual intercourse with a member of the opposite sex. About 1% of both males and females reported homosexual activities. Most of the sexual acts reported are vaginal intercourse among heterosexual couples, oral sex (28% of males and 24% of females reported having oral sex often), and anal sex (2% of men reported having anal sex often).

Thirty-five per cent of men and 14% of women reported that they had two or more sexual partners in the past five years. About one quarter of all men and 7% of women had three or more partners, and about 15% of the men and 3% of the women reported six or more partners in the same period. Aside from gender, the only factors affecting the number of sexual partners were marital status and age (single and younger tending to have more partners). Education and other socioeconomic measures had no effect.

Among respondents with two or more partners in the previous five years, 6% of men and 2% of women reported that they had sex without using a condom with someone [they] thought might be a carrier of the AIDS virus" and 41% of the men and 27% of the women reported that they had "had sex without using a condom with someone [they] did not know very well". Changes in behaviour to avoid contracting AIDS were reported by 54% of the men and 41% of the women. Of both these groups, 70% said they had reduced the number of partners; about 90% said they were "more cautious"; 60% had started to use condoms or used them more often; and about 40% said that on at least one occasion they had not had sex because of fear of exposure to AIDS. Condoms were "never" used by 44% of the male respondents with two or more partners, 24% used them "sometimes" or "seldom", 13% "almost every time", and 19% "every time" they had sex. Among the women, 62% reported never using a condom, and only 12% used them every time (see Chapter Five and Seven).

3.8. PREVENTIVE HEALTH PRACTICES

3.8.1. Recent Measures to Improve Health

In 1990, the Health Promotion Survey reported that 49% of Canadians had made at least one change to improve their health in the year prior to the survey. More women

(52%) than men (46%) reported doing something to improve their health. The most frequent measure taken by the men (42%) and women (33%) to improve their health was to increase the amount they exercise. Only 12% reported attempts to improve eating habits, which is of concern considering the prevalence of diets not in accordance with current nutrition recommendations. Nine per cent of Canadians had attempted to lose weight recently. In terms of substance abuse, only 2% of all adult Canadians had recently reduced the amount smoked, and only 1% were attempting to reduce alcohol use in the year preceding the survey.

3.8.2. Immunization

In 1994/95, almost all (95%) of children between ages of two and three were likely to be immunized against measles, mumps, and rubella, followed closely by three doses of diphtheria, pertussis, tetanus, and poliomyelitis (83-85%), and *Haemophilius influenzae* type b (71.5%) (52). In the 1991 General Social Survey, half of the seniors (51%) reported having a flu shot recommended by a health care professional and close to half (46%) actually received the vaccination (see Chapter Eight).

3.8.3. Screening for Blood Pressure

The National Population Health Survey examined certain preventive health practices among Canadians. With regard to screening for hypertension, 68% of all Canadians over age 12 reported that they had their blood pressure checked within the 12 months preceding the survey. For both sexes the frequency of blood pressure monitoring increases with age. Men under age 45 were the least likely to have had their blood pressure checked during the six preceding months; across all ages women were more likely than men to have theirs checked regularly. According to Canada's Health Promotion Survey, the frequency of blood pressure monitoring was affected by education, stress, body weight, personal beliefs about diet, attitudes toward hypertension as a public health issue, and perceived need for information on hypertension. The majority of the population understood the importance of blood pressure screening in the absence of overt disease; only 17% believed it important only if there is a problem. Of the total population, 10% wanted more information on high blood pressure. The Canada Heart Health Survey indicated that 16% of men and 13% of women had diastolic blood pressures greater than 90 millimetres of mercury (mm Hg) (28) (see Chapter Seven).

3.8.4. Screening for Cervical Cancer

Regarding female preventive health practices, the 1994/95 Population Health Survey found that most (85%) of Canadian women over the age of 15 reported that they had a Pap test at some point in their life. Just over 80% of adult women reported having had one within the three years of the survey (in accordance with the recommended screening guidelines), and 15% had never had one. Those women who never had Pap smear were most likely to be under age 19 or 75 and over (see Chapter Seven).

3.8.4. Screening for Breast Cancer

Breast examination is frequently done by doctors and less frequently by women themselves. According to the Health Promotion Survey of all adult women, 65% have had their breasts examined by a doctor or nurse during the year prior to the survey. Examination was more frequent among younger women and declined with age, even though the risk of breast cancer increases with age. Breast examination was most frequent in women aged 20 to 24 (71.9%), declining to 56.9% and 49.7% in women aged 55 to 64 and 65 and over, respectively. Seventy-three per cent of all women reported having been shown how to do breast self-examination, yet only 27% of all women examine their own breasts every month.

In 1994/95, among women aged 50 to 69, for whom routine screening mammography is recommended every two years, 72% reported having had a mammogram within the two-year period prior to the survey. It is of interest to note that of women aged 35 to 39, 30% had received a mammogram, as had 61% of those between ages 40 and 59 (see Chapter Seven).

3.8.5. Dental Hygiene

The vast majority of Canadians (97%) brush their teeth at least once a day and 79% brush their teeth twice a day. This preventive practice is more widespread among women, younger Canadians, and those with a higher education and income.

3.9. USE OF HEALTH CARE SERVICES

3.9.1. Contact With Health Care Professionals

According to the 1994 National Population Health Survey, the most frequently consulted health care professionals are physicians and dentists. Seventy-seven per cent of Canadian adults reported seeing a physician in 1993, compared to 55% who had consulted a dentist. It is worth noting that the presence of chronic condition was a powerful predictor of the number of physician consultations. Men were less likely than women to consult nurses, physicians, and other specialists (72% of men versus 83% of women consulted physicians). Relatively small differences existed between the proportions of men and women who consulted dentists, physiotherapists, occupational therapists, and psychologists. In 1994, the likelihood of visiting a physician in the previous year had little relationship with income, compared to the proportion who had visited a dentist, which increased with their household income (see Chapter Five).

3.9.2. Prescription and Over-the-Counter Medications

In 1994, in the month prior to being interviewed, 17.5 million people (77% of the population) aged 15 and over reported taking at least one prescription or over-the-counter medication. Not only did a greater proportion of women use some kind of medication (83% of women versus 71% of men), but on average women reported using more medications than men (1.9 and 1.3 respectively). This was still the case even after birth control and menopausal hormones were excluded. Pain relievers (headache medication and other analgesics) were most commonly used (62%), followed by cough and cold remedies (15%), and allergy medications (10%). Overall, 21% of women aged 15 to

39 reported using birth control pills in the month prior to interview, with the highest rate of use among women aged 20 to 24 (38%). Approximately 15% of women aged 45 and over reported using menopausal hormones, with the rate peaking among those aged 50 to 54 (31%) (see Chapter Five).

3.9.3. Alternative Medicine

Alternative medicine refers to a range of services offered outside of the conventional health care system. For the purposes of this section chiropractors are included among alternative health care providers. In 1994/95, an estimated 15% of Canadians aged 15 and over (3.3 million people) used some form of alternative health care in the year preceding the survey (53). In general, alternative medicine use was the highest among those aged 25 to 44 for both sexes. Women generally use alternative medicine more than men (16% and 13% respectively), except for among those aged 15 to 19; in this group the proportion of use by both sexes is approximately the same (11%). The most commonly sought alternative health care service was chiropractic services. In the previous year, 11% of the population had consulted a chiropractor, 2% used homeopathy, and 2% consulted a massage therapist. Alternative medicine was observed to be highly associated with conditions such as back problems (34%), food allergies (25%), urinary incontinence (20%), and stomach and intestinal ulcers (17%).

4.   SUMMARY

This chapter dealt with the determinants of health and disease in the Canadian population. The determinants of health include human biology, environment (psychosocial and physical), lifestyle, and behavioural and risk factors, and health care organizations (which are discussed elsewhere in this book).

The genetic potential of the individual is a major aspect of human biology and has an impact on health.

Sociodemographic and socioeconomic indicators represent the interaction of demography with social and economic conditions. In May 1996, Canada's population was 29.9 million, which has more than doubled since 1941. The ratio of males to females has remained roughly constant, but there has been a definite change in the age distribution. With the availability of better contraception, more liberal abortion laws, and more women participating in the labour force, the proportion of children under age 14 decreased since 1971, while at the same time there was an increase among those aged 65 and over.

Geographic distributions also affect the health status of a population. Three quarters of the population live within 320 kilometres of the border between Canada and the United States, with the remaining population spread across a vast land mass. This creates a substantial challenge to providing health care services, particularly with regard to the northern areas of Canada.

Life expectancy at birth has increased significantly in Canada between 1941 and 1996, mainly due to the significant decline in infant mortality. Life expectancy has increased significantly more for females than for males. The life expectancy in 1996 for males is 75.7 years and for females it is 81.4 years.

Sociodemographic indicators include aging, immigrant population, language, and family environments. An important demographic change is the rise in the proportion of the population over age 65. In 1996, seniors represented 12.2% of the population. The composition of the Canadian population is also changing in relation to ethnicity and is expected to continue changing as more immigrants from non-European countries are allowed into Canada. As an example of Canada's ethnic diversity, 4.7 million people reported a first language other than French or English. Family violence plays a role in the health of the individual family members. Family violence, prevalent among Canadians, takes the form of child abuse, wife battering, and elder abuse.

The composition of the population in terms of education, income, and employment influences health. The proportion of the population aged 15 and over with fewer than 11 years of education is an indicator of socioeconomic status. One in six adults (16.6%) in Canada had literacy limitations in 1994. These limitations may affect health directly in terms of the inappropriate use of medicines, difficulty communicating with health care workers, and difficulty in following instructions.

Income is another major socioeconomic indicator. A family that spends 56.2% of its income on the basic needs of accommodation, food, and clothing is defined as living in poverty. In 1996, 17.9% of Canadian families were living in poverty. Unemployment rates in Canada are high, although they have decreased from over 11% in 1993 to just under 9% in 1998.

Homelessness is associated with many health risks. Many homeless persons are ex-patients of mental health institutions, runaway teenagers, alcoholics, or Aboriginal peoples.

Environmentally caused health problems include acute poisoning, chronic irritation, cancer, and genetic damage.

Occupational hazards can also affect the health of an individual. For example, grain workers and swine and poultry producers have been found to be at a significant risk for respiratory disorders. As well, occupational exposure to chemicals such as solvents and fungicides has been linked with neurodegenerative disorders.

The lifestyle of Canadians is also a major factor in determining their health. Chronic stress, substance abuse, compulsive gambling, nutrition, use of protective devices, activity and fitness levels, sexual practices, and preventive health practices are behaviours and risk factors that affect the health of an individual.

Chronic stress has a significant impact on Canadians. Not only is it related to smoking, but also as stress increases, so does family dysfunction.

Substance abuse refers to the problems associated with the use of alcohol and tobacco, overuse of tranquillisers and sedatives, and use of illicit drugs. In the last two decades, the proportion of Canadians who smoke tobacco has decreased. However, the smoking rates of males and females have converged, as the number of male smokers has been declining. Large decreases in tobacco consumption in Canada have been recorded recently. In the last decade, there has been a 35% decline in tobacco consumption. However between 1990 and 1994, no differences were reported. With respect to alcohol, trends indicate that fewer adults are drinking, more have stopped drinking, and those who drink are consuming less. Alcohol remains an important factor in health problems such as cirrhosis, and in motor vehicle accidents, family violence, and violent deaths. The National Alcohol and Other Drugs Survey indicated that cannabis is the most commonly used illicit drug in Canada. The Ontario Student Drug Use Survey found an increase in use of illicit drugs.

Over the past few years, gambling has become common in Canadian society. This must now be recognized for the serious negative personal and societal consequences that are a result of problem gambling, which is a form of addiction.

Good nutrition is fundamental to good health and to the prevention or reduction in severity of disease. The Nutrition Survey in Quebec revealed that in most groups over age 18, calorie intake is less than recommended, except for males aged 18 to 34. With regard to total fat intake, it was higher for all age groups and in both sexes. Iron intake was found to be lower among females aged 18 to 49. According to the Population Health Survey in 1994, 43% of Canadians have an acceptable weight (according to the Body Mass Index), 9.0% are underweight, 16.0% are potentially overweight, and 23.0% are overweight. Young women tend mostly to be in the underweight group, whereas middle-aged men constitute a large proportion of the overweight group.

Seat belts and bicycle helmets are examples of protective devices. Even though the established role of seat belts in the reduction of fatalities has been well publicized, only 79% of Canadian drivers wear them all or most of the time. The effectiveness of wearing bicycle helmets in the prevention of serious head injury and death has also been demonstrated.

Frequency of exercise is categorized into three groups: physically active, moderately physically active, and inactive. According to the National Health Population Survey, 17% of Canadians were physically active, 27% were moderately active, and 56% were inactive. The proportion of individuals who carry out regular exercise decreases with increasing age.

According to AIDS-related research, many of today's adolescents are beginning their sexual experiences by age 14. Thirty-five per cent of men and 14% of women reported having two or more sexual partners in the past five years. Factors affecting the number of sexual partners were an individual's marital status and age. Education and socioeconomic status had no effect.

Canada's Health Promotion Survey and the National Population Health Survey examined certain preventive health practices among Canadians. Sixty-eight per cent of respondents reported that they had their blood pressure checked within the last 12 months. Frequency of blood pressure monitoring is affected by education, stress, body weight, personal beliefs about diet, attitudes toward hypertension, and perceived need for information on hypertension. The survey also found that more than 80% of all women had regular Pap tests. However, breast self-examination is done less frequently, and approximately three in four (72%) women aged 50 to 69 had received a mammogram in the past two years. Contact with health care professionals includes many different facets, including prescription and over-the-counter medicine use, and alternative medicine, as well as contact with conventional forms of health care professionals.

Health care organization is also a determinant of health (and is discussed elsewhere in this book). The major feature is the availability of universal health insurance for all Canadians, which has significantly contributed to reducing the inequities in access to health care within the population. While most Canadians visited their doctors in the past year, one in six also consulted alternative health care providers, with visits to chiropractors being the most frequent.

5. REFERENCES

1. Jaworski M, Severini A, Mansour G, et al. Genetic Conditions Among Canadian Mennonites: Evidence for a Founder Effect Among the Old Colony (Chortiza) Mennonites. Clinical and Investigative Medicine 1989;12(2):127-141.

2. Yorke D, Mitchell J, Clow C, et al. Newborn Screening for Sickle Cell and Other Haemoglobinopathies. Clinical and Investigative Medicine 1992;15(4):376-383.

3. Statistics Canada. 1996 Census Canada: Age and Sex. Ottawa: The Daily, 1996.

4. Statistics Canada. 1996 Census Canada: Marital Status/Common Law Families. Ottawa: The Daily, 1997.

5. Statistics Canada. 1996 Census Canada: Immigration and Citizenship. Ottawa: The Daily, 1997.

6. Statistics Canada. 1996 Census Canada: Mother Tongue: Home Language and Official and Non-Officials Languages. Ottawa: The Daily, 1997.

7. Statistics Canada. 1996 Census: Education, Mobility and Migration. Ottawa: The Daily, 1998.

8. Statistics Canada. 1996 Census Canada: Aboriginal, Ethnic Origin and Visible Minorities. Ottawa: The Daily, 1998.

9. Community Health System Working Group, Chevalier S. Community Health Indicators: Definitions and Interpretations. Ottawa: Canadian Institute for Health Information, 1995.

10. Statistics Canada. Projections of Households and Families for Canada, Provinces and Territories 1994-2016. 1995.

11. Ford D, Nault F. Changing Fertility Patterns, 1974 to 1994. Health Reports 1996;8(3):39-45.

12. Nault F, Wilkins K. Deaths 1993. Health Reports 1995;7(1):51-60.

13. Statistics Canada. The Violence Against Women Survey. Ottawa: The Daily. 1993.

14. Trudeau R. Transition Homes. 1995.

15. MacMillan HJ, Fleming JE, Trocme N, Boyle MH, Wong M, et al. Prevalence of Child Physical and Sexual Abuse in the Community. Results from the Ontario Health Supplement. Journal of the American Medical Association 1997;278(2):131-135.

16. Podnicks E. National Survey on Abuse of the Elderly in Canada. Journal of Elder Abuse Neglect 1992;4:5-58.

17. Statistics Canada. Births and Deaths, 1993. Ottawa: Government of Canada, 1996.

18. Statistics Canada. Literacy, Economy and Society: Results of the First International

Adult Literacy Survey. Ottawa: Government of Canada, 1994.
19. Canadian Public Health Association. Homelessness and Health, Position Paper. Ottawa: Canadian Public Health Association, 1997.
20. Worker's Compensation Boards of Canada. Work Injuries and Diseases: 1994-96. 1997.
21. Health Canada Communications and Consultation Directorate. Federal, Provincial, Territorial Advisory Committee on Population Health. 1996.
22. Ministry of Supply and Services. A Vital Link. Health and the Environment in Canada. Ottawa: Canada Communication Group, 1992.
23. Minister of Health, Health Canada. Health and Environment, Partner for Life. Ottawa: Minister of Public Works and Government Services Canada, 1997.
24. Zedja J, Semchuk K, McDuffie H, Dosman J. A Need for Population-Based Studies of Health and Safety Risks in Canadian Agriculture. Canadian Medical Association Journal 1991;145(7):773-775.
25. do Pico GA. Hazardous Exposure and Lung Disease Among Farm Workers (Review). Clinics in Chest Medicine 1992;13(2):311-328.
26. Canadian Council on Social Development, The Progress of Canada's Children 1996. Ottawa: 1996.
27. Stephens T, Fowler-Grahman D. Canada's Health Promotion Survey 1990: Technical Report. Ottawa: Ministry of Supply and Services, Health and Welfare Canada, 1993.
28. Canadian Heart Health Surveys Group. Canadian Heart Health Surveys: A Profile of Cardiovascular Risk. Canadian Medical Association Journal 1993;146(11):1969-2029.
29. Addiction Research Foundation. Facts on Tobacco 1996. Toronto: The Ontario Tobacco Research Unit, 1996.
30. Ministry of Health. Ontario Health Survey 1990. Toronto: Premier's Council on Health, Well-Being and Social Justice, 1992.
31. Trends in Canadian Tobacco Consumption, 1980-89. Canadian Medical Association Journal 1990;143(9):905-906.
32. Kaiserman MJ. Tobacco Production, Sales and Consumption in Canada, 1991. Chronic Disease in Canada 1992;13(4):68-71.
33. Addiction Research Foundation. The Ontario Student Drug Use Survey. Trends Between 1977 and 1991. Toronto: Addiction Research Foundation, 1991.
34. Addiction Research Foundation. Drugs in Ontario. Toronto: Addiction Research Foundation, 1991.
35. Chen J, Ng E, Wilkins R. The Health of Canada's Immigrants in 1994-95. Health Reports 1996;7(4):33-45.
36. Poulin C, Webster I, Single E. Alcohol Disorders in Canada as Indicated by the CAGE Questionnaire. Canadian Medical Association Journal 1997;157(11):1529-35.
37. Mao Y, Johnson R, Semencins R. Liver Cirrhosis Mortality and Per Capita Alcohol Consumption in Canada. Canadian Journal of Public Health 1992;83(1):80-81.
38. Canadian Centre on Substance Abuse, Addiction Research Foundation of Ontario. Canadian Profile: Alcohol, Tobacco and Other Drugs 1995. Ottawa: Addiction Research Foundation, 1995.
39. Williams B, Chong K, Truong MV. Alcohol and Other Drugs: Ontario Profile 1994. Toronto: Addiction Research Foundation, 1994.
40. Poulin C, Elliot D. Alcohol, Tobacco and Cannabis Use Among Nova Scotia Adolescents: Implications for Prevention and Harm Reduction. Canadian Medical Association Journal 1997;156(10):1387-93.
41. Statistics Canada. General Social Survey Analysis Series. Health Status of Canadians. 1994.

42. Statistics Canada. Health and Welfare Canada, The Health of Canadians, Report of the Canada Health Survey. Ottawa: 1981.

43. Ministry of Supply and Services Canada. Gambling in Canada: A Report by the National Council of Welfare. Ottawa: 1996.

44. Statistics Canada. Per Capita Food Consumption 1996. Ottawa: The Daily, 1997.

45. Gouvernement du Québec, Bertrand L (Ed.). Rapport de L'Enquête québécoise sur la nutrition 1990. Montréal: Government of Quebec, 1995.

46. McIssac J, Tucker K, Gray-Donald K, Stafford-Smith B. Nutritional Status of Single Male Government-Sponsored Refugees from Ethiopia. Canadian Journal of Public Health 1991;82(6):381-384.

47. Transport Canada, Road Safety. 1995.

48. Ministry of Health Ontario. The 1991 Ontario Ministry of Transportation and Communication Seat Belt Survey: Some Interesting Findings. Public Health and Epidemiology Reports Ontario 1992;3(11):168-174.

49. Statistics Canada. The Daily. 1995.

50. Ornstein M. AIDS in Canada: Knowledge, Behaviour and Attitudes of Adults. Toronto: University of Toronto Press, 1989.

51. King A, Beazley RP, Warren WK, et al. Canada Youth and AIDS Study. Kingston: Queen's University, 1988.

52. Health Canada. Childhood Vaccination Coverage Levels in Canada, 1994-1997: Progress Towards National Targets, Update: Vaccine-Preventable Diseases. (www.hc-sc.gc.ca/main/lcdc/web/publicat/vacprev/vol6-1/index.html), May 1998.

53. Millar. WJ. Use of Alternative Health Care Practitioners by Canadians. Canadian Journal of Public Health 1997;88(3):154-158.

5

Health Status
and Consequences

The previous chapter examined aspects of Canadian life that affect health. But how does one identify health status and assess its relative significance? The two health status indicators, namely mortality and morbidity, and the ensuing disability and economic burden, are the most commonly used measures of health in Canada. Much information is available on death in Canada, but morbidity, which encompasses all other health outcomes, is more difficult to assess. Several different approaches to the assessment of morbidity are outlined in this chapter. Other outcomes, such as human suffering or quality of life, are of no less importance but as the methodologies for their measurement are difficult and evolving, they are not used extensively in assessment of health and planning of health care.

1. HEALTH STATUS

1.1. SELF-ASSESSED

1.1.1. Perception of Health
The most fundamental health outcome is the perception of well-being by the individual. This may or may not lead to other outcomes such as limitation of usual activities, consultation with a health care professional, hospitalization, or death. The National Population Health Survey (1994) (1) asked individuals age 15 and over the following question: "In general, compared to other persons your age would you say your health is ... excellent, very good, good, fair or poor?" It also asked questions related to long-term activity limitations and level of happiness. The highlights of the study included:
- Just over nine out of ten Canadians (92%) assessed their health to be good, very good, or excellent, compared with the health of others their age.

- Less than one in ten people (8%) reported either fair or poor health.
- Older Canadians were more likely to report poorer health. Between the ages of 65 and 74, 24% reported that they were in fair or poor health; this number reaches approximately one in three (31%) among those age 75 and over.
- Almost all (95%) of those university educated Canadians assessed their health to be good, very good, or excellent compared with those who had less than a high school education (85%).

Perception of Ill Health

Few data are available on this subject, but the National Population Health Survey has afforded us a look at Canadian perceptions. Inquiries were made about all health problems at the time of the survey, and more than half of the respondents identified one or more health problems. Fewer than half of the problems reported did not induce the individuals to limit their activity, visit a health care professional, or treat themselves with a commercial remedy. The survey identified people with chronic health problems as a proportion of the total population. Of all adults surveyed, 35% (12.5 million) had at least one chronic condition: approximately 28% reported one, 13% reported two, and another 13% three or more. The leading health problem was skin diseases and allergies, reported by 20% of adults, followed by back problems (15%), arthritis and rheumatism (13%), and high blood pressure (9%). It was also observed that chronic health problems were more prevalent among women and that women were also more likely to report multiple chronic conditions. One of the most common psychiatric disorders is depression. In 1994, 5.7% of the population aged 15 and over reported having had a depressive episode in the year preceding the survey. Twice as many women reported depression than men (7.6% and 3.7% respectively). High levels of chronic stress and relatively lower incomes were also associated with depression. Although some of this subjective morbidity may be minor in nature it is worthy of examination to learn more about the relationship between perceived ill health and the pursuit of health care, and the potential role of health education in this process.

In 1967, Robert Kohn estimated the health of a standardized population of 100,000 Canadians based on the following outcomes: individuals perceiving themselves to have at least one health problem or disability, whether individuals consulted health professionals or were admitted to hospital for these problems, and the number of deaths. It is possible to create similar estimates based on information from the National Population Health Survey and other recent sources. Figure 5.1 illustrates these estimates, which give a glimpse of the health of an average group of Canadians on an average day. It is notable that the recent statistics do not differ significantly from those of Kohn 30 years earlier (2). With the exception of death, these outcomes do not necessarily reflect disease; healthy people may feel ill, see a doctor, and even be admitted to hospital. All of these outcomes do, however, have consequences for health care and its planning.

Figure 5.1:   Health of a Population of 100,000 Canadians on an Average Day

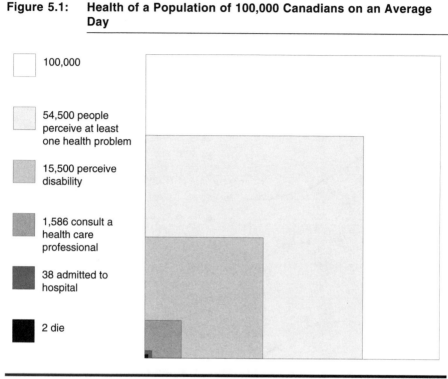

100,000

54,500 people perceive at least one health problem

15,500 perceive disability

1,586 consult a health care professional

38 admitted to hospital

2 die

Source: Adapted from R. Kohn, Royal Commission on Health Services: *The Health of Canadian People*, Ottawa, 1967.

1.2. OBJECTIVE INDICATORS

1.2.1. Mortality

The crude mortality rate in Canada was 7.1 deaths per 1,000 population per year in 1994. This number is important, but much more information is gained by examining mortality in more detail. Mortality may be expressed in terms of life expectancy, age- and sex-specific death rates, causes of death by age and sex, and potential-years-of-life-lost. Most of these terms are explained in Chapter Three. Each yields different useful information about Canadian health. Life expectancies for the Canadian population were discussed in Chapter Four.

Trends in Age- and Sex-Specific Death Rates (1951-1994)

Figure 5.2 illustrates age-specific mortality rates for both sexes from 1951 to 1994 (3). Among those under the age of one year, there has been a steady decline in mortality rates throughout this period, which appears to be continuing. In 1995, the overall infant mortality rate was 6.1 per 1,000 live births; rates for male and female infants were 6.7 and

Figure 5.2:   Trends in Age-Sex Specific Mortality Rates per 1,000 Population in Canada, 1951-1994

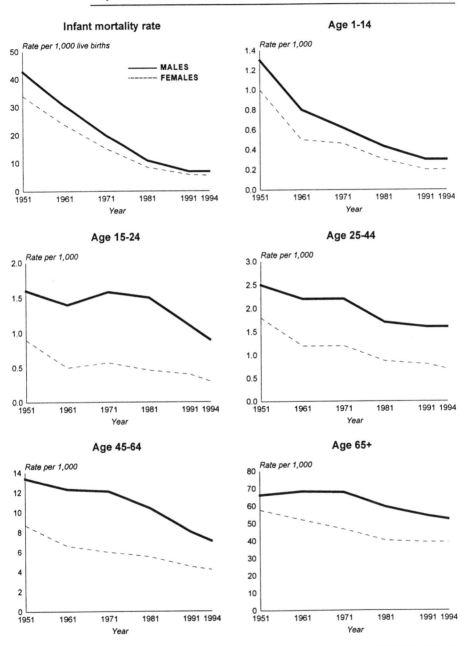

Source: Adapted from *Health Field Indicators*. Health and Welfare Canada, 1986 and *Statistics Canada*.

5.5 respectively. The overall rate has remained the same since 1992. Internationally, among the developed countries, three — Japan (4.2), Australia (6.1) and Canada — had the lowest infant mortality rates while New Zealand, the United States, and the Russian Federation had the highest rates (7.3, 8.3, and 18.1, respectively). The majority of these deaths occur during or shortly after delivery and are due to congenital anomalies and conditions specific to the perinatal period, such as hypoxia or placental anomalies. After the first week of life (the postneonatal period), most infant deaths are due to congenital anomalies, sudden infant death syndrome, respiratory tract infections, or accidents. There is room for improvement in infant mortality, as the success of Japan shows (4).

From 1 to 14 years of age, mortality rates continue to decline slowly to very low levels. More than half of these deaths are due to motor vehicle and other accidents, and are potentially preventable.

Among those aged 15 to 24, a very serious trend developed in the late 1960s and early 1970s with a sharp increase in death rates, especially among young men. The gap between male and female rates widened so that the mortality among males was about three times that for females. In this age group, the most significant causes of death are motor vehicle and other accidents, and suicide.

Recently, however, there has been a significant drop in the death rate for this group, especially for males. This was due mainly to a decrease in mortality from motor vehicle accidents, which may have been a result of the introduction of lower speed limits and increased seat belt usage. In spite of this favourable trend, most of the deaths in this age group must be regarded as preventable, and there is much room for improvement.

Among those aged 25 to 44, mortality rates were relatively stable throughout the 1960s and early 1970s, with a slight decline. Male rates in this and the next age group, 45-64 years, remain about double the female rates. The excess male mortality at these ages is largely due to accidents, ischemic heart disease, suicide, and cancer of the lung, each of which is determined to some extent by lifestyle.

Among those age 45 to 64, female rates have been slowly declining for several decades. Male rates on the other hand were relatively stable until the mid 1970s and have fallen since. This is, in part, due to the decline in mortality from ischemic heart disease, the leading cause of death in men at these ages.

Beyond age 65, there remains a wide gap between male and female death rates, although both rates now appear to be on the decline. The major causes of death for both men and women are ischemic heart disease, cerebrovascular disease, and respiratory illness.

Causes of Death by Age and Sex

As listed in Table 5.1, the leading causes of death ranked by number of deaths for men are cancer, coronary heart disease, stroke, respiratory diseases, and accidents; for women, they are cancer, coronary heart disease, stroke, respiratory disease and pneumonia and influenza (4). Based on current knowledge of the aetiology of these health problems, many of these deaths could be prevented or delayed by lifestyle modifications.

Table 5.1:   Leading Causes of Death and Death Rate by Sex, Canada, 1994

| | | | Rate per 100,000 | | |
Cause	Number	Percent	Total	Males	Females
Cancer	57,324	27.7	188.3	239.0	153.9
Heart disease	56,960	27.5	184.2	245.0	137.8
Stroke	15,306	7.4	49.1	54.3	45.2
Respiratory diseases	8,920	4.3	28.9	46.4	18.3
Accidents	8,687	4.2	29.1	40.9	18.1
Pneumonia & influenza	7,302	3.5	23.3	30.6	18.8
Diabetes mellitus	5,165	2.5	16.8	20.0	14.4
Suicide	3,749	1.8	12.7	20.6	5.2
Kidney diseases	2,480	1.2	8.0	10.6	6.4
Cirrhosis of liver	2,208	1.1	7.3	10.7	4.4
AIDS	1,628	0.8	5.5	9.9	0.9
Other causes	37,348	18.0	121.9	142.9	105.0
All causes	**207,077**	**100.0**	**675.0**	**870.8**	**528.5**

Source: *Statistics Canada, Health Statistics Division.*

When Canadian mortality is examined from this point of view, it becomes clear why the Lalonde report placed emphasis on the lifestyle element of the health field concept.

Figure 5.3 (3) provides a broad overview of the prevailing causes of death by sex and age group in Canada in 1994. It demonstrates the relative contribution of our lifestyle to mortality up to middle age and emphasizes differences in causes of death between males and females. Highlights of this figure are as follows:

- In children, perinatal disorders and congenital anomalies account for a significant proportion of total mortality because of the concentration of deaths in infancy. Accidents and suicides, however, account for 41% of deaths of young men between the ages of 15 and 24 and 27% of young female deaths in the same age group.
- Among those aged 25 to 44, accidents, suicide, cancer, and heart disease are important causes of death for both sexes. Over the last decade, AIDS has become one of the major causes of death among males.
- In mid-life, the leading causes of death are cancer and coronary heart disease. Cancer takes a particularly large toll among women, accounting for 56% of deaths between ages of 45 and 64. Coronary heart disease and cancer are each responsible for approximately 61.5% of deaths among men in this age group.
- At older ages, coronary heart disease and cancer continue to be the leading causes of death, but the proportion of deaths due to coronary heart disease increases, especially among women, while the relative importance of cancer declines. Stroke becomes a significant cause of death after age 70.

Figure 5.3:   Causes of Death by Age and Sex, Canada, 1994

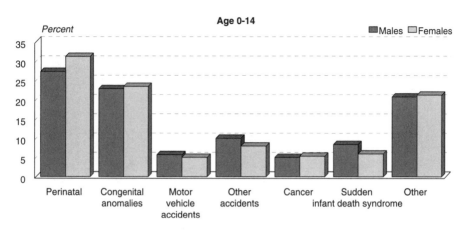

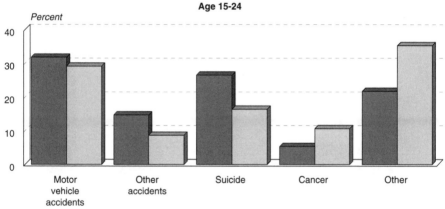

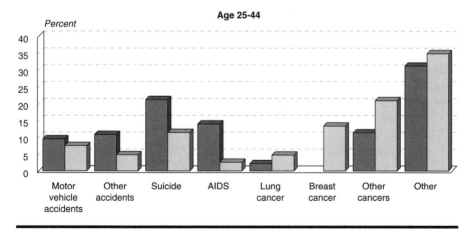

Figure 5.3:   Causes of Death by Age and Sex, Canada, 1994 *(con't)*

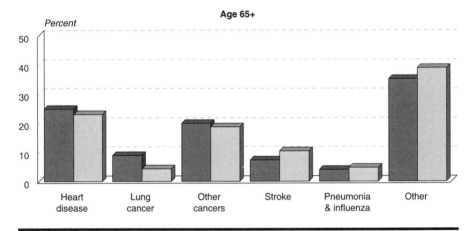

Source: *Deaths 1994*. Statistics Canada (CAT 84-208), Ottawa.

A comparison of the 1991 and 1994 rates reveals changes in the relative importance of leading causes of death: coronary heart disease has remained stable in relative
importance at 23% from 1991 to 1994, decreasing from 29% in 1981 for all ages and both
sexes combined. In addition:

- the proportion of deaths due to cancer has increased slightly for all ages and both
  sexes combined; it was 28.2% in 1994 compared with 27% in 1991;
- among cancer deaths, lung cancer increased in relative importance dramatically
  among women, now ranking first among those aged 25 to 44;
- motor vehicle accidents have decreased in relative importance overall (from 3% of
  all deaths to 1%);
- AIDS has become one of the leading causes of death among males aged 25 to 44
  (14% of all deaths in this age range).

Figure 5.4:   Potential-Years-of-Life-Lost (PYLL) per 100,000 Person-Years, by Leading Causes of Death, Canada, 1994

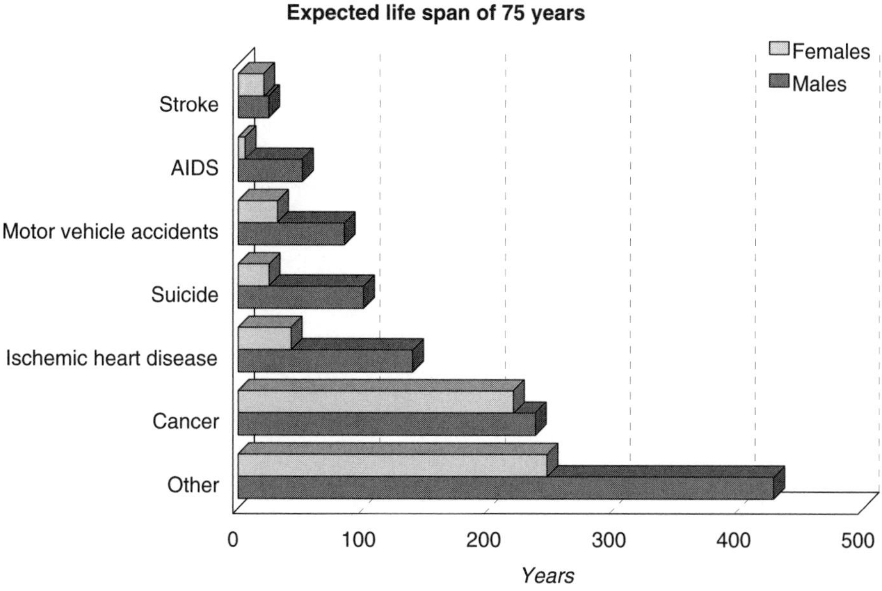

Expected life span of 75 years

Source. *Statistics Canada*

Potential-Years-of-Life-Lost

For any cause of death, the potential-years-of-life-lost (PYLL) is calculated by totalling the years of life remaining until age 75 for each person who dies of that cause between birth and age 75, within a given period, using the midpoint of a five-year interval. Thus, a person who dies at age 21 would contribute 54 years to the total. This indicator has the main effect of assessing premature mortality, which may be useful for setting priorities for prevention. The first five causes listed in Figure 5.4 are responsible for approximately 55% of PYLL (5). Immediately apparent is the importance of motor vehicle accidents, ischemic heart disease, suicide, and cancer. Males lose approximately three times as many years as females due to these causes of premature mortality.

Quality of Life

The concept of measuring quality of life is becoming popular in the health care sector as an outcome measure of a procedure, drug, or service provided, reflecting the importance of quality not merely quantity of life. **Health-related quality of life (HR-QOL)** refers to the measurement of health status of an individual (6); domains may include health perceptions, functional status, cognitive function, pain, impairments or symptoms, and opportunity influenced by disease, injury, treatment, or policy. The Health

Utilities Index (HUI) (7) developed at McMaster University is a HR-QOL index that combines both a description of health status (based on attributes of vision, hearing, speech, mobility, emotional state, thinking and memory, dexterity, and level or pain or discomfort) with a value of the preference for different state of health.

Health-adjusted life expectancy (HALE) is a population health indicator that modifies life expectancy by a value-weighted index such as the Health Utility Index. Monitoring HALE answers whether we are achieving the goal of the World Health Organization's Healthy People 2000, namely "to add life to years and years to life". In Canada between 1990 and 1992, the difference in HALE between men and women aged 15, is 3.7 years, smaller than the 6.3-year difference in life expectancy, and largely attributed to increased functional disability of women in their older ages (8).

Cancer

Reporting cancer cases to provincial cancer registries is voluntary but results in a valuable database for the investigation of potential causes of malignancies through case-control studies, and allows the long-term evaluation of the effect of new therapies, early detection programs, and changes in environmental and lifestyle factors. It was estimated that in 1997, 130,800 new cases of cancer (approximately 61,000 cases excluding non-melanoma skin cancer) would be diagnosed in Canada. Deaths from cancer in 1997 were estimated at 60,700. Lung cancer in males and females, followed by prostate cancer in men and breast cancer in women, are the most frequent cancers, in terms of incidence and deaths, followed by colorectal cancer. Table 5.2 illustrates the frequency of the sites of cancer (9).

1.2.2. Morbidity

Mortality, although of great importance, is clearly only one part of the health status of a population. Morbidity, which includes all health outcomes other than death, is difficult to quantify due to a paucity of accurate information. No single source of information reflects all morbidity, but by looking at several sources, one can gain an appreciation of the nature and extent of morbidity and detect trends. It is also important to remember that in examining a particular health problem, some aspects of morbidity may be more relevant than others. For example, time off work may be a better reflection of morbidity associated with the common cold than hospital admission rates, which might more appropriately be used to assess the morbidity of bleeding duodenal ulcer. Each of the sources of information described in this section is of value in assessing some aspect of morbidity.

Communicable Diseases

As described in Chapter Three, selected diseases in Canada are reported to central authorities on a voluntary or mandatory basis. These centralized reports constitute an important source of information on morbidity. The disease-specific case definitions set out in the Canadian Communicable Disease Surveillance System are used for federal surveillance (10). Most provinces provide annual summaries of reportable disease experience incorporating time trends.

Table 5.2:   Percent Distribution of Estimated New Cases and Deaths for Major Cancer Sites, Canada, 1997

Site	Males Incidence n=70,200	Males Mortality n=60,700	Females Incidence n=60,600	Females Mortality n=28,100
Lung	17.8	32.5	12.9	22.4
Breast	-	-	30.4	18.1
Prostate	28.2	12.6	-	-
Colorectal	12.7	9.8	12.4	9.6
Leukemia & lymphoma	7.3	7.1	7.0	7.2
Bladder	4.8	2.8	1.8	1.6
Uterus & cervix	-	-	7.1	3.5
Stomach	2.5	3.2	1.7	2.6
Kidney	3.4	2.5	2.5	1.8
Pancreas	1.9	4.1	2.6	5.3
Ovary	-	-	3.6	4.8
Oral	3.1	2.2	1.6	1.0
All others	18.3	23.2	16.4	22.1

Source: Canadian Cancer Statistics 1997, National Cancer Institute of Canada.

Most of the communicable diseases for which reporting is mandatory are reasonably well controlled, and appear in the population with low frequency, which is not true for the major sexually transmitted diseases (STDs). Data from Health Canada indicating the incidence of notifiable diseases and notifiable diseases requiring vaccination in Canada in 1991 is shown in Table 5.3.

Occupational Injuries and Illness
Since the advent of widespread financial compensation for injuries and illness in the working environment, a quasi-voluntary reporting system has developed. Figure 5.5 illustrates the incidence of occupational injuries and diseases from workers' compensation board records for all of Canada, 1994. There was a total of 429,758 work-related lost-time claims reported for the year 1994, of which 99.8% related to injuries. The most common injuries were strains and sprains (which accounted for about half), and contusions and wounds. Occupational diseases are infrequent compared with injuries. The most common diseases were tenosynovitis, chemical burns, welder's flash, poisoning, and dermatitis. The permanent disabilities related to occupational exposure were chronic back problems, strains, and hearing loss. Despite safety programs to reduce work injuries and increasing awareness of occupational illness, the incidence of these important health problems has changed little (11).

Table 5.3:   Incidence of Notifiable Diseases and Notifiable Diseases Requiring Vaccination (per 100,000 Persons), Canada, 1991

Disease category	Crude rate per 100,000 people
Incidence of notifiable diseases requiring vaccination	
Diphtheria	0.01
Whooping cough	10.10
Tetanus	0.01
Measles	22.90
Rubella	2.60
Mumps	1.50
Poliomyeletis	0.00
Haemophilus influenzae type B	1.40
Incidence of notifiable diseases	
Early symptomatic syphilis	1.40
Syphilis, other	3.90
AIDS	3.80
Gonococcal infections	46.00
Chlamydia infections (1993)	154.06
Hepatitis A	11.20
Hepatitis B	9.90
Meningoccal infections	1.60
Tuberculosis	7.60

Source: Working Group on Community Health Information Systems et al. Directions de la santé publique, Quebec. *Community Health Indicators. Definitions and Interpretations*. Ottawa, June 1995.

Causes of Hospitalization

General Hospitals. Hospitalization may vary according to availability of beds and local medical practice. Although hospitalization data omit important information about morbidity in outpatients, they do reflect the magnitude of serious illness and use of vital resources. Figure 5.6 indicates the pattern of major causes of hospitalization in general hospitals in Canada (in 1992/93) in descending order of importance. Expressing hospitalization in terms of patient-days inflates the importance of illness requiring longer hospital stays; conversely, using separations emphasizes shorter stays, such as for obstetrical admissions. In 1994/95, Canadians spent over 43 million days in general and allied hospitals, a figure that represents a rate of fewer than 1,500 days per 1,000 population. The average length of hospital stay for 1994/95 was 11.1 days including chronic care and long-term psychiatric cases, or 7.0 days if only acute care is considered. Females use more hospital days than males, but much of this excess is due to obstetrical admissions and

Figure 5.5:   Percentage Distribution of Occupational Injuries as Causes of Temporary Disability among Workers, Canada, 1994

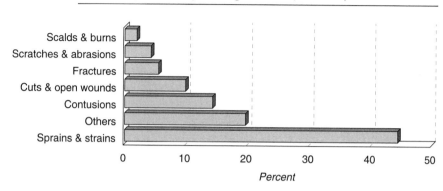

Source: *Work Injuries, 1992-1994*, Labour Division, Statistics Canada: 14-19, 1995.

the health care utilization by the preponderance of elderly females. The five leading causes of hospitalization shown in Figure 5.6 were also represented in the list of common causes of death. Mental illness, with low mortality, accounted for the second highest total number of hospital days in 1992/93. For the same period, obstetric admissions also accounted for a significant proportion of hospitalizations (over half a million). Delivery without complication is not true morbidity but must be considered in planning for hospital services.

Mental Hospitals. Figure 5.6 also shows the significant contribution of mental illness to patient days even in general hospitals. When all institutions that provide psychiatric care are taken into account, including special mental hospitals and psychiatric units in general hospitals, the tremendous hospital morbidity associated with mental illness is apparent. In 1993/94, these institutions provided 15.9 million patient days of care for the 204,617 cases of mental disorder in which the patient was either discharged or died.

The development of new therapies for mental disorders since the early 1980s (for example, improved drugs) and the establishment of alternative facilities in the community have meant that only the more serious cases are hospitalized. Since 1982 there has been a slight shift in the hospitalization of mental disorder cases toward treatment in general hospitals (from 82% in 1982/83 to 85% of separations in 1993/94) (12). The average length of stay in psychiatric hospitals increased (from 193 to 316 days), and that of psychiatric patients in general hospitals rose (from 27 to 33 days); this trend reflects the tendency to admit patients with the most serious diagnoses to psychiatric hospitals.

Table 5.4 illustrates the separations and days of care and average length of stay secondary to mental disorders in both general and psychiatric hospitals. To some

Figure 5.6:   Leading Causes of Discharges and Number of Days in General Hospitals, Canada, 1992-1993

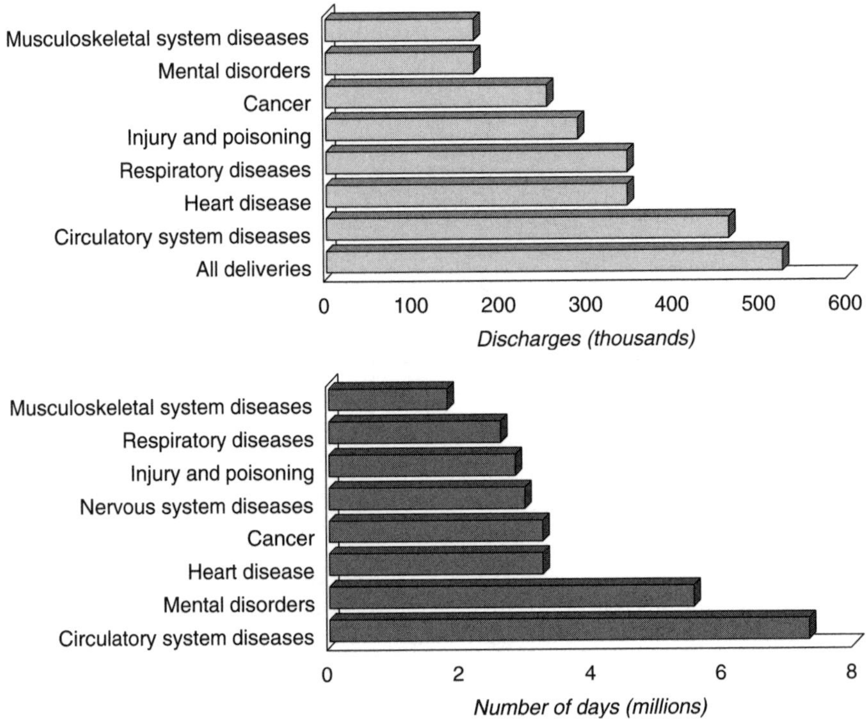

Source: *Hospital Morbidity 1992-1993*, Health Statistics Division, Statistics Canada: 2-9, 1995.

extent, the increase in the number of patient-days provided for mental disorders is attributable to the time required for the treatment of disorders such as schizophrenia and affective psychoses despite the declining separation rates. The leading cause of separations among males was schizophrenia disorder, affective psychoses, and alcohol dependence syndrome (19.2%, 14.8%, and 10.8% respectively), as compared to females where the principle causes of separations were affective psychoses, neurotic disorder, schizophrenia, adjustment reaction, and depressive disorder (23.4%, 12.2%, 11.7%, 8.9%, and 7.9% respectively). The chief cause of days of care among males and females were schizophrenia disorder and affective psychoses (72.2% and 16.6% for males and 58.3% and 28.4% for females respectively), as well as neurotic disorder in females (4.9%). The average length of stay among both sexes was found to be similar (13).

Table 5.4:   **Separations, Days of Care, and Average Length of Stay in Psychiatric and General Hospitals by Diagnosis, 1993-94, Canada**

Type of mental disorder	Separations (%) n=204,617	Days of care (%) n=8,705,337	Average length of stay (days)
Affective psychoses	19.4	22.2	47.8
Schizophrenia disorder	15.2	65.7	179.5
Neurotic disorder	9.5	3.8	16.3
Adjustment reaction	7.9	2.8	15
Alcohol dependence syndrome	6.9	2.3	13.7
Depressive disorders	6.4	3.1	20.8
Other	34.7	0.1	-
Total	**100**	**100**	**42.5**

Source: *Mental Health Statistics, 1993-94*, Health Reports 7(4), 60, 1996. Statistics Canada.

Dental Morbidity

Dental illness is considered separately in this chapter to emphasize its significance. Dental diseases are associated with a great deal of morbidity. The recent Health Promotion Survey indicated that overall, 84% of Canadian adults reported having one or more of their natural teeth. This proportion was fairly consistent throughout all provinces, with the exception of Quebec, where 73% of the population were dentate. The proportion of toothless persons increased with age; 35% of those aged 55 to 64 and 50% of the those over age 65 are toothless. This measure may be said to reflect dental disability, and is useful in planning dental care. In 1994, 10.3% of Ontarians aged 12 years and over reported being edentulous (toothless). Gender differences were very small in each age group, with slightly more women than men living with this condition (14).

As there is no large-scale reporting by dental health professionals and hospitalization is infrequent, the only information on dental morbidity comes from studies and surveys (15-17). Dental caries and periodontal disease were assessed by means of indices based on a dental examination. The index for caries, for example, was the DMFT (decayed, missing, or filled teeth) or DEFT (decayed, extracted, or filled teeth) score, which identifies the number of teeth involved with caries. The rate of dental caries in elementary school children in Canada, and particularly in Ontario, shows a steady long-term decline, which appears to be continuing (18). The Canadian average of DMFT at age 13 is 3.1. Ontario has the lowest (1.7); British Columbia (2.9) and Alberta (3.1) are in the middle; while Quebec (4.2) and the Atlantic provinces (5.5) have the highest DMFT index in 13-year-old children. When Canadian DMFT rates are compared to those of other developed nations, Canadian children rated very favourably. It must also be noted that the prevalence of dental morbidity is un-

Table 5.5:   Disability Rates in the Canadian Population, 1991

Population	Number with disabilities	Disability rate (%)
Both sexes	4,184,685	15.5
Age 0-14	389,355	7.0
Age 15-64	2,346,455	12.9
Age 65+	1,448,875	46.3
Females	2,217,640	16.2
Age 0-14	156,365	5.7
Age 15-64	1,182,145	12.9
Age 65+	879,130	48.4
Males	1,967,045	14.8
Age 0-14	232,990	8.1
Age 15-64	1,164,310	12.8
Age 65+	569,745	43.4

Source: *The Daily*, October 13, 1992, Statistics Canada.

evenly distributed, with immigrant children having the highest levels of caries: 52.4% of Canadian-born children have a DEFT/DMFT score of 0 compared to 37.6% of those born outside of Canada (18).

2.   CONSEQUENCES

The consequences of illness are personal disability, impairment, or handicap, as well as the utilization of health care resources in the management of the condition, and the economic burden to the community.

2.1. DISABILITY

Disability as a measure of morbidity (see Chapters One and Three) has been defined in various ways. All definitions include the notion of the inability to carry on usual functions of living and working. All attempts subdivide disability by degree of severity. Sources of disability information include surveys, disability pension plans, and records of time lost from work due to ill health. Data from several different surveys serve here as examples.

The National Population Health Survey examined both short-term and long-term disability. Short-term disability was based on the individual's experience during the previous two weeks; disability days were recorded if the individual was unable to do things he or she would normally do for all or most of the day. One or more disability days were reported by 15% of Canadians in 1994/95. For Canadians aged 15 and older, this is a substantial increase from 1991 and is the highest average value recorded in surveys over almost 20 years. Females aged 15 and older reported more disability days than males, and were somewhat more likely to report one or more days. With increasing years beyond the teens, there is also a steady increase in two-week disability days, reaching a maximum of 1.72 days for Canadians age 75 and older.

The Health and Activity Limitation Survey 1991 (19) used the international definition of disability and handicap and found that over 4.1 million Canadians or 15.5% of the population reported some level of disability. Disability rates increased with age (see Table 5.5). Two thirds of disabled individuals aged 15 and over reported more than one type of disability. The prevalence of multiple disabilities increased with age: of the disabled population aged 15 to 34, 46% reported having more than one disability, increasing to 76.0% in the population aged 65 and over. Among those over age 15, 60% of all disability problems identified in the survey related to mobility or agility, 16% related to hearing and 8.6% related to eyesight. The National Population Health Survey reported higher prevalence (20%) of activity limitation or handicap in 1994; however, the actual questions asked to determine the level of activity limitation may have overestimated the rates of disability.

2.2. PHYSICIANS' SERVICES

Since the advent of government health insurance in Canada, it has been possible to acquire information about the kinds and numbers of illnesses treated by physicians outside hospitals. National data are unavailable, and provincial comparisons are difficult due to differences in reporting, but an example of data from the Saskatchewan Health Care Commission for 1994/95 is shown in Table 5.6. These data indicate that the largest numbers of services were related to health check-ups, respiratory conditions, cardiovascular, urinary conditions, and diabetes. In Canada overall, for all physicians' services, whether inside hospitals or in the community, 10.6% were for well-patient care, followed by respiratory diseases (9.1%), cardiovascular diseases (8.9%), and nervous system and sense organ diseases (8.2%).

A study conducted in Manitoba reported that in 1991/92, 60% of total physician utilization in the form of visits or expenditures was accounted for by people who contacted a physician eight or more times. Overall, general practitioners were seen most frequently in terms of speciality (74.8% of all visits), followed by medical specialists, including general internists as well as those with a subspeciality such as geriatrics or neurology (6.7%) and pediatricians (6.6%). Surgical specialists — including all specialists such as thoracic and cardiovascular, plastic, or urology — accounted for 5% of all patient visits followed by psychiatrists, obstetrician/gynecologists, and general surgeons (2.7%, 2.1%, and 2.1% respectively) (20).

Table 5.6:   Utilization of Physician's Services by Common Medical Conditions, Saskatchewan, 1994-95

Conditions	Number of services (thousands)
Acute upper respiratory infection (except influenza)	566
General medical examination	518
Hypertension	274
Diseases of genitourinary tract	248
Otitis media	228
Ischemic heart disease	225
Asthma	210
Bronchitis	200
Chronic sinusitis and other respiratory symptoms	170
Rheumatic disease	166
Diabetes mellitus	159
Arthritis	158
Neurosis	146
Hay fever	143
Others	1,475
Total	**4,886**

Source: *Annual Statistical Report, 1994-95*, Saskatchewan Health, Government of Saskatchewan, 1996.

2.3. PRESCRIPTION DRUG USE

The prevalence of drug use is a relatively new area of investigation. Large-scale data are available from Saskatchewan and so are reported here (21, 22).

- In 1994/95, 93% of Saskatchewan's total population was eligible to receive benefits under the Prescription Drug Plan. Certain classes of individuals, such as those on social assistance or residing in special care homes were exempted from the deductive program.
- There were 5.7 million prescriptions processed during the fiscal 12-month period.
- An average of 10.1 prescriptions were dispensed to each active beneficiary exempted from the deductible program. An average of 6.7 prescriptions were dispensed to each active beneficiary under the deductible program.
- An average of 14.7 prescriptions were dispensed to each family unit exempt from the deductible program. An average of 11.0 prescriptions were dispensed to each family unit under the deductible program.
- The average drug cost of a prescription was $17.94.
- Sixty-nine per cent of the population was prescribed at least one drug during 1994.

- The average number of prescriptions per patient was 6.0, with females receiving notably more prescriptions than males, particularly for cardiovascular drugs and sedatives/antidepressants.
- Amoxicillin was the most commonly prescribed drug overall.
- Benzodiazepines were still being prescribed on a long-term basis.

2.4. USE OF DENTAL CARE SERVICES

The recent Health Promotion Survey indicated that three out of four Canadians aged 15 and over (75%) visited a dentist in the 12 months prior to the survey. This proportion fluctuates from 80% in Ontario to 58% in Newfoundland. Whereas the highest proportion of Canadians reporting a dental visit is among those aged 15 to 19 (81%), rates were at their lowest among those aged 20 to 24 (67%). The rates then slightly increased among those aged 35 to 44 and levelled off. With few exceptions, these trends were fairly consistent from one province to another. There is a positive association between income and dental visits: 69% of very poor Canadians went to a dentist in the previous 12 months compared with 86% of rich people. The common reasons for visits to a dentist by Canadians aged 15 and over were for check-ups or cleaning, tooth filling, or extraction, to have crown or bridge work done in order to replace, repair, or maintain missing or damaged teeth, and to have periodontal treatment.

2.5. ECONOMIC BURDEN

In Canada in 1993, the total burden of ill health was defined as that created by illness, disability, and premature death on individuals and on Canadian society; it was estimated to be $156.9 billion (compared to $97 billion in 1986), of which $72 billion were direct costs and $85 billion were indirect (23). The two leading causes of direct expenditure were hospital care costs (16.6%), and professional services, which are medical and other health care practitioner services (10.5%). Drug costs accounted for 6.3% of total direct costs. For indirect costs, premature mortality accounted for 18.7% and chronic disability 24.4%. The remainders of the indirect costs were for short-term disability. Cardiovascular disease, injuries and violence, cancer, and arthritis and related conditions accounted collectively for half of the total costs. Cardiovascular disease was the leading cause of both direct ($7.4 billion) and indirect costs ($12.4 billion), making it the most expensive category overall. Musculoskeletal disorders and injuries ranked next (total cost of $17.8 and $14.3 billion respectively), followed by cancer (total cost of $13.7 billion). Overall, chronic conditions were responsible for the major economic burden. Figure 5.7 illustrates the economic burden of illness in Canada.

Figure 5.7:   Cost of Illness by Disease Category, Canada, 1993

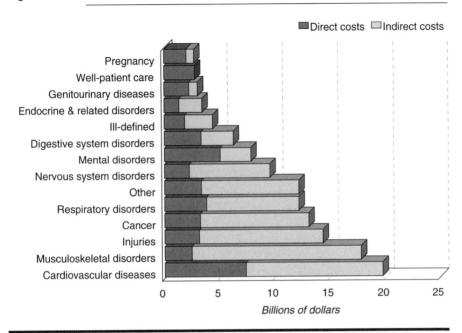

Source: *Economic Burden of Illness in Canada, 1993.* Health Canada, 1997.

3. SUMMARY

The two health status indicators, mortality and morbidity, are the most commonly used measures of health in Canada.

The trend in age- and sex-specific death rates between 1951 and 1994 indicates that over a 40-year period death rates have been declining at different rates for different age groups. Among those under age one year, there has been a steady decline in mortality rates. In 1995, the infant mortality rate per 1,000 live births was 6.1. The majority of these deaths occur due to congenital anomalies, sudden infant death syndrome, and perinatal problems. Between 1 and 14 years of age, mortality rates continue to decline slowly. More than half of these deaths are due to motor vehicle and other accidents, and are preventable. Among those aged 15 to 24, the most significant causes of death include motor vehicle and other accidents, and suicide. Recently, a significant drop in the death rate for this age group occurred, especially for males. Among those aged 25 to 44, mortality rates have recently begun to decline slightly. Male rates in this age group and those aged 45 to 64 remain about double the female rates, being largely due to accidents, ischemic heart disease, suicide, cancer of the lung, and AIDS (particularly among those aged 25 to 44). For those between the ages of 45 and 64, both male and female mortality rates are on the decline. Although there is a wide gap between male and female death rates beyond the age of 65, both rates are now declining. The major causes of death for both men and women are ischemic heart disease, cancer, cerebrovascular disease, and respiratory illness.

The leading causes of death for men ranked by number of deaths are cancer, coronary heart disease, stroke, respiratory diseases, and accidents. For women, the leading causes are cancer, coronary heart disease, stroke, respiratory disease, and pneumonia. Many of these deaths could be prevented or delayed by lifestyle modifications. Lung cancer in males and females is the most frequent cancer, in terms of both incidence and deaths, and exceeded breast cancer as the leading cause of death in women in 1997.

No single source of information reflects all morbidity. There are several useful sources of information for assessing some aspect of overall morbidity such as communicable diseases or injuries. Centralized reports of communicable diseases indicated that the crude rate for vaccine-preventable diseases is low except for tuberculosis. However, the crude rates for sexually transmitted diseases and hepatitis are high, and chlamydia and gonorrhoea have the highest crude rate. With regard to injuries, the most common causes of temporary disability as a result of workplace accident were strains and sprains, followed by contusions. Occupational diseases are infrequent compared with injuries.

Another aspect of morbidity that has been documented is hospitalization. The main causes of hospitalization are mental disorders, heart disease, injury and poisoning, cancer, and respiratory diseases. In 1994/95, Canadians spent 43.0 million days in general hospitals. As a result of obstetrical admissions and longer longevity, females have a higher use of hospital days than males. In 1993/94, these institutions provided 15.9 million patient days of care for the 204,617 cases of mental disorder in which the patient was either discharged or died. The leading cause of separations among males was schizophrenia disorder, affective psychoses, and alcohol dependence syndrome (19.2%, 14.8%, and 10.8% respectively), as compared to females where the principle causes of separations were affective psychoses, neurotic disorder, schizophrenia, adjustment reaction, and depressive disorder (23.4%, 12.2%, 11.7%, 8.9%, and 7.9% respectively).

Morbidity is also associated with dental disease. Dental caries in elementary school children has been declining steadily.

The consequences of illness are disability, impairment, or handicap, as well as the utilization of health care resources and economic burden to the community. Over 4.1 million Canadians in 1991, or 15.5% of the population, reported some level of disability, with females having a slightly higher rate than males. The prevalence of multiple disabilities increases with age, with loss of mobility or agility being the largest form of disability, followed by hearing and eyesight problems. The largest number of services rendered by physicians were related to routine check-ups, respiratory conditions, cardiovascular diseases, urinary conditions, and diabetes. The total burden of ill health for Canada in 1993 was estimated to be approximately $156.9 billion, of which $72 billion was direct costs and $85 billion was indirect costs. Hospital care costs, professional services, and drugs constitute the three leading causes of direct expenditures. Premature mortality, chronic disability, and short-term disability primarily account for the indirect expenditures. Cardiovascular disease is the leading cause of both direct and indirect costs.

4. REFERENCES

1. Statistics Canada. National Population Health Survey Overview. Ottawa: Government of Canada, 1995.
2. Kohn R. Royal Commission on Health Services: The Health of the Canadian People. Ottawa: Queen's Printer and Controller of Stationary, 1967.
3. Statistics Canada. Deaths 1994. Ottawa: Government of Canada, 1995.
4. Nault F, Wilkins K. Deaths 1993. Health Reports 1995;7(1):51-60.
5. Statistics Canada. Statistics Canada 1994. Ottawa: Government of Canada, 1994.
6. Patrick D, Erickson P. Health Status and Policy: Quality of Life in Health Care Evolution and Resource Allocation. New York: Oxford University Press, 1992.
7. Torrance G, Zhang Y, Feeny D, Furlong W, Barr R. McMaster University Centre for Health Economics and Policy Analysis Working Paper. 1998.
8. Wolfson MC. Health-Adjusted Life Expectancy. Health Reports 1996;8(1):41-45.
9. National Cancer Institute of Canada. Canadian Cancer Statistics, 1997. Toronto: National Cancer Institute of Canada, 1997.
10. Health and Welfare Canada. Canadian Communicable Disease Surveillance System: Disease-Specific Case Definitions and Surveillance Methods. Canadian Disease Weekly Report 1991;17 (Supplement 13):35-36.
11. Statistics Canada. Work Injuries 1992-1994. Ottawa: Government of Canada, 1995.
12. Statistics Canada. Mental Health Statistics, 1993-1994. Ottawa: Government of Canada, 1996.
13. Randhawa R, Riley R. Mental Health Statistics, 1982-83 and 1993-94. Health Reports 1996;7(4):33-45.
14. Jokovic A, Locker D. Oral Health Status of Ontarians Aged Twelve Years and Over. North York: North York Public Health Department, 1995.
15. Public Health Branch. Dental Health Indices 1987/88 Survey. Toronto: Ontario Ministry of Health, 1990.
16. Payette M, Brodeur JM, Lepage Y, Plante E. Enquête Santé Dentaire Quebéc, 1989-90. Montreal: Department de Santé Commuataire, Hôpital Staint-Luc, 1991.
17. Gray H, Gunther D. A Comprehensive Review of Dental Caries Experience Shown by Grade 7 Students in the Provincial Health Units of British Columbia. Victoria: Dental Health Branch, Minister of Health, Government of British Columbia, 1987.
18. Mair P. Preliminary Findings from the 1994 Ontario Children's Dental Health Survey. Canadian Journal of Community Dentistry 1995;10(2):38-43.
19. Statistics Canada. The 1991 Health and Activity Limitation Survey — Highlights. Ottawa: Government of Canada, 1992.
20. Tataryn DDJ, Roos DN, Black DC. Utilization of Physician Resources. Vol. 1: Key Findings. Winnipeg: Manitoba Centre for Health Policy and Evaluation, Department of Community Health Sciences, Faculty of Medicine, University of Manitoba, 1994.
21. Saskatchewan Health Prescription Drug Services Branch. Annual Statistical Report 1994-1995. Regina: Saskatchewan Health, Government of Saskatchewan, 1996.
22. Saskatchewan Health Medical Care Insurance Branch. Annual Statistical Report 1990-1991. Regina: Government of Saskatchewan 1996.
23. Economic Burden of Illness in Canada, 1993. Chronic Disease in Canada 1996 (Special Supplement).

Chapter

6

Health of
Special Groups

The previous two chapters outlined the determinants of health, health status, and consequences in the Canadian population as a whole. This chapter examines the health of certain segments of the population: Aboriginal peoples, seniors, poor children, and people with disabilities. The health of each of these groups reflects the influence of the determinants of health. For the first three groups, the determinants are race, age, and psychosocial factors. The fourth group, people with disabilities, has been chosen as an example of how the determinants of health frequently interact and compound further the inequities in health relative to the rest of the population.

1. THE HEALTH OF ABORIGINAL PEOPLES

According to the census, Aboriginal peoples, also known as the First Nations peoples or Native Canadians, fall into four groups; Status Indians, non-Status Indians, Mètis, and Inuit. In this chapter, the term "Aboriginal peoples" is used to designate Status and non-Status Indians. "Status Indian" has specific legal connotations and is defined as Aboriginal peoples registered under the *Indian Act* (1). This group has signed treaties with the federal government that accord them certain privileges to be compensated for having relinquished certain land rights. Four centuries of colonization — being subjugated and stripped of their land, religion, culture, language, and autonomy — have taken their toll on the physical, mental, emotional, and spiritual health of the Aboriginal communities. The present-day determinants of health reflect these injustices.

1.1. DETERMINANTS

Most of the data on health determinants and status for this section are derived from *Trends in First Nations Mortality 1979-1993* (2), published by the Medical Services Branch of Health Canada, *Summary of First Nations Health Status, 1995*, published by Statistics Canada (3), and a background paper on the health of Aboriginal people by Postl et al (4).

Although information is lacking about off-reserve Aboriginal people, it is believed that their health status is actually worse than the health status of on-reserve groups. This may be due to the additional stresses of the urban environment, particularly a very high unemployment rate (28%) (5), racial discrimination, and lack of a social support network. Non-status Indians are often ineligible for government benefits, which may afford a modicum of relief for Status Indians (6). Up to 70% of Aboriginal peoples may be ineligible for federal programs, making access to some services such as alcohol and drug rehabilitation programs difficult for off-reserve Aboriginal groups (7).

1.1.1. Psychosocial Environment

At the time of Confederation, there remained roughly 102,000 Aboriginal people (8) (down from the approximately 222,000 in the 16th century). By 1941, estimates of the Aboriginal population fluctuated between 100,000 and 122,000, representing approximately 1.1% of the total Canadian population. Since then, the Aboriginal population has grown, and the 1996 census, which asked respondents to specify whether they were North American Indian, Métis, or Inuit, found that 799,010 or 2.8% of Canadians reported that they were Aboriginal. Of these, about two thirds or 554,000 people were North American Indian, one quarter (210,000) were Métis, and 1 in 20 (41,000) were Inuit.

This population growth is solely due to natural increase. While the crude birth rate per 1,000 population declined from 44.3 in 1965 to 27.3 in 1993, it is still almost double the Canadian rate. Similarly, Aboriginal death rates have declined, although they are still higher than the rates for other Canadians. In 1993, life expectancy at birth for Aboriginal males was 67.0 years and 74.9 years for females, while it was 73.7 years for Canadian males, and 80.6 years for females. Life expectancy is lowest for Status Indians living on reserves: 62 years for men and 69.6 years for women.

The high birth rate of Aboriginal people, coupled with a consistently lower life expectancy than the general population, ensures a relatively young population compared to the general population: in 1996, 35% were aged 0 to 14 years, 61.5 % were aged 15 to 64, and 3.5% were aged 65 years and over. Although the proportion in the youngest age group had declined slightly since 1979, the predominance of younger Aboriginal people is in contrast to the total Canadian population (20.7% of population aged 0 to 14). The gender distribution (49:51 male:female) is approximately the same as for all Canadians.

Of the total Aboriginal population in 1996, 17.7% lived in Ontario, 8.9% in Quebec, 4.7 % in the Atlantic region, and 68.7% lived in the four western provinces. However, when viewed as a percentage of the total provincial or territorial population, Aboriginal peoples constituted 61.9% of the Northwest Territories and 20.1% in the Yukon Territories. Ontario had more North American Indians than any other province. Alberta had the largest Mètis population, while the Northwest Territories had the largest Inuit population. Most Aboriginal people live off reserve; however, 59% of Status Indians lived on reserves (also known as the First Nations communities), with the proportion of the off-reserve Status Indians increasing from 29% in 1985 to 41% in 1991. There are 2,284 reserves in Canada, with 65% of the Aboriginal population living in either rural or remote locations; those who live in the city lived mainly in Winnipeg, Edmonton, Vancouver, Saskatoon, Toronto, Calgary, and Regina. The labour force participation rates were 47% for Status Indians living on reserves, 57% for off-reserve Indians and Inuit each, and 59% for Mètis, compared to the national rate of 68%. Most Aboriginal peoples are employed in low-paying service industry jobs. The average Aboriginal income in constant 1986 dollars increased in the 1991 census but was still almost half the Canadian mean.

1.1.2. Physical Environment

On and off reserves, relative homelessness has been well documented by both government and other sources including the Royal Commission on Aboriginal Peoples (7). Houses occupied by Aboriginal people are twice as likely to need major repairs as those of all Canadians, and 90 times more likely to be living without piped water supply. On reserves, 14% of all dwellings have no indoor plumbing, 12.5% have no central heating, 6.5% have no electricity, and approximately 11.4% of dwellings have more than one person per room, which is eight times the Canadian rate. There are few recreational facilities for children or adults. Many northern Aboriginal communities have no potable water supply (9).

1.1.3. Lifestyle and Behavioural Risk Factors

Alcohol, Smoking, and Substance Abuse

While there are no useful national trend data for alcohol use among Aboriginal people, the 1991 report by Statistics Canada on alcohol and drug abuse provides some suggestive information (3). Alcohol use among adults over age 15 years indicated that approximately 70% reported drinking alcohol in the past year; 15% indicated they never drink alcohol, and 15% reported not using alcohol in the past year. Of those who reported drinking in the previous year, 4.5% reported drinking either every day or four to six times a week; 11% reported drinking two to three times a week and 19% at least once a week.

The same survey also found that 61% of the respondents indicated that alcohol abuse is a problem in their community. While the levels of drinking are not very different from those reported for the general Canadian population (see Chapter Four), other studies suggest that alcohol abuse levels were between 35% and 40% for the adult population and between 10% and 15% for Aboriginal adolescents. The prevalent drinking patterns for Aboriginal adults were periodic, high-volume drinking (binge drinking) and problem drinking (trouble with the law, fighting, or family problems while drinking)

(10). An Ontario Needs Assessment Survey of Aboriginal children and youth also indicated a high prevalence of alcohol abuse: 10% of children in grades three to eight reported drinking enough to get "high" at least once in the past year, while 53% of youth in grades 7 to 13 reported the same (11). For the latter group, this is about double that of non-Aboriginal youths in Ontario and New Brunswick.

Statistics Canada data indicated that 45.2% of Aboriginal adults smoke daily, 11.6% smoked occasionally, and 43.1% of these people reported not smoking at the time. The rate was higher among males. A 1988 survey indicated that 48.2% of Aboriginal mothers smoked during and after pregnancy. While no specific national data are available, gasoline and glue sniffing appear to be common among Aboriginal teenagers (12) and two surveys in the mid 1980s have indicated continued use of solvents at a prevalence of 6% and 9%, respectively. Twenty per cent of the Manitoba youth and 15% of the Quebec youth reported solvent abuse. The 1993 Ontario First Nations AIDS and Health Lifestyle Survey found that in the month prior to the survey 17.4 % of respondents reported use of one or more of marijuana, cocaine, crack, LSD, glue, or gasoline (13).

Nutrition

Data from Nutrition Canada from 1972 indicate that Aboriginal peoples were at high risk for deficiency of nutrients such as iron, vitamins, and protein (14). Prevalence of obesity is marked in females aged 30 and over (more than 70%), and about 40% of males aged 40 and over are obese. Overall physical activity levels among Aboriginal peoples is low, although not dissimilar to that for the general Canadian population.

Sexual Practices

According to the Ontario First Nations Healthy Lifestyle Survey (13), knowledge about AIDS was consistently high among on-reserve Aboriginal peoples, although there were reported deficits in knowledge among the older members of the communities, some of whom practise high-risk behaviour. In this study, two out of every five males and one out of every five females reported multiple sexual partners in the 12 months prior to the survey; 15.4% of respondents reported having sexual partners both within and outside the community; 56.9 % of respondents reported having unprotected sexual intercourse at least some of the time, and only 13.3% of respondents reported protected intercourse only. About two thirds of Aboriginal women surveyed by the Aboriginal Nurses Association of Canada indicated that they did not use condoms (15). A relationship with a steady sex partner was the most common reason for not using a condom at any age, and younger respondents were more likely to be influenced by a partner and the availability of a condom than older respondents.

1.1.4. Health Care Organizations

The federal government is responsible for the health care of Aboriginal peoples on reserves, and the provincial government for those off the reserves. Two thirds of Aboriginal peoples live in rural or remote areas, and health care services, which are less than optimal, are provided by nurses or community health workers supplemented by infrequent visits from physicians. Admission rates for general and mental hospitals, usually located at great distances from the communities themselves, are high compared with other Canadian rates (16). With the exception of immunization, public health programs and rehabilitation services are poor. Nurses working directly on Aboriginal reserves or, by agreement with Band councils, provide some community health care services. Some bands operate their own services and, in a few places, provincial health units provide services under contract (17). Geographic isolation also makes it difficult to provide appropriate services to northern communities. The priorities set by Aboriginal people are frequently at variance from those developed by the government, and hence there are inappropriate strategies for delivering health programs. However, in recent years, many of Aboriginal communities have assumed the administration and management of health care in their own communities.

1.2. HEALTH STATUS AND CONSEQUENCES

1.2.1. Mortality

In the past 10 to 20 years, there has been a substantial decline in Aboriginal mortality; however, the gap in mortality between the Aboriginal and general Canadian population remains wide. Between 1979 and 1993 the overall Aboriginal mortality rate declined by 21.4% from 7.0 deaths per 1,000 to 5.5 deaths per 1,000. This gain has remained fairly constant since the early 1980s. Due to the high proportion of Aboriginal young people, age-standardized death rates are more useful for comparison purposes. In 1993, the Aboriginal mortality rate, standardized to the 1991 Canadian population, was 10.8 per 1,000 (1.6 times the Canadian rate of 6.9).

Infant Mortality

In 1993, the average Aboriginal infant mortality rate was 10.9 per 1,000, compared with 6.3 per 1,000 Canadian average, which represents a 16.7 % decrease in Aboriginal infant mortality between 1979 and 1993 compared with a 4.6 % decrease during the same period for the Canadian average.

Age-Specific Death Rates

As seen in Figure 6.1, age-specific Aboriginal death rates were much higher than the Canadian rates, except among those aged 80 and over.

Causes of Death

Between 1979 and 1993, the four leading causes of death in order of decreasing frequency were unchanged: injury and poisoning, diseases of the circulatory system, neoplasm (cancer), and diseases of the respiratory system. For Canada as a whole, the four leading causes of death were circulatory diseases, neoplasm, injuries and poisoning, and respiratory diseases. Although there has been a 36.6% improvement in mortality rates from injury and poisoning, the age-standardized death rate for that category remains four times higher in Aboriginal people. The overall risk of suicide among Aboriginal people is about 2.5 times that of the general population (18), while the rate for

Figure 6.1:   Age-Specific Indian Death Rates as a Percentage of Canadian, 1989-1993.

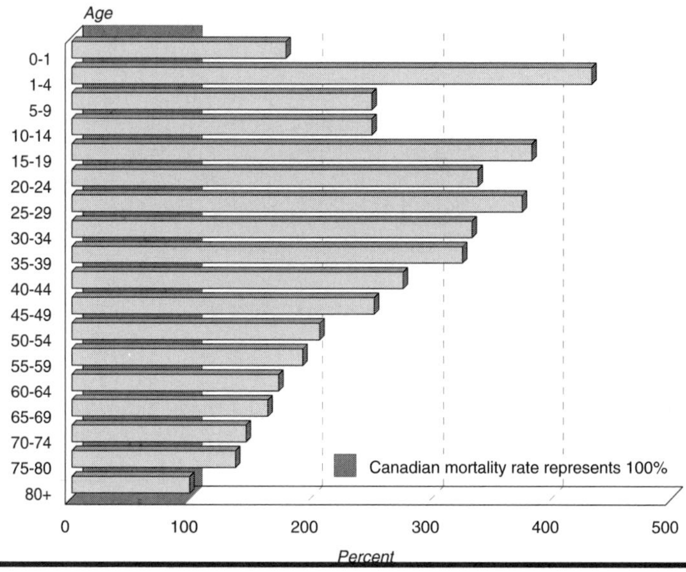

Source: Adapted from Trends in First Nations Mortality.

Aboriginal people aged 15 to 24 was up to eight times higher than that of other Canadian youth. The differences between Canadian and Aboriginal suicide rates disappear with age, and, among those aged 65 and over, the Canadian rate exceeds that of the Aboriginal population. The Aboriginal death rates due to circulatory diseases do not differ much from Canadians overall, especially for those over age 65, although the cardiovascular mortality rate has been declining more slowly than that of Canadians overall and now slightly exceeds the national average.

Potential-Years-of-Life-Lost (PYLL)

In 1993, the PYLL among Aboriginal people was approximately 46,037, of which 25,031 were contributed by males. The ratio of the Aboriginal PYLL to the Canadian PYLL was two times higher. The main causes were injury and poisoning, ill-defined symptoms (mainly due to sudden infant death syndrome), congenital anomalies, and perinatal conditions.

1.2.2. Morbidity
Infectious Diseases

Among Aboriginal people there is a high incidence of gastroenteritis, diphtheria, rheumatic fever, respiratory problems, and infectious hepatitis. Data from the Pacific region indicated that in 1983 to 1984 infectious and parasitic diseases were responsible for 3.4% of all Aboriginal hospitalization and 10.2% of hospitalization of infants under age one year. Botulism, sometimes fatal, occurs in Aboriginal (and more frequently, Inuit) communities due to ingestion of fermented marine mammal meat, raw or parboiled fish, or salmon eggs. The incidence of meningitis among Aboriginal peoples and Inuit under age eight years in the Northwest Territories is 7%, 200 times that of the general population (19); however, it is declining due to widespread use of Haemophilus influenzae type b vaccine. The incidence of pneumonia among Aboriginal children is about 8.3 times higher than the general population (20). It is difficult to estimate the prevalence of HIV-infected Aboriginal people; as of September 1996, Health Canada reported 210 Aboriginal AIDS cases, a number that has grown from 25 in 1992 (21).

Chronic Conditions

Among the Aboriginal population aged 15 and over, 31% were told by their health care provider that they had a chronic health problem, specifically, in order of frequency, arthritis and rheumatism, high blood pressure, bronchitis, heart problems, diabetes, asthma, and tuberculosis (22). Chronic conditions among Aboriginal children were primarily chronic otitis media and psychomotor developmental delay. The incidence rates of all these conditions far exceeded the Canadian norms. The presence of diabetes was reported by 6% of Aboriginal adults, compared with 2% of Canadian adults aged 15 and over, and while the average age of onset is about 43 years, onset is occurring earlier. Heredity, obesity, lack of physical activity, and poor diet, which vary from one age group to another, influence the prevalence of diabetes. Both new and reactivated tuberculosis is also of concern; rates for all age groups far exceed the Canadian average. The rate among Status Indians in 1994 was 47 cases per 100,000 persons, compared to the rate of 7 per 100,000 for total Canadian population (23). Other indicators, such as dental caries and nutritional disorders, are also higher than in the general population.

Disability

In 1991, disability rates among Aboriginal people aged 15 and over were high compared with the total Canadian population: 31.4% versus 12.6% (24). Compared to women, men had lower rates (29.6% versus 32.8%). Disability rates increased with the age: rates for those aged 15 to 24, 25 to 34, 35 to 54, and over age 55 were 21.7%, 23.6%, 35.5%, and 66.5%, respectively — almost two to three times higher than those for the total Canadian population. In northwestern Ontario, the disability rate was found to be 13.3% among Aboriginal children under age 14, almost double the corresponding rates for the rest of the Canadian population (25). The major disabilities for people age 15 and over were in the areas of mobility, agility, and hearing.

1.3. FUTURE DIRECTIONS

Aboriginal health is likely to continue to improve if appropriate attention is paid to the determinants of health. Misinterpretation of the Aboriginal peoples' active struggle against colonization has led to the paternalistic imposition of ineffective public health interventions, coupled with a lack of comprehension of the measures that could well improve Aboriginal health. Waldram et al. (26) advise that five basic areas must be addressed, namely health research, a greater sensitivity to Aboriginal culture, a continuing process of control of health service transfer to the communities, increased opportunities for Aboriginal peoples' success in various health care professions, and an overall improvement in the socioeconomic status of Aboriginal Canadians. To achieve this end, several efforts are currently underway to establish areas of Aboriginal self-government, and the federal government is transferring control of health care services to the local level of Aboriginal government or band councils. Ultimately, self-determination remains the best hope for improving Aboriginal peoples' health.

In 1996, the Royal Commission on Aboriginal Peoples delivered the most comprehensive report on all aspects of the Aboriginal peoples' life, including their health, and made over 400 recommendations (7). It called for a partnership based on the principles of mutual respect, recognition, responsibility, and sharing. The federal government responded in January 1998 (27), stating four objectives: to renew the partnerships, to strengthen Aboriginal governance, to develop a new fiscal relationship, and to support strong communities, people, and economies. To underscore this commitment, it pledged $350 million to support the development of community-based healing for "the legacy" of the residential school. In March 1998, the Aboriginal Healing Foundation was established. It is a non-profit corporation, independent of both government and the representative Aboriginal political organizations, created to address the healing needs of all Aboriginal peoples. This may well prove to be the turning point in Canadian history.

2. THE HEALTH OF SENIORS

Seniors are a heterogeneous group, each generation having a different social history. However, for the purpose of comparison, numbers of seniors is divided into three sub-groups, 65 to 74 years, 75 to 84, and 85 and over; these sub-groups are also referred to as the young elderly, middle elderly, and old elderly. The number of seniors and their proportion in the population of Canada continue to grow, particularly the number of the old elderly.

This section identifies some characteristics relevant to the health of seniors. Many stereotypical notions about seniors and the so-called limitations of advanced age need to be abandoned. For example, even though disability increases with age, aging and poor health are not synonymous.

Aging is a lifelong process, encompassing a series of transitions from birth to death. Reaching the age of 65 does not therefore herald old age. Although functional disability appears to accompany aging, it is not clear how much is intrinsic to the aging process or whether death is always the result of a disease process. This is the prevalent biomedical model. The degree of handicap also depends on society's response. Successful aging has been defined in terms of retaining the ability to function independently, remaining mobile, and undertaking all the activities of daily living (e.g., dressing, bathing, using stairs, getting in and out of bed, eating). In addition to age itself and measures of physical and mental health status, two major social predictors of successful aging have been identified: not having one's spouse die and not entering a nursing home. These indicate the interaction of biological and psychosocial factors (28).

There is controversy about the biological process of aging. On one hand, the organism can be viewed as having a preprogrammed life span after which natural death occurs (due possibly to a general decline in withstanding external stressors). As increasing proportions of the population age to the natural limit of about 85, survival tends to "rectangularize" the mortality curve. The onset of chronic disease may be postponed (29, 30), thus compressing the period of disability, a concept known as "compressed disability" (31). On the other hand, it is argued that life expectancies can increase almost indefinitely. Some studies (32, 33) suggest that the average period of decreased vigour will probably increase if life expectancy increases indefinitely, and that chronic diseases will occupy a large proportion of the life span. There may be a biological basis for the female health advantage related to the genes in the X chromosome that surpasses lifestyle and environmental influences (34).

2.1. DETERMINANTS

2.1.1. Psychosocial Environment

Demography

Information in this and the next section is derived from the 1996 census (35), the *Report on the Health of Canadians* (36), and *The Active Health Report on Seniors* (37).

On May 14, 1996, there were 3.5 million Canadians over the age of 65 years constituting approximately 12.2% of the population — 2,040,000 women and 1,487,000 men. It is estimated that by 2021, there will be 7.5 million seniors, more than 15% of the population. This increase is attributed to an increase in average life expectancy, the aging of the baby boomers, and the projected decline in fertility (38). Older Canadians are more likely to be of British origin (55% of those over 80 are of British origin compared with 39% under 65). A sizeable proportion (11%), however, speak neither English nor French at home.

Another striking trend is the expanding population of senior women, particularly among those aged 80 and over. There were 787,00 people in that age group in 1996, a 19.3% increase from 1991 census and over twice the level of 25 years ago. In 1996, two thirds of people aged 80 years and over were women. The female proportion of the population over age 65 has increased from 49% in 1951 to 57% in 1991 and will likely be approximately 60% in 2001, due to the increased longevity of women on average and the gain in female life expectancy relative to males. Approximately 57.4% of senior women were single, whereas 77% of senior men were married. Widows constitute 50% of the senior female population, whereas widowers are only 13% of senior men. Widows account for a greater proportion because women tend to marry older males and then outlive them.

Income

Seniors' incomes have increased substantially over the last few years, narrowing the gap between seniors and the rest of the population. In 1980, 34% of seniors met the criteria for poverty, compared to 21% in 1992 (36). This number increased slightly to 22% in 1993, when seniors were still more likely to have lower incomes than any other age group. Interestingly, 51% of unattached senior individuals fell below the poverty line, while only 8% of those in families did. Currently, seniors depend heavily on public pension and income security plans (particularly security plans), which comprise their single largest source of income. However, because 64% of seniors own their own home, frequently mortgage-free, income is not the only relevant indicator of socioeconomic status for the elderly.

Living Situation

Seniors may be stereotyped as being passive and dependent; however, the majority are "well elderly" who remain healthy into their 80s or even 90s, needing only minimal assistance. Many seniors are active and contribute to the community. For example, 15% of seniors provide baby-sitting services to friends and family, and 80% of women over 80 and 50% of men do their own housework. Although spouses are the main source of assistance for people aged 65 and over, the fact that men tend to predecease their wives has led to a difference in assistance provision. It appears that more widows turn to others, making for a higher reliance of senior women on friends and neighbours, while senior men tend to rely most on spouses. Daughters are the main source of assistance for people aged 80 or over (37%), and grandchildren also play an increasing role. Living situations range from full independence in the community, to community living and support from family and community services, to long-term institutionalization (38).

For the demographic reasons cited above, the living situation of senior women, 34% of whom live alone, frequently differs from men, 14% of whom live alone. Surveys show that, above all else, seniors value independence and fear admission to a nursing home. In 1988, the National Advisory Council on Aging identified the barriers to independent living as follows: physical health (71%), mental health/emotional well-being (52%), transportation and mobility (50%), lack of adequate community-based support services (48%), safety and security (44%), housing (43%), and inadequate communication/information (43%) (39). The average age for entry into long-term care institutions is 82 in Canada, but there is a tendency for over-institutionalization. Eight per cent of senior Canadians live in institutions, where some custody or care is provided, compared with 5% in the U.S. The proportion of seniors in institutions is actually higher due to the seniors occupying acute hospital beds while awaiting transfer to long-term care facilities.

Elder Abuse

Elder abuse can encompass physical, psychosocial, and financial abuse or neglect (see also Chapter Four) (40). A 1989 survey found that 4% of community-dwelling seniors had experienced some form of abuse within the preceding 12 months (41). The most common form was financial or material, experienced by 2.5%, usually perpetrated by a neighbour, friend, or acquaintance, followed by a son or daughter or a more distant relative. The next common forms were chronic verbal abuse (1.4%) and physical abuse (0.5%), both usually perpetrated by the spouse. Accurate estimates of the prevalence of elder abuse within institutions are not available. Abuse within institutions can include the inappropriate or excessive use of physical or chemical restraints, such as restrictive "gerry chairs", bed railings, or sedatives. Strategies to combat elder abuse are aimed at increasing public awareness, enhancing the training and working conditions of those employed at institutions, providing support services for abusers, further research, and prevention by fostering independence for seniors through adequate housing and income.

2.1.2. Physical Environment

With advancing age there is less ability to tolerate hazards in the physical environment, which may be exacerbated by wandering and forgetfulness associated with dementia. There is also increasing prevalence of visual, auditory, and locomotive disability, predisposing seniors to possibly serious falls, and gait disorders may result in also falls and subsequent injury. In fact, falls in the elderly are a threat to health. Approximately 800 male and 1,100 female over age 65 die every year in Canada as a direct or indirect result of falling (42). While many falls among seniors are due to intrinsic changes such as decreasing visual acuity and osteoporosis, they are also caused by preventable extrinsic factors such as poor lighting and loose rugs (43). In elderly women, the most common injury is a fracture of the neck of the femur.

Motor vehicle crashes are another cause of mortality and morbidity among seniors. Deteriorating visual acuity and contraction of the visual field are among the principle contributing factors. Many provinces require mandatory vision and written tests every one to two years for all drivers aged 80 and over, and physicians and optometrists are required to report people with conditions that may make driving dangerous. However, concerns over road safety must be weighed against the desire to maintain the mobility of seniors. Driving provides a sense of personal control, can allow timely access to means of ensuring well-being, and can reduce social isolation in municipalities with limited public transit systems.

2.1.3. Lifestyle and Behavioural Risk Factors

Alcohol, Smoking, and Drug Use

In 1994/95, 56% of men and 36% of women aged 65 to 74, as well as 45% of men and 23% of women aged 75 and over, consumed one or more drinks of alcohol per month, compared to 55% of all Canadians over age 12 (36). More seniors (15%) drank daily, as compared to 11% of those aged 45 to 64 and 4% of those aged 25 to 44. There was no appreciable difference between seniors and other adult age groups in the percentage (4-7%) who drank four to six times per week. While 50% of all drinkers had consumed five or more drinks on one occasion in the previous year, only 19% of those over 65 had done so. The National Alcohol and Other Drugs Survey in 1989 found the average drinker consumed 2.8 drinks per occasion, while the average senior consumed 1.7 (44). Seniors were, however, most likely to be former smokers, including 46% of those aged 65-74 and 43% of those 75 and over, yielding a quit rate of 72% for those aged 65 and over.

Prescription drug use is much more common among seniors than among younger Canadians. According to Bergob (45), 18% of senior women and 14% of senior men had taken three or more prescription drugs within the month prior to the survey. Senior men were less likely than senior women to be taking multiple prescription drugs. Heart and blood pressure medications were most common, followed next by prescription pain relievers, and then stomach remedies or laxatives. About half the seniors surveyed had taken a pain reliever, either prescription or non-prescription medications, within the month prior to the survey, making this the most commonly used class of medication overall. Twelve per cent of seniors use tranquillizers and 21% use sleeping pills, a greater percentage than younger Canadians (44); women aged 65 and over were more than twice as likely then men to have used tranquillizers in the month prior to the survey. Individuals over age 75 have a high rate of hospitalization due to drug psychosis (9.7 per 100,000), poisoning due to analgesics, antipyretics, and antirheumatics (10.2 per 100,000), and sedatives and hypnotics (7.0 per 100,000). Doses of medication not geared to seniors can result in adverse drug effects, which are responsible for a significant proportion of hospitalizations.

Nutrition

A review of recent surveys concluded that 10-28% of elderly Canadians were at risk for deficiencies of calcium, beta-carotene, and vitamins A, C, and D (46). Protein, zinc, iron, and vitamin B6 were also frequently deficient. Based on light activity requirements and basal metabolic rates in a 1990 Quebec survey, senior females consumed only 77% of predicted energy requirements, while senior males consumed 92%; 55% of senior males, and 53% of senior females consumed more than 30% of their energy requirements as fat, the level recommended by Canada's Food Guide to Healthy Eating. Both senior men and women were deficient in calcium, and senior women were also mildly deficient in folate. Considering food intake alone, no other micronutrient deficiencies were identified.

Exercise and Other Activities

Many able-bodied seniors exercise regularly; this proportion increased from 50% to 60% between 1976 and 1981. In 1994/95, 17% of seniors aged 65 to 74 described themselves as "active", and 22% stated they were "moderately active" (36). Among those 75 and older, 12% identified themselves as "active" and 16% reported moderate physical activity. In the period of a month, over 50% of those aged 65 or more travelled outside their neighbourhood, attended entertainments, or participated in group activities.

2.2. HEALTH STATUS AND CONSEQUENCES

2.2.1. Mortality

From 1964 to 1993, mortality rates among seniors steadily decreased 0.5% per decade, particularly among women (47). The trend for women may have been due to a decline in infectious disease and cardiovascular mortality (48). However, for males, the negative impact of lifestyle behaviours may have outweighed the decline in infectious disease mortality. Common causes of death among seniors is shown in Figure 5.3, in Chapter Five.

2.2.2. Morbidity

In 1991, the Canadian Study of Health and Aging identified a prevalence of dementia of 8.0% — approximately a quarter of a million (252,500) Canadians — with rates similar across 36 Canadian cities (49, 50). The prevalence increased sharply with age: 2.4% of those aged 65 to 74 had dementia, 11.1% of those aged 75 to 84, and 34.5% of those aged 85 and over. About half these people lived in institutions, and approximately two thirds of these cases were due to Alzheimer's disease. Alzheimer's disease caused dementia in more women (69%) than men (53%), and whose dementia was more likely to have a vascular cause (30% versus 14% for women). Women with dementia were also more likely to be institutionalized, attributable to the fact that they are less likely to have a spouse to care for them at home.

The annual net cost of dementia in Canada has been estimated at over $3.9 billion, $2.18 billion of which goes towards long-term institutionalization (51). The burden on society is not strictly economic, however. Of those with dementia living in the community, 92% have either a family member, relative, or friend as an unpaid care giver (49). These care givers rarely have access to community support services, and are more vulnerable to chronic health problems and depressive symptoms than are those caring for the non-demented elderly.

2.2.3. Consequence

Disability

The 1994/95 National Population Health Survey reported that 19% of those aged 65 to 74 and 35% of those aged 75 and over had functional status score of less than optimal daily functioning due to health limitations; and 28% of those aged 65 to 74 and 36% of those 75 and over reported long-term activity limitation at home (36). The primary conditions responsible for activity limitation in seniors were arthritis, heart problems, central nervous system problems such as vision or hearing loss, back problems, limb problems, and respiratory or digestive problems. Annual disability days for those aged 65 to 74 were 32.0 for men and 37.7 for women, while for those 75 and over they were 36.7 for men and 49.9 for women. Disability rates are also listed in Table 5.5 in Chapter Five.

Dental Health

Approximately half of Canadians aged 65 and over retain none of their natural teeth (36), and in 1990 approximately 77% of seniors had not seen a dentist in the preceding year (52). In Ontario, 48% of the edentulous (toothless) and 15% of those with teeth reported a limited ability to chew. The dental health of seniors living in institutions was poorer; 25% of those in collective living centres required dental treatment urgently and 75% required preventive dental services. Almost 30% of seniors (the proportion increasing with age) reported that because of dental problems they avoid eating with other people, avoid laughing or smiling, are embarrassed with the appearance of their teeth or condition of their mouth, or avoid conversation with others (53). Low income was associated with edentulousness and with less likelihood of having visited a dentist within the previous year.

2.2.4. Health-Care Utilization

Hospitalization

Between 1974 and 1993, the five leading causes of hospitalization for Canadian males aged 65 and over were coronary heart disease, stroke, system-related symptoms (e.g., abdominal pain), chronic obstructive lung diseases, and accidental falls (47). For females, they were coronary heart disease, accidental falls, system-related symptoms, stroke, and fracture of the lower limb.

Hospital use rises dramatically with age. The old elderly use approximately 10 times more hospital days than any other age group under 60 (54). Seniors make only 1.7 more physician visits per year than those aged 25 to 44 and only 0.9 more visits than those aged 45 to 64. An analysis of hospital use in Manitoba showed that 42% of seniors were never admitted to hospital; however, 2% of the senior population used 20% of total hospital days, with most of this being in the last year prior to death. Ontario data show that from 1982 to 1983, seniors constituted 10% of the population and consumed 40% of acute care hospital days (55). In 1994/95, men and women aged 65 to 74 who were admitted to hospital had an average length of stay of 14 and 16 days respectively, which increased to 21 and 29 for those aged 75 and over, compared to 8 and 5 days for men and women aged 25 to 44 (36). Per capita health expenditures in Canada for senior males and females in 1994 were $7,879 and $8,206, compared with an average for all age groups (males, $2,228 and females, $2,722).

The elderly are the major consumers of home care services, with 6% of those aged 65 to 74 and 18% of those aged 75 and over using some form of home care at least once in 1994/95, compared to only 1-2% of the younger population (36).

2.3. FUTURE DIRECTIONS

Most jurisdictions in Canada have recognized the need for improved geriatric services. Many have planned for the expected increase in the number of seniors by increasing funding for gerontology programs, and some are considering innovative ways of program delivery, which are discussed in Chapter 17. Health promotion for seniors is becoming an important approach to the development and maintenance of optimum levels of functioning as aging occurs. These approaches may incorporate physical activity, social support, awareness of adverse drug response, nutrition counselling, and programs to prevent falls. Future cohorts of seniors will not be the same as current ones, as they will be better prepared for retirement. They will also depend less on government transfer support, thanks to private pension plans and the increase in the number of women entering the work force.

3. THE HEALTH OF CHILDREN LIVING IN POVERTY

Over the last two decades, the proportion of Canada's youth who live below the poverty line has increased dramatically. Canada has no official poverty line. However, Statistics Canada uses a low income cut-off (LICO) to identify those who are "substantially worse off than the average"; a family at or below the LICO is one that spends 56.2% or more of its gross income on food, shelter, and clothing. In 1981, 12% of Canadians less than 18 years of age were living in poverty. This increased to 16% by 1987, to 18% by 1991, and to 20.5% by 1995 (56, 57).

3.1. DETERMINANTS

3.1.1. Psychosocial Environment

Poverty disproportionately affects the children whose parents are young, single, and female and of a lower level of education. In 1991, 43% of young families lived in poverty, compared to 15.6% of all families. The rate of poverty among families with children under age seven was as follows: 81% for single-mother families, 100% for families of single mothers who have never been married, 38% for single-father families, and 13% for the families of couples (58). Single-mother families also suffer the most severe degrees of poverty: their household income was on average 59.6% of the poverty line in 1991. Data from 1995 indicate that the poverty rate for single-mother families in which the mother is under age 25 is 83% (57). Poverty rates in children under age seven in Canada in 1991, listed by the level of education of the family head, are as follows: 37% for those with less than high school completion, 22% for high school graduates, and 11% for the graduates of post-secondary school. Employment status is not always predictive for family poverty, as the employment rates are similar for poor and non-poor families (58).

Aboriginal populations experience some of the highest rates of poverty and ill health of any group in Canada. Child-poverty issues are no exception to this. The potential impact of high child-poverty rates in this group is significant when considering that they are a young population.

Immigrant families have always had higher rates of poverty than those of the general Canadian population. In 1995, 20.3% of families with a foreign-born household head were living below the poverty line, compared to 12.9% for those with a Canadian-born family head (57). Immigrants make up a substantial proportion of families with young children within Canadian society.

Among the industrialized countries Canada's overall poverty rate is now second only to that of the United States (59). A report published in 1994 by the Canadian Institute of Child Health indicated that Canada's rate of poverty for families with children is 15.7%, compared to 23% in U.S., 7.3% in the Netherlands, and 5.1% in Sweden (58).

Child-poverty rates in Canada vary considerably among the provinces. In 1995 the prevalence of poverty for families with children of all ages ranged from 9.3% in Prince Edward Island to 19.2% in Newfoundland (57). The nature of communities affects child poverty rates. In general, larger, more populous communities have more poverty. According to 1991 Canadian data, on average the poverty rate for children under age seven increases with community size, from 14% for populations less than 2,500 to 25% for cities with populations of 500,000 or more (60). Thus child poverty is a more pressing issue for large cities.

3.1.2. Physical Environment

Poor children often live in social and low-rent housing located very close to industrial areas. Housing is often inadequate due to chronic poor maintenance and faulty design. This leads to a variety of indoor air-quality hazards including mould growth or the presence of toxic substances such as lead paint or asbestos. Poor housing conditions create chronic cockroach problems, increasing antigen exposure and the possibility of ongoing exposure to pesticide residues. Urban poor children may have higher exposures to benzene, a known carcinogen, from automobile traffic, tobacco smoke, or industrial activity. In fact, streets with heavy traffic, where poor children often live and play, have been shown to be correlated with benzene exposure (61).

3.1.3. Lifestyle and Behavioural Risk Factors

Children who live in poverty are more likely to adopt behaviours that are a risk to their health and that put their social and future economic well-being in jeopardy. Considering the relationship between health and income, poor academic performance or dysfunctional social behaviour can ultimately threaten the well-being of impoverished children.

Risk behaviours are more prevalent among poor children. In 1990, among Ontarian children under age 15, 48.9% of poor children smoked, compared to 20.7% of well-off children, and 46% of sexually active adolescents from low-income families reported never using a condom, versus 32% of those of high-income families (58).

Parental depression and family dysfunction have important effects on the development of children. When parents have difficulty coping with life, work, family, or parenting, they may be unable to provide their children with the necessary emotional, social, and physical support. A poorly functioning family deprives children of a supportive home atmosphere and positive relationship. Data from the 1994 National Longitudinal Survey of Children and Youth show that nearly 20% of children in low-income families lived with a parent who had depressive tendencies, compared with less than 5% of children in high-income families (62). Similarly, one in seven children from low-income households lived within two-parent dysfunctional families, compared with 1 in 20 children from high-income families.

3.1.4. Health Care Utilization

Lower consumption of medical care may also contribute significantly to the negative impact of poverty on health. Canadian studies have shown conflicting results on this issue because of differing definitions of benefits and services, differing population units (families compared with per capita), and lack of controls for confounding factors such as age and sex (63). Per capita costs of medical services in Ontario did not vary significantly with income. Low-income families had a greater number of physician visits, but less costly services were provided per visit, and a greater proportion of visits were hospital rather than office-based. With regard to children, except for the lowest income group, benefits and average cost of services increased with increasing income. Rates of health care system utilization are higher among poor children than those who are better off. In Ontario in 1990, 14% of children up to age 19 on family benefits had been admitted to hospital in the preceding year, compared to 8% of those not on family benefits, and 35% of those on family benefits had visited an emergency department in the preceding year (versus 27% of children without benefits) and 33% have at least one chronic health problem (versus 26% of children without benefits) (58). Poor children also have less access to dental care than those children from more affluent families; according to the National Longitudinal Survey 56% of poor children under age 12 did not visit a dentist in 1993, compared to 37% of children in non-poor families.

3.2. HEALTH STATUS AND CONSEQUENCES

3.2.1. Mortality

As in the case of adult poverty, the association between childhood poverty and increased disease and death has been well documented. The following sections rely on data from four major studies: Wigle and Mao (64) (for 1971 data), Dougherty (65) (1981), Wilkins (66, 67), and a report published by the Canadian Institute of Child Health. In these studies, data from Canadian urban census tracts were grouped according to median household income. Income levels were divided into quintiles, level 1 being the highest and level 5 the lowest. Mortality rates were compared among these quintiles.

Infant Mortality

In Canada in 1986, the infant mortality rate in families of the poorest quintile was double that of the richest quintile (68). The effects of poverty on mortality begin before birth and may predate conception. Low birth weight (LBW) (less than 2,500 grams) is the single most important cause of infant mortality, especially in the neonatal period (0 to 28 days), and is strongly associated with poverty. Infants with low birth weight account for 75% of all deaths within the first year of life (69). LBW children also have higher rates of physiologically and intellectually delayed development: 31% have delayed development before age three years, compared to 13.5% of those with normal birth weight (56). Furthermore, LBW infants born to low-income families in Canada fare much worse than do infants of similar weight born to higher income families (70). The rate of LBW infants is an important population health indicator that links family poverty with poor infant and child health and increased early mortality (71). In Canada in 1995, 5.8% of all live-born children were of low birth (72), whereas the LBW rate was 6.5% for infants with family incomes under $30,000 and 4.2% for those with incomes over $60,000.

In Canada, the death rate for infants younger than 28 days was 1.5 times greater in the poorest quintile than in the richest quintile, and the death rate for infants aged 28 days to 1 year was over twice as high in the poorest quintile than the richest quintile. The mortality rate for children in families with the lowest income level was higher for all major causes of death in infancy, including pneumonia, respiratory distress syndrome, immaturity, difficult labour/birth injury, and congenital anomalies of the nervous system and circulatory system. In 1986, it was estimated that at birth, males born into the highest income group have a life expectancy 5.6 years longer than those in the lowest income group, and affluent females have a 1.8-year longer life expectancy than poor females.

Overall mortality was higher in 1971 and 1986 for poor children than for those who are not poor. Total mortality in boys aged 1 to 14 years was 2.0 times higher in the lowest income level than in the highest. The mortality rate for girls who were poor was 1.5 times higher in both 1971 and 1986.

Poverty has a marked impact on the health of Aboriginals and their children. Death rates from accidents, suicide, homicide, cancer, and infections are higher among poor children.

3.2.2. Morbidity

General measures of health status are usually directly related to social class: the higher the social class of the children, the better their health is. The U.S. National Health Interview Survey found that low-income children had lower parental ratings of general health and slightly more restricted activity days, more bed disability days, and a higher rate of school absenteeism (73). The Ontario Child Health Study found that the prevalence rates of chronic health problems per 1,000 children who were below the poverty line was 237, compared with 183 per 1,000 children above the poverty line (74).

Mental Health

A landmark study, the 1989 Ontario Child Health Study (75), provides a good insight on the effect of poverty on the mental health of children. The study was a cross-sectional, province-wide survey of the mental and physical health of a randomly selected sample of more than 3,000 children aged 4 to 16 years.

For children living on social assistance, compared with those not on social assistance, the risk of developing a psychiatric disorder was 2.8 times higher (31.2% compared with 18.8%). Similarly, the risk for children living in one-parent families was 1.7 times higher (21.7% compared with 14.2%) than for two-parent families; for children living in subsidized housing, the risk was 2.6 times higher than those in non-subsidized housing (30.4% compared with 14.2%).

The National Longitudinal Survey of Children and Youth, currently being done by Statistics Canada, has found that 7.0% of very poor children have impairment in social relationship, compared to 1.9% of those who are well off (56). Children of low socioeconomic status also have higher mean aggression scores than do children of high socioeconomic status (56). The study done by Lipman et al. of data from the Ontario Child Health Study found that children of low-income families were 2.5 times mores likely to have poor school performance, and 3.4 times more likely to have social impairment (76). Adolescent crime has been found to be associated with child poverty (62).

Academic performance tends to be compromised among poor children. The school dropout rate for 16- to 17-year-olds in Canada in 1991 was 12.9% for those of poor families and 5.1% for those whose families were better off (58).

Nutrition

Low-income children are at greater risk for nutritional disorders. Poor children are more likely to develop iron-deficiency anaemia. Iron-deficiency anaemia was found in 25% of 218 infants aged 10 to 14 months whose mothers lived in the five poorest districts of Montreal (77). Low-income mothers tend to discontinue breast-feeding early and switch to using cow's milk (which is known to cause occult intestinal bleeding and possibly contribute to iron-deficiency anaemia in infants). A follow-up evaluation of infants whose iron status and treatment were known demonstrated lowered scores on mental and developmental tests at five years of age, raising the issue of whether iron-deficiency anaemia, even if treated, causes irreversible defects (78).

Dental Health

Two surveys of randomly selected 13- and 14-year-olds in Alberta (79) and Quebec (80) found that dental caries, as measured by the decayed/missing/filled teeth (DMFT) index, varied inversely with social class. The ratio of filled teeth to the DMFT index, which reflects the amount of dental care received, was directly related to social class. The social class gradient was largest in Quebec, with an F/DMFT ratio of 65.1% for the highest socioeconomic group and only 17.4% for the lowest.

3.2.3. Disability

The rate of childhood disability in 1986 was more than twice as high among children from poor families compared with affluent ones. Seven per cent of children from the poorest quintile had some degree of disability, compared with 3.5% from the richest. The differences between income quintiles were even more pronounced when only severe disability was considered, in which case the rate was 2.7 times higher among the poor compared with the rich.

3.2.4. Illness and Well-being in Later Life

Some researchers propose the idea that an impoverished early childhood results in developmental changes that determine one's health and well-being throughout life. "Programming" and " latency" are terms that have been used to describe this concept (81-83). In essence they state that those who experience inadequate nurturing and stimulation in the earliest years of life (0 to 6 years of age, and under 3 years in particular) will suffer higher rates of ill health and poor intellectual, social, and economic performance through their entire lives. This effect is proposed as being independent of their socioeconomic status in later life.

Birth weight, as indicated above, is closely linked with socioeconomic status. A number of ecological studies from the Environmental Epidemiology Unit at Southampton, England (84), suggest that fetal and early childhood growth (reflected by birth weight and weight at one year of age) correlate with such adult conditions as coronary heart disease, stroke, hypertension, diabetes mellitus, chronic obstructive lung disease, ovarian cancer, suicide, autoimmune thyroiditis, abdominal obesity, atopy, and renal failure. The authors hypothesize metabolic or physiologic programming that occurs at critical periods of early development (84).

3.3. FUTURE DIRECTIONS

Government programs are an essential means of preventing child poverty in Canada. The federal government plays a critical role in the well-being of families and children, and the $6 billion reduction in federal transfer payments for social programs between 1995 and 1998 constitutes a major threat to the health and welfare of Canadian children, even though for many children even this assistance is inadequate.

The federal government recently pledged to increase spending on low-income families by $850 million, in keeping with the Canadian Council on Social Development's call for a more coordinated national child benefit system (85). Federal efforts to improve the unemployment rate, for example by extending job creation programs, are also expected to alleviate child poverty (85). A number of provincial governments, including Quebec, Saskatchewan, and British Columbia, have also taken action to improve the well-being of children (62).

The actions taken by both levels of governments have been critically appraised by interested organizations, which have in turn made recommendations for further interventions needed. For example, the National Forum on Health has called for societal resolutions that recognize the supreme value of children, and establish community supports for children and families in need (86). The provincial governments recently called upon the federal government to increase child benefit expenditures by $2.5 billion by the year 2000 (87). A federal-provincial government task force has recommended that high-quality child care be available 24 hours a day (88).

Governments at the federal and provincial levels have pledged to address the issue of child poverty directly even though many critics consider the government's financial commitment inadequate. Any such programs to improve the well-being of children must be part of a greater societal approach that includes strategies to promote economic growth in all areas of the country, reductions in unemployment, wage increases, accessible and affordable high-quality child care, and the removal of other barriers that prevent economically disadvantaged, vulnerable groups from gaining employment.

4.   THE HEALTH OF PEOPLE WITH DISABILITIES

4.1.   EXTENT AND TYPES OF DISABILITIES

As indicated in Chapter One, the World Health Organization defines disability as "any restriction or lack ... of ability to perform an activity in the manner or within the range considered normal for a human being". This definition applies to individuals whose conditions have existed for more than six months and whose limitations were not completely eliminated by the use of a technical aid. Disability is distinguished from impairment and handicap (see Chapter One). There are seven categories of disabilities (89):

- *Mobility*: limited ability to work, move from room to room, carry an object for 10 metres, or stand for long periods.
- *Agility*: limited ability to bend, dress or undress oneself, get in and out of bed, use fingers to grasp or handle objects, reach or cut one's own food.
- *Sight*: limited ability to read ordinary newsprint or see further than 4 metres even when wearing glasses.
- *Hearing*: limited ability to hear what is being said in a conversation with one other person or two or more people, even when wearing a hearing aid.
- *Speaking*: limited ability to speak and be understood.
- *Other*: limitations because of a learning disability, an emotional or psychiatric disability, or developmental delay.
- *Unknown*: unspecified nature of limitation.

Causes of Disability

There are a number of causes of disabilities, and age plays an important role in determining the cause. Among those aged 15 and older with disabilities, the most common disabilities were in mobility, agility, hearing, speaking, and seeing. The medical conditions that most frequently cause disability are diseases of the musculoskeletal system (connective tissue, arthritis, and rheumatism) and hearing disorders. Among children, the major causes were due to developmental delay, and hearing or vision problems. For individuals over 50 and those who are not institutionalized, a disease is reported as the most common cause of disability; however, those under 50 were usually born with their disability or cited accidents as the major cause of their disability.

Male respondents more than females reported that their disability was the result of a disease or accident. For example, in Ontario, 21% of males with disabilities cited accidents as a cause, compared with 14% of females; 36% of males cited disease as a cause, compared with 25% of females. Among those living in institutions, 45% reported disease as the main cause; for 30% aging or the effects of stroke were reported as the cause of their disability (90). Among those aged 15 to 34 living in institutions, mental retardation, diseases of the nervous system, and diseases of the sense organs were reported as the main causes of their disability. However, among those aged 55 years and over, diseases of the musculoskeletal system and connective tissue were cited as the main causes.

Approximately 4% (8,700) of children with disabilities between the ages of 5 and 14 had a diagnosis of cerebral palsy; 2,000 were diagnosed as having spinabifida, 3,400 as having muscular dystrophy, and approximately 35,500 had hearing impairments.

Disability Rate

Most of the statistical information in this section is derived from the Health and Activity Limitation Survey for Canada (HALS) (89, 91), the National Population Health Survey (NPHS) (36) and the Statistical Profile of Disabled Persons in Ontario (92).

In 1986, 3.3 million or 13.2% of Canadians had some level of disability. While this had grown to 15.5% of the population in 1991 (4.2 million), most of the increase was due to mild disability. One reason for this was a change in survey methodology, which incorporated more learning disabilities. An analysis of disability by sex and age is given in Table 5.5 in Chapter Five. As the rate of disability in the population increases with age, these data support the hypothesis that disability increases proportionally with age. The 1994 NPHS found that almost 5 million Canadians aged 12 and older reported a disability or handicap, or limitation on a continuing basis because of a health problem, but the methodology of that survey precludes comparison with previous figures. The disability rate for females in 1994 was 21%, slightly higher than the male rate of 20%. The higher female rate reflects the longer life span of women.

In 1991, 7% or 389,355 of children under age 15 years had disabilities. The majority of the disabilities for children of all ages were mild although long-term health conditions such as asthma and cerebral palsy were reported for more than half of the disabilities. Apart from these health conditions, speech difficulties were the most common disability in those under age 9 years, hearing difficulties the next most common and occurring slightly more frequently in the older age groups, and vision difficulties the least common sensory disability. Psychiatric conditions as a cause of disability were most frequent among those aged five to nine years.

4.1.1. Psychosocial Environment

Education

Disabled respondents to the HALS tended to have less formal education than those with no disabilities, as disabilities often interfered with their education. Among individuals with disabilities, those individuals with mild disabilities were more likely to have attained a higher level of education than those with moderate or severe disabilities. Nearly half (45%) of respondents with severe disabilities had eight years of education or less, compared with 25% of those who had mild disabilities, and 21% of respondents said that their education was interrupted for lengthy periods of time causing them to change schools or alter courses. Six per cent stated that they started school later than most children with no disabilities. The more severe the disability, the greater effect it had (e.g., in beginning school, changing schools, changing course of study). Of the children with disabilities between the ages of 5 and 14 years, almost 30% attended a special school or special classes within regular schools. Aboriginal people with disabilities aged 15 to 64 who resided off-reserve tended to have a higher level of education than their on-reserve counterparts. On the reserves, 65% reported having 0 to 8 years of education, 22% reported having some secondary education, and 13% reported having postsecondary education.

Income

Ontarians with disabilities from age 15 to 64 (inclusive) had gross incomes 46% lower than those without disabilities. However, the income of seniors with disabilities was only 18% lower than those of seniors without disabilities. Aboriginal adults with disabilities living on reserve tended to have lower incomes than either those living off-reserve or non-Aboriginal adults with no disabilities. The most common sources of additional income reported by people under age 65 with disabilities were the Canada Pension Plan (CPP) (45%) and workers' compensation (32%). For those over age 65 with disabilities, the veterans' disability pension provided 35% of their income, CPP provided 32%, and workers' compensation contributed 25%.

Of the 2.3 million people with disabilities aged 15 to 64 in Canada who were living in private households in 1989, 48% were employed, compared with 72.9% of people without disabilities. Of those working, over half reported a work limitation due to their disability.

Substance Abuse

It is sometimes assumed that adults with severe physical disabilities are susceptible to alcohol and drug abuse due to low self-esteem, social isolation, and other problems caused by their physical conditions. However, a recent survey of college students in wheelchairs found that the rate of alcohol and illicit drug use was similar to the general college population. Approximately 20% of students with disabilities are considered "problem users" of drugs and alcohol. Another survey administered to university students with disabilities found 40% drinking alcohol one or more times a week and 14% smoking marijuana one or more times a week. Again, however, these rates are similar to the general college population (93). As with young adults in general, drug usage among students with disabilities is correlated with a previous history of drug usage.

Nutrition

Children with disabilities are at risk for malnutrition, attributable either directly or indirectly to several factors: physical disability, cognitive delay, altered nutrient requirements caused by their medical condition, and drugs used to treat their medical condition. Children with severe developmental disabilities are significantly below their expected weight. Evers et al. (94) found that one third of children with disabilities were below the third percentile for weight, primarily the result of eating dysfunctions, which affect a notable portion.

4.1.2. Physical Environment

Nine per cent of women with disabilities and 6% of men with disabilities live in institutions. Of those living in the community, many report difficulty in moving outside of their neighbourhood, especially for long-distance travel, and 5% reported using special facilities such as access ramps where provided. Three quarters of women with slight to moderate disabilities were able to prepare meals for themselves, compared with only half of those with severe disabilities. In relation to personal care such as feeding, the proportion of people with severe disabilities requiring assistance was 24%, compared with 1% of those with mild disabilities.

4.2. HEALTH STATUS AND CONSEQUENCES

4.2.1. Morbidity

In 1986, 45% of the population with disabilities indicated that they had a mild disability, 32% a moderate disability, and 23% a severe disability. Slightly less than 66% cited restricted mobility as the most frequent disability, followed by limitations in agility. Aboriginal people also reported limited mobility as the most frequent disability. In the 1986 HALS, 43% of people between the ages of 15 to 34 with disabilities reported a mobility disability, compared with 75% of people 65 and over with disabilities; 18% (552,580 persons) of the population aged 15 years and older with disabilities reported a visual disability, and 973,830 individuals 15 and older reported a hearing disability. In the general Canadian population, 66% of people aged 15 and older with disabilities reported having more than one type, with the prevalence of multiple disabilities increasing with age. In addition, over 75% of off-reserve Aboriginal people with disabilities reported having only one or two disabilities, compared with about 65% of those living on-reserve.

4.3. FUTURE DIRECTIONS

As indicated in Chapter One, the impairments and handicaps related to disability are mediated by the social context of the person. Societal attitudes toward people with disabilities, and the degree of modification of the physical and psychosocial environment to accommodate them, have a great impact on their quality of life. There has been a consumer movement in recent years to enhance the quality of life of people with disabilities. An example of response has been the increased number of access ramps and toilet facilities for people with disabilities in public buildings. Some long-term care facilities have recognized that they are in fact "home" for their residents, with consequent changes in how they function as institutions. With the growth in the elderly segment of the general population and the survival of people who have been seriously injured and have major disabilities (particularly neurological damage), this movement will likely gain momentum in changing the sociopolitical context of disability and health organizations.

5. SUMMARY

This chapter examined the health of certain groups in the Canadian population in terms of the determinants of their health, health indicators, and consequences. The groups considered were Aboriginal peoples, seniors, poor children, and people with disabilities.

Aboriginal people include Status Indians, non-Status Indians, Mètis, and Inuit, although this chapter only discussed the health of Status and non-Status Indians. In 1996, there were 554,000 North American Indians in Canada, of which 35.0% were under age 14 years, 61.5% between ages of 15 and 64, and 3.5% aged 65 and over. The high proportion of young people in the Aboriginal populations is different from the Canadian population, and life expectancy for males is 67.0 years and for females 74.9 years, significantly shorter than for the general Canadian population.

Approximately 62% of Status Indians live on reserves. Their incomes are approximately two thirds that of the non-Aboriginal average. Most of their employment is in the service industry and is low paying. In 1984, almost half of Aboriginal housing failed to meet basic standards. Alcohol abuse levels have been estimated at between 35% and 40% for the adult Aboriginal population and between 10% and 15% for Aboriginal adolescents. Smoking is also prevalent among children and adults. Aboriginals are at high risk for obesity and deficiency in nutrients such as iron, vitamins, and protein.

The federal government is responsible for the health care of Aboriginal people on reserves, and the provincial government for those off reserves. Since two thirds of Aboriginal people live in rural or remote areas, health care services are less than optimal. On many remote reserves, primary care is provided by nurses or community health workers.

In the last 20 years there has been a substantial improvement in Aboriginal mortality, although the gap in mortality between Aboriginal people and the general Canadian population is still wide. In 1993, the Aboriginal mortality rate standardized to the Canadian population was 10.8 per 1,000, which is 1.6 times the Canadian rate. The four leading causes of death in order for the Aboriginal population were injury and poisoning, diseases of the circulatory system, neoplasm, and diseases of the respiratory system. Aboriginal people have a high incidence of gastroenteritis, diphtheria, rheumatic fever, respiratory problems, and infectious hepatitis. Hospitalization rates for Aboriginal people are high compared with Canadian rates, and the disability rates are almost double the corresponding rates for the rest of the Canadian population. The major disabilities for Aboriginal people 15 years and over were in the areas of mobility, agility, and hearing.

One of the major solutions proposed by Aboriginal people to improve their health status is to gain control over their health, social, and educational programs. Another solution is to settle the unresolved land claims and have their rightful place in Canadian society recognized.

The conventional definition of a *senior* is someone aged 65 years or over. The number and proportion of seniors in the population continues to grow with a tendency toward an increasing proportion of the very elderly (over age 85). In June 1996, seniors accounted for 12.2% of the population. It is estimated that by 2021, 15% of the population will be elderly. It is also interesting to note that in 1996 there were 1.2 times the number of 65- to 84-year-old women than men in the same age group. Seniors' income has increased substantially recently, with the gap narrowing between them and the rest of the population. Seniors depend on public pension and income security plans for their income. Many are predisposed to falls and injuries due to increased rate of visual, auditory, and locomotive disabilities. As well, they have low tolerance levels to the presence of hazards in the physical environment.

Successful aging has been defined in terms of retaining the ability to function independently, remain mobile, and undertake all the activities of daily living. The predictors of successful aging include a surviving spouse, having not entered a nursing home, and age. Over 50% of seniors drink alcohol, while less than 20% smoke regularly. Many are malnourished. The majority of the population aged 65 years and over have diets deficient in nutrients such as protein, iron, calcium, and thiamin.

Mortality rates for senior women are lower than those for males. The leading health problems include arthritis, rheumatism, hypertension, limb and joint disease, respiratory and heart diseases, and diabetes; Alzheimer's disease represents the most frequent dementing illness. The overall disability rate for seniors was 45%, increasing to 80% for the very elderly. The major types of disability reported were in mobility, agility, vision, and hearing. Hospital usage rises dramatically with age. The old elderly use approximately 10 times more hospital days than any other age group under age 60.

It has now been recognized that there is a need for improved geriatric services. Health promotion for seniors is becoming important to the development and maintenance of optimum levels of functioning as aging occurs. These approaches include physical activity, social support, nutrition counselling, and programs to prevent falls.

A family that spends over 56.2% of their income on the basic needs of accommodation, food and clothing lives in poverty. In Canada in 1995, there were one in five (20.5%) *children living in poverty*. Several groups are at particular risk for poverty, particularly single mothers, immigrants, and Aboriginal people. These children face both short-term and long-term social, educational, and health disadvantages. It is well documented that poor children have poor health, although the exact mechanisms of how poverty affects health is not clear.

The effects of poverty on mortality begin before birth and may predate conception. Low birth weight is the single most important cause of infant mortality and is inversely related to social class. Hence the effects of poverty on neonatal mortality are mediated through low birth weight. Overall mortality among those aged 1 to 14 was higher in 1986 for poor children than for those who were not poor. Accidents are the major cause of death in children. Children from low-income families are also at a greater risk for infectious diseases, chronic health problems, dental caries, and nutritional disorders. The rate of childhood disability in 1986 was over twice as high among children from poor families compared with rich families. Children whose parents were living on social assistance had a 2.8 times higher chance of developing a psychiatric disorder.

The federal government has taken new initiatives to address the problems of children living in poverty. They include the implementation of a new child benefit program to supplement the income for low-income working families.

The World Health Organization defines *disability* as "any restriction or lack ... of ability to perform an activity in the manner or within the range considered normal for a human being". Seven categories of disabilities have been identified: mobility, agility, sight, hearing, speaking, other, and unknown. In 1994, 20% of the population or 5 million Canadians had some level of disability. Mobility is cited as the most frequent form of disability, followed by agility as the next most frequent type. In 1991, 7% of children under the age of 15 had disabilities. Individuals with disabilities tended to have less formal education than those without disabilities, as disabilities often interfered with education. Gross incomes of people with disabilities between age 15 and 64 are likely to be as low as 46% less than the income of people with no disabilities in the same age group.

There are a number of causes of disability, and age plays an important role in determining the cause. Medical conditions that lead to disability most often are diseases of the musculoskeletal system and hearing disorders. Among children, the major causes of disability were developmental delay and hearing or vision problems. Among individuals over 50, diseases were the leading cause of the disability, whereas for under 50, accidents were the major cause of the disability. Children with disabilities are at a risk for malnutrition, due to physical disabilities, cognitive delay, altered nutrient requirements caused by medical condition, or drugs used to treat the medical condition accordingly.

There is a consumer movement to enhance the quality of life of people with disabilities, and institutions are beginning to recognize that they are in fact "home" to their residents and are changing.

7.   REFERENCES

1.   1996 Census: Aboriginal Data (www.statcan.ca/Daily/English/980113/d980113.htm), May 1998.
2.   Lemchuck-Favel L. Trends in First Nations Mortality 1979-1993. Ottawa: Ministry of Public Works and Government Services Canada, 1996.
3.   Statistics Canada. Language, Tradition, Health, Lifestyle and Social Issues. 1991 Aboriginal Peoples Survey. Ottawa: Statistics Canada, 1993.
4.   Postl B, MacDonald S, Moffat M. Background Paper on the Health of Aboriginal Peoples in Canada. In Canadian Medical Association Submission to the Royal Commission on Aboriginal Peoples, Bridging the Gap, Promoting Health and Healing for Aboriginal Peoples in Canada. Ottawa: Canadian Medical Association, 1994.
5.   Shah CP, Dubeski G. First Nations Peoples in Urban Settings: Health Issues. In Masi R, Mensah L, McLeod KA, Oakville K, eds. Health and Cultures: Exploring the Relationships. Oakville: Mosaic Press, 1993:71-93.
6.   Health in Canada: Perspectives of Urban Aboriginal People. Ottawa: Canadian Nurses Association, 1995.
7.   Report of the Royal Commission on Aboriginal Peoples; Gathering Strength. Volume 3. Ottawa: Canada Communication Group, 1996.
8.   Siggner AJ. The Socio-Demographic Conditions of Registered Indians. Statistics Canada: Canadian Social Trends 1986;1(1):1-9.
9.   Young TK, Bruce L, et al. The Health Effects of Housing and Community Infrastructure on Canadian Reserves, Prepared for Department of Indian and Northern Affairs, Government of Canada. Winnipeg: Northern Health Research Unit, University of Manitoba, 1991.
10.   Alcohol and Drug Abuse Among Treaty Indians in Saskatchewan: Needs Assessment and Recommendations for Change. Saskatoon: Federation of Saskatchewan Indian Nations and Health and Welfare Canada, 1984.
11.   Brief to the Standing Committee on Health and Welfare, Hearings Concerning Resources Required to Address Substance Abuse [unpublished]. Ottawa: Union of Ontario Indians, 1987.
12.   Health Status of Canadian Indians and Inuit: Update 1987. Ottawa: Medical Services Branch, Minister of National Health and Welfare, 1988.
13.   Myers T, Calzavara LM, Cockerill R, Marshall VW, Bullock SL. Ontario First Nations AIDS and Healthy Lifestyle Survey. Toronto: LB Publishing Services, 1993.
14.   Nutrition Canada: National Survey. Ottawa: Information Canada, 1973.
15.   HIV/AIDS and the Impact on Aboriginal Women in Canada. Aboriginal Nurses Association of Canada, 1993.
16.   Postl B. The Health of Canada's Native People: An Overview. Canadian Family Physician. 1988;34(11):2413-2419.
17.   Epidemiology and Community Health Specialities Indian and Northern Health Services. Overview of Health Services for First Nations provided by Medical Services Branch, Health Canada. Ottawa: Health Canada, 1994.
18.   Task Force on Suicide in Canada. Suicide in Canada. Ottawa: Minister of National Health and Welfare, 1994.
19.   Report of the Subcommittee on Indian Health Care to the Health Services Review Committee. Winnipeg: Chairman, Postl, B.D. University of Manitoba, 1985.

20. Evers SE, Rand CG. Morbidity in Canadian Indian and Non-Indian Children in the Second Year. Canadian Journal of Public Health 1983;74(3):191-194.

21. McLeod A. Aboriginal Communities and HIV/AIDS. A Joint Project with the Canadian AIDS Society and the Canadian Aboriginal AIDS Network. Final Report. Ottawa: Canadian AIDS Society, 1997.

22. 1991 Aboriginal People Survey. Ottawa: Statistics Canada, The Daily, 1993.

23. Wilkins K. Tuberculosis. Health Reports 1994. 1994;8(1):33-39.

24. Ng E. Disability Among Canada's Aboriginal Peoples in 1991. Health Reports 1996;8(1):25-31.

25. Shah CP, Park IR, Casson I. Prevalence of Disabilities in Two Native Communities in the Sioux Lookout Zone of Northwestern Ontario. Proceedings of Canadian Association of Physical Anthropology. Vancouver, 1989.

26. Waldram JB, Herring DA, Young TK. Aboriginal Health in Canada: Historical, Cultural and Epidemiological Perspectives. Toronto: University of Toronto Press, 1995.

27. Minister of Indian Affairs and Northern Development. Gathering Strength: Canada's Aboriginal Action Plan. Ottawa: Government of Canada, 1997.

28. Roos P, Havens B. Predictors of Successful Aging: A Twelve-Year Study of Manitoba Elderly. American Journal of Public Health 1991;81(1):63-68.

29. Barer ML, Evans RG, Hertzman C, Lomas J. Aging and Health Care Utilization: New Evidence on Old Fallacies. Social Science and Medicine 1987;24(10):851-862.

30. Fries JF. Aging, Natural Death and the Compression of Morbidity. New England Journal of Medicine 1980;303(3):130-135.

31. CMA Committee on the Health Care of the Elderly. Health Care for the Elderly: Today's Challenges Tomorrow's Options. Ottawa: Canadian Medical Association, 1987.

32. Ableson J, Paddon P, Stohmenger C, eds. Perspectives on Health. Ottawa: Statistics Canada, Queen's Printer, 1983.

33. Schneider E, Brody, JA. Aging, Natural Death and the Compression of Morbidity: Another View. New England Journal of Medicine 1983;309(14):854-856.

34. Wylie CM. Health-Related Contrasts Between Older Men and Women. In Issacs B, ed. Recent Advances in Geriatric Medicine. Number Three. Melbourne, Australia: Churchill Livingstone, 1985.

35. Statistics Canada. 1996 Census Canada: Age and Sex. Ottawa: The Daily, 1997.

36. Federal, Provincial and Territorial Advisory Committee. Report on the Health of Canadians: Technical Appendix. Ottawa: 1996.

37. Health and Welfare Canada. The Active Health Report on Seniors. Ottawa: Ministry of Supply and Services, 1989.

38. Ministry of Supply and Services. Canada's Seniors. A Dynamic Force. Ottawa: Government of Canada, 1988.

39. National Advisory Council on Aging. Understanding Seniors' Independence. Report No. 1: The Barriers and Suggestions for Action. Ottawa: Minister of Supply and Services Canada, 1989.

40. Wigdor B. Elder Abuse: Major Issues for a National Perspective. Ottawa: National Advisory Council on Aging, Government of Canada, 1991.

41. Podnicks E. National Survey on Abuse of the Elderly in Canada. Journal of Elder Abuse Neglect 1992;4:5-58.

42. Wilkins K. Causes of Death: How Sexes Differ. Health Report 1995;7(2):33-43.

43. Tinetti M, Speechley, M, Ginter SF. Risk Factors for Falls Among Elderly Persons Living in the Community. New England Journal of Medicine 1988;319(26):1701-1707.

44. Eliany M, Clarke J. The Use of Alcohol and Other Drugs by Older Canadians and Its Consequences: Highlights. 1992. (www.hc-sc.gc.ca/hppb/alcohol-otherdrugs/pub/use/use2.htm), May 1998.
45. Bergob M. Drug Use Among Senior Canadians. 1996. (www.statcan.ca/Documents/English/SocTrends/drugs.html), 1998.
46. Chandra R, Imbach A, Moore C, Skelton D, Woolcott D. Nutrition of the Elderly. Canadian Medical Association Journal 1991;145(11):1475-1487.
47. Stokes J, Lindsay J. Major Causes of Death and Hospitalization in Canadian Seniors. Chronic Disease in Canada 1996;17(2):63-73.
48. Health and Welfare Canada. Mortality of the Elderly in Canada. Chronic Disease in Canada 1990;11(1):1-3.
49. Canadian Study of Health and Aging. Patterns of Caring for People with Dementia in Canada. Canadian Journal on Aging 1994;13(4):470-487.
50. Hill G, Frobes W, Berthelot J, Lindsay J, McDowell I. Dementia Among Seniors. Statistics Canada: Health Reports 1996;8(2):7-10.
51. Ostbye T, Crosse E. Net Economic Costs of Dementia in Canada. Canadian Medical Association Journal 1994;151(10):1457-1464.
52. Locker D, Leake JL, Lee J, Main PJ, Hicks T, Hamilton M. Utilization of Dental Services in Four Ontario Communities. Journal of Canadian Dental Association 1991;57(9):879-881.
53. Locker D, Leake JL, Hamilton M, Hicks T, Lee J, Main PJ. Oral Health Status of Older Adults in Four Ontario Communities. Journal of Canadian Dental Association 1991;57(9):727-732.
54. Roos NP, Shapiro E, Roos LL. Aging and the Demand for Health Services: Which Aged and Whose Demand? Gerontologist 1984;24(1):31-36.
55. Horne RV. A New Agenda: Health and Social Service Strategies for Ontario's Seniors. Toronto: Government of Ontario, 1987.
56. Growing Up in Canada: National Longitudinal Survey of Children and Youth. Ottawa: Human Resources and Development Canada: Statistics Canada, 1996.
57. Report Card 1997. Child Poverty in Canada. Toronto: Campaign 2000, 1997.
58. Chapter 6: Poverty. The Health of Canada's Children: A Statistical Profile. 2nd ed. Ottawa: Canadian Institute of Child Health, 1994.
59. Higher Poverty Rate Clouds Child's Day. Canadian Medical Association Journal 1996;155(10):1468.
60. Monsebraaten L. 36%: That's the Percentage of Metro Children Who Live in Poverty. They and the Rest of the Urban Poor May Not Be Dying in the Streets, But They Are Suffering in Ways That the Well-off Don't Imagine. The Toronto Star 1997 August 2, 1997:D1, D9.
61. U.S. Department of Health and Human Services. Healthy Children — Toxic Environments — Acting on the Unique Vulnerability of Children Who Dwell Near Hazardous Waste Sites. Atlanta, Georgia: Agency for Toxic Substances and Disease Registry, 1996.
62. Canadian Council on Social Development. The Progress of Canada's Children 1997. Ottawa: Canadian Council of Social Development, 1997.
63. Manga P. Equality of Access and Inequalities in Health Status: Policy Implications of an Apparent Paradox. Ottawa: University of Ottawa, 1986.
64. Wigle DT, Mao Y. Mortality by Income Level in Urban Canada. Ottawa: Ministry of National Health and Welfare, 1980.
65. Dougherty GE. Social Class and the Occurrence of Traffic Injuries and Deaths in Urban Children. Canadian Journal of Public Health 1990;81(3):204-209.

66. Wilkins R, Adams O, Brackner A. Changes in Mortality by Income in Urban Canada from 1971 to 1986. Health Reports 1989;1(2):137-174.
67. Wilkins R, Sherman GJ. Birth Outcomes and Infant Mortality by Income in Urban Canada, 1986. Health Reports 1991;3(1):7-31.
68. The Health of Canada's Children: A CICH Profile. Ottawa: Canadian Institute of Child Health, 1989.
69. Chance G. A Warning for the Cradle? Because They May Signal a Deterioration in the Nation's Health, Trends in Infant Mortality and Low Birth Weight Bear Watching. Canadian Medical Association Journal 1997;157(5):549-551.
70. Health Canada. Bureau for Reproductive and Child Health. Pregnancy and Child Development. 1996. vol 1-4. (www.hc-sc.gc.ca/main/lcdc/web/publicat/aphe/newsld_e.html).
71. Aber JL, G. BN, Conley DC, Li J. The Effects of Poverty on Child Health and Development. Annual Review of Public Health 1997;18:463-483.
72. Nault F. Infant Mortality and Low Birthweight, 1975 to 1995. Statistics Canada: Health Reports 1997;9(3):39-45.
73. Kovar MG. Health Status of U.S. Children and Use of Medical Care. Public Health Reports 1982;97(1):3-15.
74. Cadman D, Boyle MH, Offord DR. Chronic Illness, Function Conditions and Limitations in Ontario Children: Findings of the Ontario Child Health Study. Canadian Medical Association Journal 1986;135(7):761-767.
75. Ontario Child Health Study: Children at Risk. Toronto: Queen's Printer for Ontario, 1989.
76. Lipman EL, Offord DR, Boyel MH. Relation Between Economic Disadvantage and Psychosocial Morbidity in Children. Canadian Medical Association Journal 1994;151(4):431-437.
77. Lehmann F, Gray-Donald K, Mongeon M, Di Tommaso S. Iron Deficiency Anaemia in 1-Year-Old Children of Disadvantaged Families in Montreal. Canadian Medical Association Journal 1992;146(9):1571-1577.
78. Lozoff B, Jimenez E, Wolf AW. Long-Term Developmental Outcome of Infants With Iron Deficiency. New England Journal of Medicine 1984;325(10):687-694.
79. Stamm JW, Lizaire A, Fedori D, et al. Dental Health Status of Alberta School Children. Canadian Dental Association Journal 1980;46(2):98-107.
80. Stamm JW, Dixter CT, Langlair RP. Principal Dental Health Indices for 13-14 Year Old Quebec Children. Canadian Dental Association Journal 1980;46(2):125-137.
81. Mustard F. Ideas, Collaboration and Healthy Children. Ideas 1996;3(1):3-8.
82. Joseph KS, Kramer MS. Recent Trends in Infant Mortality Rates and Proportions of Low-Birth-Weight of Live Births in Canada. Canadian Medical Association Journal 1997;157(5):535-541.
83. Hertzman C, Wiens, C. Child Development and Long-Term Outcomes: A Population Health Perspective and Summary of Successful Interventions. Social Science Medicine 1996;43(7):1083-1095.
84. Joseph K, Kramer, MS. Review of the Evidence on Fetal and Early Childhood Antecedents of Adult Chronic Disease. Epidemiologic Reviews 1996;18(2):158-174.
85. Canadian Council on Social Development. Position Paper: CCSD's Response to the 1997 Federal Budget. (www.ccsd.cas/budgt97.htm), May 1998.
86. Steinhauer P. Summary of Developing Resiliency in Children from Disadvantage Populations. 1996. National Forum on Health.

87. Greenspon E. Provinces Want More Federal Funds for Child-Benefit Plan: Social Services Ministers Meeting in St. John's to Work Out Details of New National Program to Aid Low-Income Working Families. The Globe and Mail 1997 October 7, 1997:A8.
88. Philp M. Task Force Aiming to Give Children Head Start. The Globe and Mail. 1997:A:9.
89. Hamilton M. The Health and Activity Limitation Survey. Health Reports 1989;1(2):175-187.
90. Dowler J, Jordon-Simpson D. Canada's Disabled Population in Institutions. Health Reports 1990;2(1):27-36.
91. Statistics Canada. Health and Activity Limitation Survey. The Daily 1992 .
92. Ministry of Citizenship: Office for Disabled Persons. Statistical Profile of Disabled Persons in Ontario. Vol 2. Toronto: Queen's Printer for Ontario, 1990.
93. Science News. Substance Abuse among the Disabled. Science News 1989 .
94. Evers S, Munoz MA, Vanderkooy P et al. Nutritional Rehabilitation of Developmentally Disabled Residents in a Long-Term Care Facility. Journal of American Dietetic Association 1991;91(4):471-473.

Chapter

7

Chronic Diseases and Injuries

The major causes of mortality, morbidity, and the burden of illness in the Canadian population are discussed in Chapter Five. Overall, cardiovascular disease and cancer are the leading contributors to **chronic disease**, which is usually defined as a condition lasting three months or longer. A significant proportion is due to injuries, either unintentional (e.g., motor vehicle accidents) or intentional (e.g., suicidal attempts). The economic and personal burden of chronic illness to Canada is substantial. There are number of risk factors that influence the development of chronic diseases. Some of these are modifiable such as those related to lifestyles whereas others such as age, sex or genetic make-up are not amenable to change. Substance abuse (predominantly smoking and problematic alcohol use) and improper diet are major risk factors of chronic illness and play a part in a number of diseases; hence they are discussed first to avoid the repetitiveness in terms of preventive strategies.

This chapter presents detailed information on the burden of illness caused by chronic non-communicable diseases, emphasizing current approaches to prevention and control. As many chronic illnesses are preventable and few are curable in the traditional medical model, the roles of primary and secondary prevention and, more recently, health promotion have emerged as increasingly important. The reader is referred to Chapter One for the underlying principles of disease prevention and health promotion that provide the framework.

Most of the data presented here come from published studies, government sources, and non-governmental organizations. Data, particularly percentage figures for risk factors and economic estimates of the burden of illness, quickly become out of date. Also, due to differences in methods, definitions, and time of data collection, incidence and cost figures vary slightly from report to report. Readers are directed to the methods section of the reports cited below to determine how estimates were made. The organizations cited here, such as the Heart and Stroke Foundation, Statistics Canada, and the National Cancer Institute of Canada, produce annual or semi-annual compilations of statistics. Updates can be listed on the World Wide Web. Suggested web sites are found at the end of this book.

1.   MAJOR MODIFIABLE LIFESTYLE ISSUES

The major underlying cause of many chronic diseases is substance abuse in the form of tobacco use, excessive alcohol use, or improper diet. As mentioned above, in order to avoid repetitiveness, the strategies for primary prevention of major diseases are described in the sections on substance abuse and diet.

1.1. SUBSTANCE ABUSE

Although much attention focuses on illicit drugs, the major burden of illness caused by substance abuse is due to use or abuse of **tobacco and alcohol**, which are readily available, socially sanctioned, and promoted widely. These substances are discussed separately in the context of the burden of illness caused by each, and then together in the context of control and prevention of the consequences of their use and abuse. A risk continuum framework of the spectrum of problems arising from use and abuse of these substances and the appropriate level of response are provided in Chapter One (see Figure 1.1 in Chapter 1).

1.1.1. Tobacco
Tobacco smoking is the most important preventable cause of death in Canada. The trends and prevalence rate of smoking are discussed in Chapter Four. In 1992, 33,498 people were estimated to have died as a result of exposure to tobacco (1). The effects of smoking contribute to several major health problems: lung cancer, where smoking is responsible for 80% of cases, chronic obstructive lung disease, and cardiovascular illness. The population attributable risk (PAR, see Chapter Two) for smoking in relation to cancer deaths is 29% and for cardiovascular deaths, 17%. Women over age 40 who are on the birth control pill and who smoke are at particular risk. Smoking also contributes to the incidence of a number of other cancers and consequently tobacco use constitutes the major preventable cause of cancer. The age-standardized mortality rates for lung cancer per 100,000 persons have increased from 40 for males and 6 for females in 1970 to an estimated 77 for males and 34 for females in 1996 (2). The overall cancer death rates of male smokers are double those of non-smokers. Female deaths, while much lower in number than males, have risen proportionately at a greater rate than for males within the last 15 years, parallelling the increase in female smoking. The overall cancer death rate of female smokers is 30% greater (and rising) than that of non-smokers. Maternal smoking is the major preventable cause of low birth weight, which, in turn, is the major risk factor of infant mortality in Canada. Infants born to women who smoke, on average, weigh 200 grams less than those of non-smoking mothers.

Smoking also affects the mortality rates for chronic obstructive pulmonary disease (COPD), which includes bronchitis, emphysema, and asthma. In 1992, there were an estimated 208,095 hospitalizations and more than 3,000,000 bed days related to tobacco use in Canada. COPD was the largest contributor with 21% of the hospital days followed by stroke (19%), ischemic heart disease (15%), and lung cancer (14%). In terms of economic burden, the costs to society attributable to tobacco use (for premature mortality, hospitalization, physician services, and fires) were estimated at approximately $9.56 billion in direct costs. This represents 51.8% of the costs associated with substance abuse in Canada. Lost productivity due to illness and premature death account for $6.8 billion of these costs. The remaining $2.67 billion represent the direct costs for health care (1). The costs in terms of quality of life and disability-free life expectancy are additional.

Smoking is well entrenched in our society as a symbol of sophistication and even liberation for women; however, the image of a person who smokes is changing. Smoking was widely promoted by governments in North America during World War II, and likely this promotion greatly expanded its prevalence. Recent Canadian surveys estimate the percentage of male and female regular smokers to be 28% and 25% respectively. Of the Canadian population who smoke cigarettes regularly, 13% smoke more than 25 cigarettes per day (see Chapter Four). An additional 5% smoke occasionally or are pipe or cigar smokers. For those under age 45, males and females had equal prevalence of regular smoking: for those over age 45, males were more frequently regular smokers. The age group with the highest proportion of female smokers was 25 to 34 (34%), with similar percentages for males and females between 15 and 24 and between 35 and 44. For males, the prevalence of smoking was highest also among those aged 25 to 34 (35%) (1).

Secondhand Smoke

Smoking is not only a hazard to those who smoke. The Report of the Working Group on Passive Smoking stated that there is strong evidence of an association between residential and workplace exposure to environmental tobacco smoke and respiratory illness (3). This report has been confirmed by recent studies. The relationship between environmental tobacco smoke and adverse health effects is now well accepted (4).

Secondhand smoke is a mixture of exhaled smoke (mainstream) and smoke emitted from the smouldering lit tobacco (sidestream). There are over 4,000 chemicals in secondhand smoke of which 42 are known carcinogens. Besides being a known mucous membrane irritant, secondhand smoke exposure is linked to increases in mortality from lung cancer and cardiovascular disease. Secondhand smoke has serious consequences to exposed children: smoking mothers bear children with lower birth weights, sudden infant death syndrome and children living in homes exposed to tobacco smoke have higher rates and greater severity of asthma attack, and higher rates of otitis media and respiratory tract problems (4).

Brief Interventions for Smoking Cessation by Health Care Professionals

Studies have provided evidence that health care providers, including physicians and non-physicians, can be effective in motivating patients to quit smoking by using brief interventions of smoking cessation messages reinforced on multiple occasions. Cessation techniques developed by the National Institutes of Health in the United States and by the Canadian Council on Smoking and Health (*Guide Your Patients to a*

Smoke-Free Future) can be utilized and incorporated into office procedures (5). The manual for the latter technique (available from the Canadian Council on Smoking and Health) lists the following steps: select a smoking cessation coordinator in the office, create a smoke-free office, identify all smoking patients, develop individual smoking cessation plans, and provide follow-up support. Health Canada recently piloted a clinical tobacco intervention called "Talk About Smoking" that is based on the stages of change model (see Chapter One). This strategy aims to have every chart in a physician's office colour coded as to the individual's smoking status. Consequently, smoking can be discussed at every office visit in a brief informative manner and interventions tailored to each patient's individual needs.

Legislation and Community Action

In the late 1980s, incidence and mortality rates for lung cancer in males began to level off, likely reflecting the fall in men's tobacco consumption that began in the 1960s. Well-designed health promotion strategies aimed at preventing the uptake of smoking by impressionable youth, as well as cessation in older smokers, can continue the reversal of trends in smoking prevalence. Recent findings on passive smoking have had an impact on public policies. With increased awareness of adverse effects of passive smoking in closed environments some cities have passed legislation banning smoking in the workplace. The public seems broadly supportive of initiatives to restrict exposure to environmental tobacco smoke (6). Similarly, the federal government has also banned smoking in all federal buildings and flights operating in Canada. These strategies are aspects of a comprehensive approach to tobacco use prevention that includes multiple strategies directed at multiple sites and on an intersectoral basis (discussed under the section on health promotion below). The federal government released the *Blueprint for Tobacco Control* in 1995 (7). Highlights of that document include more stringent restrictions on advertisements and sponsorship by tobacco companies. It also calls for restrictions on the access to tobacco and limits at the point of sale. Increased restrictions on packaging and labelling requirements are also recommended.

In 1996, Bill C-71 was passed to regulate the manufacture, sale, labelling, and promotion of tobacco products. The legislation further limits youth access to tobacco products, restricts the promotion of tobacco products, increases health information on tobacco packages, and establishes powers to regulate tobacco products. Specifically, there can be no self-service displays, vending machine sales, or mail-order distribution, and photo identification is required for confirmation of minimum age. Advertising of tobacco products is curtailed, and sponsorship links reduced. The logo of the company and other brand elements are limited to the bottom 10% of the display surface; sponsorship items containing brand information are restricted to publications catering to a predominantly adult audience. More detailed reporting on the sales of tobacco products, promotional activities, and distribution and manufacturing practices, as well as information on toxic substances, are required from tobacco manufacturers.

1.1.2. Alcohol

There are various diseases and injuries associated with alcohol consumption, such as cirrhosis, suicide, breast cancer, respiratory cancer, and motor vehicle and other accidents. For the trend and prevalence rates for drinking, please refer to Chapter Four. In social terms, an estimated 1.8% of all deaths are directly attributable to alcohol abuse and an estimated 10.5% of all deaths are alcohol-related. Mortality from cirrhosis of the liver has increased since the postwar period, coincident with rising levels of alcohol consumption (8). Although cirrhosis itself can be caused by several factors other than alcohol, the incidence of alcohol related cases is responsible for most of the increased death rate in Canada. It is estimated that 6,701 Canadians died as a result of alcohol consumption in 1992. Approximately 1,500 were killed as a result of impaired driving, with twice as many men as women being affected. Cirrhosis and suicide accounted for another 1,800 deaths (1).

While mortality and potential-years-life-lost (PYLL) to society are of concern, the impact of alcohol on the health of Canadians is shown more strongly in terms of morbidity. In industry, for instance, losses from reduced productivity and absenteeism due to alcohol abuse are calculated to be in the region of 1 million daily. In addition, alcohol gives rise to family and social problems. Alcoholism is also one of the leading causes of hospitalization in mental institutions. In Canada in 1992, overall costs related to alcohol abuse, i.e., health care, law enforcement, social welfare, and reduced productivity, were estimated to be $7.5 billion, of which $4.1 billion was for lost productivity. Direct health care costs alone are estimated at $1.3 billion (1).

Along the spectrum of risk are two defined groups of drinkers in whom problems most often appear. These two groups consist of "problem drinkers" and those who are "alcohol dependent" (9). **Problem drinking** does not always progress to alcohol dependence but is still associated with considerable medical and social consequences. **Alcohol dependence** is physical and psychological. It is characterized by a pattern of alcohol tolerance and symptoms, and progressive loss of control despite obvious harm and social complications. Although the most severe alcohol-related consequences occur in those with alcohol dependence, problem drinking accounts for a larger proportion of alcohol-related illness because it is more prevalent. Over 11% of Canadian men are considered heavy frequent drinkers and nearly 6% report disruption to family life. Problem drinkers outnumber those with alcohol dependence by a ratio of 4:1 (9). Problem drinkers consult their physicians twice as often as non-problem drinkers. The use of other psychoactive substances is more likely in a problem drinker or alcohol-dependent person. There are approximately 502,700 Canadians who are alcohol dependent. Five times more men than women are alcohol dependent. Men are at highest risk of becoming alcohol dependant when they are between age 35 and 64, while women are at greatest risk between age 45 and 64. Cirrhosis eventually develops in 5% to 10% of alcohol-dependent men; women, however, appear more susceptible to cirrhosis. Fetal alcohol syndrome is another adverse effect associated with alcohol consumption. It is estimated that 100 babies are born with fetal alcohol syndrome in Canada each year.

There is some evidence to suggest that alcohol consumption may reduce mortality from cardiovascular disease. The "French Paradox" relates to the observation that cardiovascular mortality rates are lower in France where wine consumption is high. There is controversy about recommending increasing alcohol consumption because of increased rates of cirrhosis found in France (9). However, the Addiction Research Foundation of Toronto recently released a brochure entitled *Alcohol and Your Health*, which recommends limiting intake of two standard drinks on any day, fewer than 14 drinks for men a week, and nine or fewer drinks for women (10).

Early Detection and Brief Interventions by Health Care Professionals

The physician is in a good position to identify problem drinking and alcohol dependence quickly and offer early intervention for patients whose drinking is at levels that increase their risks for medical and psychosocial consequences (11). Good evidence exists for the effectiveness of brief intervention programs for those at an early stage of problem drinking. Efficient approaches include behavioural self-control training (involving goal setting and self-monitoring), controlling the rate of consumption, and learning substitutes for drinking behaviour. A potential problem can be identified by asking the patient a few structured questions such as those in the Michigan Alcoholism Screening Test (12) or the CAGE questionnaire (13). Problem drinkers and alcohol-dependent people can visit their physician to have their problem diagnosed and treated appropriately. Many motivated problem drinkers and alcohol-dependent people who want to quit drinking are also being assisted by self-help groups such as Alcoholics Anonymous.

1.2. HEALTH PROMOTION IN RELATION TO SUBSTANCE ABUSE

Even though the majority of Canadians have no personal problem with the use of alcohol or other drugs, including tobacco, there remains the enormous economic burden to society in general and the suffering of those close to the people affected. Federal, provincial, and municipal governments have developed policies to reduce this burden and have tried to achieve an environment free of substance abuse for all citizens. While a plethora of information has entered the public arena, it is necessary to restructure the environment to ensure that healthy choices in relation to substance use are the easier choices and are supported by changes in community norms.

The health promotion approach provides a framework for drawing together different methods for enhancing, maintaining, or regaining the various physical, psychological, and social dimensions of health. It uses a number of policies, services, and programs designed to enhance the healthfulness of individuals and their environments, not just the physical but also the social, cultural, and economic environments. The supportiveness of environments is provided by policies and programs that help people to help themselves and build on their strengths. **Effective health promotion programs** should be **comprehensive**, dealing with all environments in which individuals work, live, and play, based on the social influences model of health promotion; **coordinated** as part of a larger framework, coalition, or partnership working toward the same goal; and **participatory**, so that the people involved in behaviour change are actively involved in identifying the problems and designing the programs. Swarbrick's Model Program for Substance Abuse Prevention gives a good guide to community participation at all levels of planning for a community program to combat substance abuse (14).

In order to reduce community influences that encourage drinking and smoking, the following strategies, incorporating education, policies and environmental support, have become established in a number of settings and are being increasingly adopted elsewhere. In the community at large, the availability of alcohol and tobacco can be reduced by federal, provincial, and municipal regulatory action. As already discussed, Bill C-17 regulates the manufacture, promotion, and sale of tobacco in an attempt to reduce cigarette consumption. However, with the recent reduction of the federal and provincial taxes, the price of cigarettes in most provinces have significantly dropped to half of its original price. This is a retrogressive step in the fight against tobacco use and has had a negative impact on its consumption.

It is established that increases in accessibility to alcohol facilitate a higher rate of consumption, and the converse is also true. Evidence indicates a positive relationship between per capita consumption and alcohol-related diseases. Alcohol consumption is related to its price. In fact, the volume of beer that cost 7% of the average weekly salary in 1944 now costs only 1.5%. This is reflected by the sales of alcoholic beverages, which have risen in recent years by as much as 40%. Measures to counter the widespread availability of alcohol include restricting the availability of alcohol by local licensing provisions for the number and location of outlets, their hours of operation and whether these are enforced, for pricing policies (using taxation), and for drinking ages. For the prevention of alcohol abuse, a number of specific strategies have been directed toward reducing drinking and driving in the community at large. Integrated drinking-and-driving plans include policies for licensed premises and server-training programs where staff learn about the effects of alcohol and the indication of intoxication, and how to try to modify the drinking behaviour. Other modalities are designated-driver programs and drinking/driving countermeasures. Visible enforcement of blood alcohol limits by way of police spot checks can increase drivers' perceived risk of apprehension.

Media campaigns such as "Break Free" (part of the national program to reduce tobacco use) (15), and "Really Me" (16) (part of Canada's drug strategy) have been conducted by Health Canada. These health promotion approaches increase awareness of substance abuse and reinforce other activities conducted by other partners such as the provinces. "Magnet events", which are events such as youth concerts that appeal to certain segments of the community, also raise awareness about substance abuse when drug-free messages are displayed.

School-based policies on alcohol, drugs, and smoking can complement integrated education and prevention programs that incorporate smoking cessation programs and drug education curricula. Peer-assisted learning uses the influence of peers in smoking prevention programs. In postsecondary schools, server intervention, designated-driver programs, and education programs should also be implemented along with campus policies. In the home setting, parents should be encouraged to discuss alcohol and smoking issues and values with children. Educational material supporting smoke-free homes and self-help smoking cessation kits can be introduced into the home. Parents can be educated about quitting smoking and alcohol use. Workplaces provide further sites for health promotion policies such as alcohol and smoke-free policies, health programs, smoking cessation programs run by trained staff and drinking driving countermeasure programs. Finally, the health care setting itself can be a useful role model by adopting smoke-free workplace policies, and providing education and smoking cessation support. Early detection and intervention programs for alcohol abuse are the responsibility of health care providers.

National programs for substance abuse have espoused the principles of health promotion. The objectives are to reduce tobacco use in Canada, protect the health and rights of non-smokers, prevent smoking (especially in the young), and smoking cessation. Canada's drug strategy initiative incorporates the concept that reduction of supply through law enforcement is not sufficient and that long-term community-based efforts are needed to control substance abuse. Alcohol is a widely available drug in our community but social norms to support its appropriate use, rather than its abuse, are appearing.

As noted in Chapter One, harm reduction programs are now recognized as important components in the reduction of risk from substance abuse.

1.3. DIET

Chapter Four, Determinants of Health and Disease, provided information on the nutritional status of Canadians. Diet, particularly fat intake, is a major factor in the development of many chronic diseases, including the two leading killers, cardiovascular disease (17) and cancer. Nutrition is also a factor in osteoporosis, chronic liver disease, and dental health. Obesity is a risk factor for diabetes and synergistic with other risks for cardiovascular disease (CVD). National guidelines for nutrition have been published by Health and Welfare Canada in the report called *Nutrition Recommendations* (18), which recommends that the Canadian diet should provide:

- Energy consistent with the maintenance of body weight within the recommended range;
- Essential nutrients in amounts recommended;
- No more than 30% of energy as fat (33 g/1,000 kcal or 39 g/5,000 kJ) and no more than 10% as saturated fat (11 g/1,000 kcal or 13 g/5,000 kJ);
- No more than 55% of energy as carbohydrate (138 g/1,000 kcal or 165 g/5,000 kJ) from a variety of sources;
- No more than 5% of total energy as alcohol, or two drinks daily, whichever is less;

- No more caffeine than the equivalent of four regular cups of coffee per day;
- A reduction in the sodium content of the Canadian diet; and
- Fluoridation of community water supplies containing less than 1 mg/L fluoride to that level.

These dietary guidelines are appropriate for the prevention of colorectal and other dietary-related cancers. In addition, there are two recommendations (19): a variety of green and yellow vegetables, tubers, citrus fruits, and whole grains and cereal should be eaten, and contamination of foods with carcinogens from any source (e.g., barbecuing) should be minimized.

The Epp framework strategies (creating healthy environments, reorienting health services, and increasing prevention, as described in Chapter One) can be applied to improving diets and reducing the burden of illness, in particular, the excessive intake of saturated fats. In encouraging healthy eating, for example, action should be directed to the community at large, involving the media and community organizations in promoting healthy-eating campaigns. Healthy food policies in schools can be introduced by healthy choices among cafeteria items. Individuals and families can receive educational material to promote healthy eating habits in home environments. In restaurants and supermarkets, labelling the content (especially fat) of grocery and menu items facilitates healthy choices at the point of purchase. Similar strategies can be implemented in workplaces and health care settings (18). Nutrition action should also include policy and regulatory changes to agricultural, marketing, and trade practices, so as to facilitate more widely available healthy choices of food.

The importance of the broader determinants of health have been recognized as crucial to the development of programs and policies to better the nutritional status of Canadians. *Nutrition for Health: An Agenda for Action* (20), which was published in 1996, describes a multisectoral collaborative vision that identifies the priorities that must be addressed to improve nutrition from the perspective of population health. Four strategic directions were identified:
- Reinforce healthy eating practices;
- Support nutritionally vulnerable populations;
- Continue to enhance the availability of foods that support healthy eating;
- Support nutrition research.

As well, the steering committee identified the need to collect data on important core indicators of population nutritional status. The indicators would systematically monitor important outcomes such as PYLL attributed to nutritional causes, determinant indicators such as estimated daily nutrient intakes of Canadians, and process indicators concerning the success of the intersectoral initiative.

2.   SPECIFIC DISEASES

2.1. CARDIOVASCULAR DISEASE (CVD)

Trends in Cardiovascular Disease

The most common forms of CVD are ischemic or coronary heart disease, particularly acute myocardial infractions ("heart attacks"), and cerebrovascular disease (stroke). Since the first national mortality statistics were published in 1921, CVD has been the leading cause of death in Canada, accounting for nearly half of all deaths each year. While CVD is still the leading cause of death, mortality rates are almost half those in 1969, having declined at a rate of about 2% per year. The CVD age-standardized mortality rates (ASMRs) per 100,000 population (standardized to the 1981 Canadian population) have shown a steady decline, which is more pronounced in men than in women. However, international comparisons indicate that ASMRs from cardiovascular disease in some countries are more favourable than in Canada, with consequent diminished burdens of premature death. In the early 1990s, Japan's ASMR for cardiovascular disease was 232 per 100,000 for males and 153.8 for females, and for France, 254 per 100,000 for males and 149 per 100,000 for females, compared to a rate of 307 per 100,000 for males and 239 per 100,000 for females in Canada. (All figures for international comparisons are standardized to European population). Unlike the ASMRs for cardiovascular disease, those for ischemic heart disease (IHD) gradually rose until the late 1960s, before declining rapidly in the early 1970s (21).

Mortality

Although CVD mortality rates have declined in recent times, the disease still poses a major burden. In 1995, the rate of death from CVD was 307 per 100,000 for men and 239 per 100,000 for women. In 1995, CVD accounted for 37% of deaths in Canada, of which IHD accounted for 21% (21). CVD is a broad term covering a number of diseases of the circulatory system. IHD and cerebrovascular disease (CBVD) accounted for 79,117 deaths in 1995, with IHD representing one quarter of all deaths. Incidence of CVD increases dramatically with age. Among those aged 35 to 44, CVD accounts for 16.1% of all deaths; the rates for those aged 45 to 54, 55 to 64, and 65 and over, are, 27%, 33.8% and 48% of all deaths respectively. The rates for women are almost half those of men, except for CBVD, where the rates are approximately equal until after age 85 when they are higher in women. The probability of a male under age 75 dying from an acute myocardial infarct is 10.2%; for a woman of the same age group 5.3%. This risk increases dramatically for females over 75, less so for males. Premature death from CVD before age 70 is the leading cause of potential life lost (294,000 years). There is an inverse relationship between socioeconomic class and incidence of CVD. The lower the socioeconomic level, the higher the incidence of cardiovascular disease. A general trend of higher to lower CVD rates from the eastern to western provinces exists. With 77% of all CVD deaths attributable to IHD and CBVD, these two manifestations have been the target of much research in the areas of public policy, screening for risk factors and clinical interventions.

Morbidity

In 1994/95, IHD and CBVD accounted for 6,522,117 million patient days in hospital. It is estimated that almost 10% of all visits to physicians each year are for cardiovascular disease. One half of these visits are related to the management of high blood pressure. As greater numbers of Canadians enter the 55 to 74 age group, it is anticipated that increases in coronary artery bypass grafting (CABG) and related procedures will occur. In 1994/95, there were 15,186 CABG operations and 16,933 angioplasties performed. Prescription drugs for management of cardiovascular disease now account for 12.8% of all prescriptions dispensed in Canada (21). The economic impact of cardiovascular disease is high, comprising 17% ($7.3 billion) of the direct costs of disease in Canada in 1995. Indirect costs, largely due to premature mortality and disability, are estimated at $12.3 billion annually; 20% of Canada Pension Plan disability payments were for CVDs, largely IHD. With this kind of impact, both social and economic, the burden of CVD deserves much attention from physicians and Canadians in general.

Risk Factors

The underlying cause of CVD is atherosclerosis. Contributing factors include smoking, high blood pressure, obesity, diabetes, lack of physical activity, high levels of dietary fat, elevated total cholesterol and low-density lipoprotein (LDL) cholesterol, and genes. Serum lipids are another risk factor. The majority of CVD deaths occur among people with moderately elevated blood cholesterol (5.2 to 6.2 mmol/L, or 200 to 240 mg/dL). A high LDL is associated with increased risk, as are high triglyceride levels. Almost half of adult Canadians (45% of males and 43% of females) fall into the range for moderately elevated cholesterol, while 18% of males and 16% of women have blood cholesterol levels above 6.2 mmol/L (240 mg/dL). For Canadians, 40% of men and 32% of women have LDL above 3.4 mmol/L, 15% have triglyceride levels above 2.3 mmol/L, and 8% have HDL-cholesterol levels below 0.9 mmol/L. These cut-off points for lipid levels have been established by the Canadian Consensus Conference on Cholesterol (22). The role of apolipoproteins, especially apoprotein b, in predisposing genetically to cardiovascular disease is currently under study.

The prevalence of these risk factors throughout the Canadian population varies among age, sex, social class, regions, and cultural groups. The role of psychosocial variables such as personality type, life stress, social support, education, and socioeconomic status has been studied in the development of coronary heart disease. According to Greenwood et al. (23), longer-term psychosocial stresses and lack of support may be influential in the development of coronary heart disease in the first place, but the magnitude of these effects remain unreliably defined. It appears that stress may have less impact than the lack of social support. People with inadequate social support are at higher risk of coronary heart disease.

Prevention

Although age and sex cannot be altered, many other CVD risk factors are amenable to preventive health practices. The following facts should be noted:

- 25% of men and 18% of women have high blood pressure (defined as systolic blood pressures above 140 mm/Hg or a diastolic blood pressure of greater than 90 mm/hg);
- 38% of Canadian consider themselves physically inactive;
- 4-5% of the population are diabetic;
- 31% of the population report a body mass index greater than 27;
- 75% of Canadians have one or more risk factors for cardiovascular disease;
- 34% of men aged 45 to 54 and 37% of women aged 65 to 74 have two or more risk factors for cardiovascular disease (21).

2.1.1. Community-Wide Approaches to Heart Health

The decline in cardiovascular mortality in Canada has been attributed, in part, to the reduction in the prevalence of smoking, reduced consumption of dietary fat, improved detection and management of hypertension, as well as improved surgical approaches to treatment of symptomatic heart disease. The current widespread prevalence of risk factors is, however, still of concern. Many Canadians, particularly those over 55, have not been persuaded to adopt a "healthy" lifestyle that includes regular check-ups for CVD risk factors, as well as attention to diet, physical exercise, and tobacco-use reduction. Physicians have played a less than optimal role in identifying and reducing risk factors through regular screening of individuals for high blood pressure and smoking cessation or dietary counselling. This situation has led to an expressed need for a public health strategy to reduce CVD mortality in Canada.

Regular screening for high blood pressure should become part of the periodic health examination for adults. Readers, however, are advised to refer to a number of recent documents that outline recommendations and issues related to clinical preventive services, particularly in relation to screening for elevated cholesterol (24, 25). Although there is an established relationship between high total cholesterol levels in populations and CVD mortality, programs for cholesterol screening do not meet the criteria for the screening program described in Chapter Two. The cholesterol screening test has poor sensitivity and specificity, as well, for most individuals it has a low predictive value. In the Framingham study (26), the level of cholesterol in the individual did not discriminate between those who would subsequently develop coronary heart disease and those who did not. Additionally, the lack of feasibility and efficiency of mass screening has been presented as a strong argument against the initial recommendation that, as resources permit, determination of lipid risk factors should become part of the routine health examination. The total cost of implementing such a program in the first year, given a prevalence of 53.5% for moderate- and high-risk cholesterol elevations among symptom-free Canadians, was estimated at approximately $500 million. Although these estimates are likely too high, given the prevalence of moderate hypercholesteraemia found in the provincial heart health surveys, they provide an order of magnitude of the costs for laboratory tests and physician visits in a mass screening program. The

Ontario Ministry of Health and the Ontario Medical Association recommended a high-risk strategy of detection and treatment of those already with cardiovascular symptoms or risk factors coupled with encouragement of community-wide dietary and lifestyle changes, given the diminishing returns of widespread screening. The Canadian Consensus Conference on Cholesterol (22) recommends screening for blood cholesterol for:

- Patients known to have coronary heart disease;
- Patients with a family history of hyperlipidaemia or early onset of coronary heart disease (heart attack in a parent, grandparent, brother, or sister before age 60 years);
- Patients with hypertension, diabetes mellitus, renal failure, or obesity, especially abdominal obesity.

It should be noted that two large clinical trials have demonstrated the benefit of drug treatment in reducing total serum cholesterol, or its sub fractions, to prevent or delay the onset of coronary heart disease in middle-aged men with very high total cholesterol levels. A note of caution, however: in both single and multiple risk-factor reduction trials, cardiovascular mortality has been reduced, but overall mortality has, in fact, been higher in those subjects in whom preventive interventions were given (25).

Community-based models for primary (and secondary) prevention of heart disease, utilizing many of the health promotion strategies described in Chapter One, have been promulgated, following the demonstration of their effectiveness for reducing cardiovascular risk in populations in a number of studies. Some limitations in evaluating community effectiveness mentioned in Chapter Two should be borne in mind.

These models used in North Karelia, Finland, and the Stanford Five-City Study (27-29) have provided the basis for the Canadian Heart Health Initiative (CHHI) currently undertaken by Health Canada in partnership with the provinces and the Heart and Stroke Foundation of Canada (30). This initiative has four phases: surveys of cardiovascular disease risk factors in all ten provinces and the development of a national database on cardiovascular risk factors; the implementation of provincial heart health demonstration program; evaluation of the demonstration heart health programs; and diffusion of the findings and interventions to communities across Canada.

The initiatives are being coordinated by departments of public health, due to their population-based (rather than high-risk) approach. They recognize the importance of social and other environmental changes that will make healthy choices easier under the rubric of the Epp health promotion framework, the appropriate referral of those detected with risk factors for follow-up, and building community-based partnerships. The initiatives are multidisciplinary, intersectoral, and part of broader health promotion programs involving multiple strategies at multiple sites. The Declaration on Heart Health (31) issued at the International Heart Health Conference in Victoria, British Columbia, in May 1992, was intended to give a sense of urgency to the prevention and control of the most important cause of death in most of the world's countries. The Declaration affirmed that effective, widely tested methods to prevent cardiovascular disease exist, and called for their translation into action that incorporates heart health into daily life. The call to initiate and support prevention directed at the entire population is made to many segments of society: health; education; social science professionals and their associations; government agencies concerned with health, education, trade, commerce and agriculture; the private sector; community health coalitions; voluntary organizations; employers; and the media. Community-based population-wide approaches, backed by research, can be expected to reduce the prevalence of risk factors for cardiovascular disease, and trends in prevalence of some risk factors, such as smoking, are encouraging. Actions to improve diet by fat reduction and to encourage active lifestyles are important strategies that need more attention.

2.2. CANCER

Trends in Cancer

Cancer is the second leading cause of death in the adult population and fourth among children. The following general trends have been observed for cancer in Canada (2).

- Cancers with stable incidence and mortality rates, including oropharyngeal cancer in males and females and leukaemia in males and females;
- Cancers where both incidence and mortality rates have been increasing, including lung cancer in females and melanoma and prostate cancers in males. Prostate cancer has risen especially sharply since 1989 with increase testing for prostate-specific antigen but mortality rates rose at a much slower rate and stabilized in the 1990s;
- Cancers where both incidence and mortality rates have decreased, including stomach and bladder cancer in both males and females, and cervical cancer in women;
- Cancers with stable or increasing incidence rates and decreasing mortality rates, including breast cancer in females, testicular cancer in males, and Hodgkin's disease in both sexes.

Mortality

In 1997, an estimated 130,800 new cases of cancer were diagnosed and 60,700 deaths occurred from cancer. Cancer deaths constituted 27% of all deaths for 1994 (2). In 1994, cancer was the leading cause of PYLL, followed closely by heart disease; an estimated 891,000 potential years of life were lost to cancer. More than one in three Canadians will develop some form of cancer in their lifetime. Up until the age of 55 years, cancer incidence and mortality are about equal in both males and females, and increases gradually. After 55 years of age, both male and female rates begin to rise at a faster rate; however, the male rate increases more sharply.

Overall, on the basis of 1993 estimates, a man had a 1 in 2.4 chance of developing cancer over a lifetime and a 1 in 3.7 lifetime chance of dying from cancer. For men, the three most common cancers are prostate, lung, and colorectal. Men have a lifetime probability of 1 in 8.6 of developing prostate cancer, 1 in 10.5 of developing lung cancer, and 1 in 15.4 of developing colorectal cancer. In 1996, a man had an estimated risk of dying of lung cancer of 1 in 11.8, for prostate cancer 1 in 26.7, and of colorectal cancer 1 in 36.2.

Based on 1993 estimates, women had a 1 in 2.7 chance of developing cancer and a 1 in 4.5 chance of dying of cancer. The three leading cancers in terms of incidence for women were breast, colorectal, and lung. Women have a lifetime probability of 1 in 8.9 of developing breast cancer, 1 in 16.1 of developing colorectal cancer, and 1 in 21.4 of developing lung cancer. The mortality risk for women for lung cancer is 1 in 23.9, for breast cancer 1 in 25.3, and for colorectal cancer 1 in 36.5.

Morbidity

Cancer was responsible for 5% of the total 3.6 million hospitalizations in 1994/95, and 8% of the total hospital days; the average length of hospitalization (18 days) was one week longer than the overall average length of stay. Cancer was the fourth most costly component of health care in 1993, with $3.2 billion in direct costs. If the ratio of direct costs to indirect costs remains the same as it was in 1986, indirect costs would exceed $13 billion. This amount indicates the enormous burden on society.

A prognostic indicator for cancer is the ratio of deaths to cases. Overall, excluding non-melanoma skin cancer, the ratio was 51% (from estimated figures for Canada in 1992). Prognosis for individual cancers varies from poor (ratios greater than 66% for lung, stomach, pancreas, and brain cancers), to fair (ratios 33% to 66% for colorectal, lymphoma, kidney, leukaemia, ovarian cancers), to very good (ratios less than 33% for breast, prostate, bladder, oral, melanoma, uterus, cervical, and testicular cancers). There has been a steady decline in mortality for childhood cancers due to improved treatment of lymphoma and leukaemia. Despite the advances and the better outlook for some cancers, the prognosis overall remains unfavourable and emphasis must be on prevention and care rather than cure.

Risk Factors

The most common causes of cancer deaths in Canada are outlined in Table 5.2 in Chapter Five. While a few cancers may be associated with inherited genetic factors (e.g., polyposis of the colon and the inherited form of retinoblastoma), environmental factors such as water and air quality, diet, and lifestyle are considered important determinants; the latter two are the most important. Smoking and alcohol are two lifestyle habits that play major roles in a number of non-occupational cancers for which multiple factors may be responsible. Variations in cancer rates in immigrants indicate possible environmental effects in the development of some neoplasms. Proportional mortality rates for cancer of the stomach and lung in Ontario show a gradient for different generations of immigrants from the same country. The highest rates are for the immigrants, intermediate for the first generation, and lowest for the second generation. Some change in lifestyle, dietary patterns or other environmental exposure may be responsible for the observed shift in rates. Exposures to high concentrations of certain chemicals in the occupational environment are associated with cancer. For example, inhalation of asbestos and chromite ore is associated with cancer of the lung, and benzidine and beta-naphthylamine with bladder cancer (see Chapter Ten).

2.2.1. General Framework for Cancer Control

An excellent planning framework for cancer control strategies in Canada has been contributed by Miller (19). On the basis of this, specific strategies for leading cancer sites are proposed (see Table 7.1). This framework could also be usefully applied to control of other chronic diseases. The steps are the following:

- *Assess the current situation:* Determine the relative importance of cancer to other diseases, determine the relative importance of different cancer sites, identify differences between provinces in the range of indicators, as well as differences between Canada and other countries, and determine the availability of resources for cancer control. Indicators may include the number of cancer cases diagnosed (incidence), number of deaths from cancer, survival, sex ratio, cumulative incidence, premature mortality, and trends.
- *Set objectives for cancer control:* Reduce morbidity from cancer, reduce mortality from cancer, and improve the quality of life of cancer patients.
- *Evaluate possible strategies.*
- *Set priorities using quantitative assessments:* Determine the potential effectiveness of different strategies, determine the potential cost of different strategies, determine the cost effectiveness of all different and competing strategies, modify the priority for action on the basis of other considerations, and monitor trends in disease to evaluate effectiveness of strategies.

2.2.2. Site-Specific Cancer Control

Since the aetiology of most cancers is unknown, emphasis on secondary and tertiary prevention is more appropriate at present, and such prevention is highly developed for certain cancers. The exception is primary prevention against smoking. The following sections discuss specific types of cancer.

Lung Cancer

Based on all the indicators previously described, lung cancer is the number-one priority. It accounted for 26% of the PYLL attributed to cancer. However, since the mid 1980s incidence and mortality rates for lung cancer in men have levelled off and shown signs of decline, although incidence and mortality rates in women have steadily climbed.

Ninety per cent of lung cancer in males, and almost the same proportion in females, is related to smoking. Passive exposure to smoke almost certainly increases the risk of lung cancer and is likely the second leading cause of lung cancer.

Lung cancer is also caused by radon, and the actual risk from exposure to radon in homes is under study, although it has been identified in less than 1% of Canadian homes (see Chapter Nine). Occupational exposures to asbestos and radiation in hard rock mining increase the risk of lung cancer. Proposed methods of early detection (such as sputum cytology, frequent chest X-rays) do not reduce mortality. No more than 10% of cases with lung cancer are cured; this does not appear likely to improve.

Table 7.1:   **Estimates of Potential Effects of Prevention or Early Detection on Cancer**

Cancer Site	Action	Incidence reduction	
		PAR (a) (%)	Potentially preventable (%)
Lung	Eliminate smoking Reduce occupational exposure to carcinogens	90	60
Colorectal	Reduce fat and increase vegetable consumption	60	77
Breast	Reduce fat and increase vegetable consumption Reduce obesity (postmenopausal women) Screen women aged 50 to 69	27	70
Prostate	Reduce fat consumption	20	78
Lymphoma	Reduce exposure to herbicides and pesticides	?	86
Bladder	Eliminate smoking and reduce dietary cholesterol Reduce occupational exposure to carcinogens	60	73
Body of the uterus	Reduce obesity Protective effect of oral contraceptives (ages 20-54)	30	82
Stomach	Reduce nitrite in cured meats and salt-preserved foods, and increase fruit and vegetable consumption	80	52
Leukemia	Reduce exposure to radiation and benzene	?	70
Oral, etc.	Eliminate smoking and reduce alcohol consumption Increase fruit and vegetable consumption	80	68
Pancreas	Eliminate smoking Reduce sugar and increase vegetable consumption	40	64
Melanoma of the skin	Reduce unprotected exposure to sunlight	20	77
Kidney	Eliminate smoking Reduce fat consumption	40	67
Brain	Reduce occupational exposure to carcinogens	?	70
Ovary	Reduce fat consumption Protective effect of oral contraceptives (ages 20-54)	30	53
Cervix	Eliminate smoking Encourage use of barrier contraceptives Screen women aged 20 to 69	23	62

(a) PAR = Population Attributable Risk. Estimates are for males, except for breast, body of uterus, ovarian, and cervical cancer.
(b) Indicates effect is on mortality, not incidence.
(?) Signifies no estimate of effect is available.

Sources: Reproduced from Miller, A. B., *Planning Cancer Control Strategies*, Chronic Disease in Canada 13(1): S36, 1992.

Colorectal Cancer

Diet, particularly saturated fat intake as well as beer drinking, has been linked to increased risk for colorectal cancer. Consumption of fresh fruits and vegetables may have a protective effect. Miller suggests that 60% or more of colorectal cancer can be prevented through dietary modification. There is no firm evidence recommending early detection by the faecal occult blood test for the general population. Those with a family history of polyposis should be under clinical surveillance.

Breast Cancer

Breast cancer is the leading cause of premature mortality from cancer in females and a little over one third of women with breast cancer die of it. Risk factors that are largely non-preventable and contribute to 17% of breast cancer include the age at first childbirth, parity (the number of stillbirths compared to live births), age at menarche, age at menopause, and occurrence of a surgical procedure that results in artificial menopause; genetic predisposition is also a factor. The presence of BRCA genes account for a small but significant proportion of inherited breast cancers.

With regard to controllable risk factors, obesity is implicated in post-menopausal breast cancer. Dietary fat makes a modest contribution to breast cancer (32), even though it may have a major impact on morbidity. Thus, prudent population-based approaches to improving nutrition should follow the guidelines similar to those for colorectal cancer and ischemic heart disease. Alcohol has been reported as a risk factor for breast cancer in a number of studies, and sensible use is encouraged.

Prolonged course of estrogens at the time of menopause increases risk of breast cancer. For oral contraceptives, however, an overall cost-benefit analysis indicates that the benefits likely outweigh the risks.

Among women aged 50 to 70, use of mammography between one and three years has resulted in early detection of breast cancer and reduced mortality; the cost effectiveness compares favourably with other medical procedures. According to the National Breast Screening Study (33), there was no benefit in reduced mortality from screening programs in women aged 40 to 49, although more tumours were detected. Nonetheless, a group co-sponsored by Health and Welfare Canada, the Canadian Cancer Society, and the National Cancer Institute of Canada has recommended mass screening programs be undertaken according to provincial policies (34). Nova Scotia, Ontario, Saskatchewan, and Alberta, have programs in place, mostly for women 50 and over; the program in British Columbia includes women aged 40 to 49. The use of a genetic screening test is under consideration, but requires systematic evaluation (35). The Canadian Breast Cancer Initiative recently issued *Clinical Practice Guidelines for the Care and Treatment of Breast Cancer,* which discuss the modalities of treatment regimes (36).

Prostate Cancer

In the 1990s, prostate cancer surpassed lung cancer as the most commonly diagnosed cancer among men, and now the second leading cause of death among men. It is not, however, a major cause of premature cancer deaths, ranking ninth in PYLL. Dietary fat is considered to play some causative role despite inconsistent evidence; hence, dietary fat reduction can be recommended. Hormonal treatment reduces symptoms and appears to prolong life.

Early detection of prostate cancer is a controversial subject. The present available methods of screening are digital rectal examination (DRE), transrectal prostatic ultra-sonography (TRUS), and serology for prostate-specific antigen (PSA). The Canadian Task Force on Periodic Health Examinations recommends DRE in men over age 40 but does not recommend PSA screening (37). Studies have shown that a substantial number of Canadian men receive screening with PSA testing despite no clear evidence as to its benefit. Part of the increase in the incidence of prostate cancer is likely attributable to more widespread use of PSA testing.

Leukaemia

These are a heterogeneous group and represent the leading cancers in children. Radiation, occupational exposure to benzene, and viruses (HTLV-I and II) are known causes. However, it is unlikely that control of currently known causes would prevent more than a fraction of these diseases.

Cancer of the Cervix

Cancer of the cervix now ranks only 16th for number of cases and deaths in Canada and 14th in terms of premature mortality, thanks to Pap test screening programs. Cancer of the cervix is strongly associated with early age at first intercourse, multiple sex partners, and smoking. There is evidence to suggest that human papilloma virus (HPV) infections of the cervix may cause cervical cancer; however, epidemiological evidence is not as yet confirmatory. A number of reviews have indicated that screening is effective in reducing incidence and mortality. However, more attention is necessary in relation to the appropriateness of screening and the organizational aspects, particularly quality assurance (38). Some groups, such as female Aboriginal people, have not benefited. Canadian programs lack two of the elements of a screening program considered essential: measures to ensure high coverage and attendance, such as a personal letter of invitation, and identification of individual women in the target population for screening. Current recommendations for the frequency of screening advises that all women over 18 who have had sexual intercourse should be encouraged to enter a cervical screening program and be re-screened every three years until age 69. Women over age 69 who have had normal cytology and at least two satisfactory smears in the previous nine years can discontinue the program. In 1995, comprehensive programs for cervical cancer control were shown to be lacking across the country except in two provinces. A workshop entitled *Interchange '95: A Canadian Forum to Collaborate on Cervical Cancer Screening Program Implementation* advocated that a cervical cancer prevention network be established in order to facilitate the development and implementation of provincial programs to ensure optimal screening (39); most provinces have submitted plans to their respective ministries of health. Safer sex practices can be recommended in general.

2.3. RESPIRATORY DISEASES

Mortality

In 1994, non-cancer respiratory diseases were the third leading identified cause of death accounting for 9% of deaths in Canada (16.3% including cancers of the respiratory tract). The overall respiratory disease death rate per 100,000 population was 65 in 1993 (40). There is a J-shaped curve to the age-specific mortality rates for both sexes with mortality higher in the very young and very old age groups. With the exception of asthma, over 60% of deaths attributed to lung cancer, pneumonia, tuberculosis, and chronic obstructive pulmonary disease occur in those over age 65.

Morbidity

Common respiratory diseases include asthma, chronic bronchitis, emphysema, and pneumonia. In Canada, the incidence, prevalence, hospitalization, and mortality rates for asthma have increased over the past two decades. The causes of these increases remain under study. The prevalence of asthma decreases with age. The highest self-reported prevalence is in young adults. The rate of hospital separations for asthma in those under age 34 tripled from 100 per 100,000 to over 300 per 100,000 in 1991, possibly due to environmental factors. More than 1 million Canadians suffer from asthma. Between 1985 and 1990, there was a 38% increase in the number of prescriptions for airway drugs (40). The economic costs in Canada in 1990 were estimated to be between $508 and $648 million. Direct costs were estimated at $306 million, of which the largest proportion related to drug expenditures ($124 million) (41).

Risk Factors

Important factors influencing respiratory disease mortality rates include smoking (active and passive), respiratory pathogens (see Chapter Eight), and indoor-outdoor air pollution (see Chapter Nine). Although smoking is considered to be an important risk factor for frequency and severity of respiratory illness, air pollution levels in a number of Canadian communities have also been found to affect hospital admissions for respiratory diseases (42, 43).

Important particulate matters are oxidants and nitrogen oxides; secondhand smoke also contributes to the level of nitrogen oxides in closed environments. While both pollutants are associated with increased admission rates for upper respiratory tract infections, bronchitis appears to be related to nitrogen oxides. Increased respiratory cancer rates have been observed in the city of Hamilton, Ontario, coincident with accelerated steel production over a 30-year period. Furthermore, the numbers affected decreased as residence became more distant from the steel plants.

Pollutants interact, and their combined effect on disease may be either additive or multiplicative (smoking and asbestos combined has a multiplicative effect). Keeping individual pollutant levels in the environment within accepted limits is not enough, since the combined effects of such pollutants may be producing disease. Also, the permitted limits may not be adhered to throughout the year. Yassi and Friesen (44) observed that oxidant levels in major Canadian cities were often over the limits in 1988.

Prevention

Approaches to prevention and cessation of smoking are discussed in the section on substance abuse. Health promotion in relation to air pollution has been discussed in Chapter Nine. More research is needed into pollutants and their effects, alone and combined, on human health. Primary prevention in this area is not as straightforward as it appears.

2.4. DIABETES

There are two types of diabetes: type 1 also known as insulin-dependent diabetes, which occurs mainly at young age; and type 2 also known as adult or maturity onset diabetes, which occurs in the older population. Type 2 diabetes is the most common, affecting up to 90% of all people with diabetes. With increases in the aging population, obesity, and sedentary lifestyle, mortality and morbidity due to diabetes have become an important health problem.

Mortality

In 1995, there were 5,496 deaths for which diabetes was certified as the underlying cause of death. This ranks diabetes as being the seventh leading cause of death in Canada. The total number of deaths due to diabetes has increased since 1950.

Morbidity

Diabetes is generally diagnosed and treated in physicians' offices, from which data collection is difficult. Therefore, hospitalization records only capture people with more severe diabetes. Prevalence data are available from national surveys such as Heart Health (1986-1992), the General Social Survey (1985, 1991), and in 1994 the National Population Health Survey (NPHS), which are discussed in Chapters Three and Four.

The incidence of type 1 diabetes ranges from 9 to 25 per 100,000 people under age 14. Incidence increases with age through childhood and adolescence but decreases during adulthood.

The most recent survey data are from the NPHS, which showed a prevalence of 3.0% mostly type 2 diabetes. Diabetes affects males and females equally. The prevalence increased with age such that the rate in those over 65 was over three times as high (over 10%) as the rate in those aged 35 to 64. In 1993, there were approximately 36,000 hospital separations and over 500,000 hospital days annually due to diabetes in Canada. The NPHS indicated that approximately 175,000 Canadians use insulin to control diabetes, 400,000 use oral medication. The present economic burden of diabetes was estimated at $1.1 billion dollars annually in 1993.

Risk Factor

Race and ethnicity are accepted risk factors for type 1 diabetes. Comparisons between countries facilitated by the World Health Organization have found the highest rates in Scandinavia, intermediate rates in Canada and the United States and low rates in Japan or Tanzania.

Known risk factors for type 2 diabetes include age, family history, obesity, physical inactivity, and ethnicity. The prevalence of type 2 diabetes increases rapidly with age; usual onset is after age 40. Increased risk of diabetes with a positive family history of diabetes is probably due to genetic and environmental factors. Gender is not a risk factor for type 2 diabetes. Obesity is a well-recognized risk factor when measured as the level of obesity, the duration of obesity, and the body-fat distribution. The prevalence of diabetes in those with an acceptable weight (Body Mass Index or BMI 20 to 24) was 1.2% compared to a prevalence of 4.0% in those classified as overweight (BMI 28 or over). Those with some excess weight (BMI 25 to 27) had a prevalence of 1.9%. Physical inactivity is a known risk factor. Prevalence rates were 2.0%, 2.6%, and 3.5% for those with active, moderately active, and inactive physical activity levels respectively.

Ethnicity has been accepted as an independent risk factor as studies of high-prevalence populations have found increased risk after controlling for all other known risk factors. There is considerable evidence that the prevalence of diabetes is much higher among Aboriginal Canadians compared to the general population. The 1991 Aboriginal Peoples Survey (45) gave a prevalence of 6.1%. This was not age-standardized, so the standardized rate is likely higher due to the young Aboriginal population distribution. The increased prevalence of diabetes was most notable in the younger age groups. For those between age 30 and 39, the Aboriginal rate of diabetes was 5%; in the NPHS it was less than 1% in the same age group. There is evidence of a decrease in prevalence as one travels north. This may be due to a more traditional diet and activity pattern in more isolated communities.

Prevention

The two main modifiable risk factors for type 2 diabetes are obesity and physical activity. Diabetes increases as physical activity decreases. The strategies needed are related to reduce obesity through healthy diets and living an active life. *Canada's Physical Activity Guide to Healthy, Active Living* provides guidelines on how to achieve health benefits by being physically active (46).

2.5. CONGENITAL AND GENETIC DISEASES

Mortality

Success in the prevention and treatment of childhood infectious diseases has reduced infant mortality rates to a level where congenital anomalies are now the second leading cause of death in infants (30% of all infant deaths). Among those aged 1 to 14 years, it is the third leading cause of death (11.5% of all deaths). The most common malformations leading to infant death were due to defects of the heart and circulatory system. Approximately 3% of newborn children have a serious congenital anomaly. Congenital heart defects are the most common congenital anomalies with an birth prevalence rate of 80 to 100 per 10,000 live births. The birth prevalence rate per 10,000 births in Ontario for the most common congenital anomalies were as follows: 11.5 for cleft lip or palate, 9.7 for hypospadias/epispadias, 8.3 for spina bifida, 6.5 for anencephaly, 4.6 for Down's syndrome, and 4.2 for hydrocephalus (47).

Risk Factors

Aetiological factors for malformations include hereditary or familial tendencies, and non-genetic factors such as maternal diabetes mellitus, anticonvulsant drug use during pregnancy, and maternal infection with herpes, syphilis, rubella, toxoplasmosis, or cytomegalovirus. Other aetiological factors associated with congenital anomalies are nutritional deficiencies (such as folic acid deficiency), exposure to external environmental agents (4), and those related to personal lifestyles (49).

Prevention

There are now more than 200 known genetic and metabolic disorders. Many, but by no means all, of these can be diagnosed prenatally. Some can cause mental retardation, for example, phenylketonuria. Many are preventable with proper counselling in susceptible populations. Certain genetic disorders have high frequencies in various ethnic groups; thalassaemia, for example, occurs once in every 25 Italian births, Tay-Sachs disease affects about one in every 1,000 births to Ashkenazi Jews, and phenylketonuria has an incidence of 1 in 10,000 live Caucasian births. Five per cent of Caucasians are carriers for cystic fibrosis. Selective screening and genetic counselling in susceptible populations are probably the most appropriate forms of primary prevention.

A number of prenatal screening methods detect congenital malformations or chromosomal abnormalities. They are the screening of maternal serum for alpha fetoprotein, human chorionic gonadotropin, and unconjugated oestriol (the triple screen for Down's syndrome and neural tube defects), chorionic villus sampling (CVS), amniocentesis, fetoscopy, and ultrasound examination. Chorionic villus sampling provides the earliest available fetal screen at 8 to 12 weeks; however, it requires considerable technical skill. Termination of pregnancy at this early stage (first trimester) is much easier for the woman. Amniocentesis, the most widely used method, is usually done at 15 to 16 weeks; it is associated with a less than 1% risk of miscarriage. Fetoscopy can be used to check for fetal malformations at 17 to 18 weeks, during which it is possible to obtain a blood sample. The final method is ultrasonography (ultrasound examination). Although this method requires a high level of skill to do well and can only identify structural abnormalities, it offers the dual advantages of being non-invasive and giving immediate results. Neonatal screening for metabolic disorders such as phenylketonuria and hypothyroidism are widely used.

Research conducted by the Royal Commission on New Reproductive Technologies showed that 5% of prenatal diagnostic tests indicated that the fetus had a serious congenital anomaly or genetic disease. In this subset, 80% of women and couples chose to terminate the pregnancy (47).

The Royal Commission comprehensively reviewed the scientific, legal, and ethical issues concerning reproductive technology and prenatal diagnosis and made a set of recommendations specifically concerning prenatal diagnosis and screening. Some have argued that the development of reproductive technologies represents a form of eugenics, in that people with potential disabilities will be screened out of the population. They argue that this is a means of sidestepping the issues of making life tolerable in society for those with disabilities. The Royal Commission recommended that prenatal diagnosis be done with adequate counselling, informed parents, and health care providers, and that people representing those with disabilities be included in the development of appropriate counselling materials. As the complete sequencing of the human genome draws near, the recommendations of the Royal Commission assume great importance, as the increase in prenatal diagnostic tests will likely increase exponentially (47).

The Canadian Task Force on the Periodic Health Examination reviewed the triple screening process for detecting Down's syndrome. It stated that there is fair evidence to offer triple-marker screening as part of a comprehensive prenatal program to women under the age of 35. There is fair evidence to offer amniocentesis or CVS to women 35 years or older and to those with a history of a Down's syndrome fetus or of a chromosome 21 abnormality (50).

Randomized control trials have demonstrated that periconceptual ingestion of at least 0.6 mg daily of folic acid is effective in reducing the rate of neural tube defects. This evidence has led to the recommendation that all women who may become pregnant supplement their diet with folic acid. A population-based strategy has been advocated that would supplement all grain products with sufficient folic acid to ensure that those who consume the recommended daily allowance of grain products would get sufficient folic acid. The strategy of food supplementation remains controversial as the addition of folic acid also raises the risk of masking B12 deficiency in the elderly. Untreated B12 deficiency is associated with irreversible neurological damage (51).

2.6. ARTHRITIS AND CHRONIC PAIN

Arthritis

Arthritis is the most frequently reported cause of physical disability in the Canadian population. The term incorporates a set of diverse but related conditions, including osteoarthritis, rheumatoid arthritis, scleroderma, and fibromyalgia. Osteoarthritis affects 10% of the population and the prevalence increases with age. Rheumatoid arthritis affects 1 in 100 Canadians. Long-term disability occurs more frequently from arthritis (2.3% of Canadians) than from circulatory or respiratory diseases. Arthritis chiefly causes morbidity and a reduction in the quality of life. Of those with arthritis, 90% report difficulty with mobility and 66% report having trouble with or being unable to climb stairs. Seventy per cent of those with arthritis report being moderately to severely disabled, and that they depend on others for care and assistance. Twenty per cent of adult Canadians with arthritis are unable to travel long distances because of their condition.

Arthritic conditions are a common cause of health service utilization. In 1990, more than 450,000 Canadians consulted health care professionals because of their condition. Medications to control the symptoms of arthritis are the third most prescribed category of medication and the second most commonly purchased non prescription medication. In 1992, 29 million prescriptions were written for arthritis medications. In 1986, the overall costs of arthritis were $5 billion; 22% or $1.1 billion were due to direct costs and 78% or $3.9 billion were due to indirect costs. With the population structure of Canada shifting towards the aged, the significance of arthritis as a public health problem will increase (52, 53).

Chronic Pain

The 1994/95 National Population Health Survey indicated that 3.9 million adults experienced chronic pain or discomfort due to physical conditions such as arthritis, injury, or migraine. The rates were higher at each age in women than men (20% versus 15%) and the incidence of chronic pain increases with age in both sexes. The highest rates are reported among those age 75, with 37% of women and 31% of men reporting chronic pain. Those reporting chronic pain report high usage of analgesics, narcotics and sedative/hypnotics, as well as high rates of health service utilization. Those reporting chronic pain average 13 physician contacts per year compared to 4 for those not reporting chronic pain (54).

2.7. MENTAL HEALTH

Psychiatric illness is responsible for a large and measurable burden of illness in the Canadian population. Affective disorders, such as depression, and psychotic disorders, such as schizophrenia, are common in the population. It is estimated that the point prevalence for depression is 5% of the adult population of Canada at any given time, and that 20-30% of the population has some symptoms of depression; 15-30% of adult men and women suffer from at least one episode of major depression in their life (55). Women are twice as likely as men to suffer from depression. Research indicates that most people, regardless of economic status, have a poor understanding about the symptoms of and treatment for depression. The cause of depression is multifactorial, representing an interplay of genetic and biological factors, including neurotransmitters and seasonal effects, cognitive and psychosocial factors, and environmental factors. The social and economic consequences of depression are immense. Depression leads to disruption of family, work, and social relationships. The most severe outcome of depression, namely suicide, is one of the leading causes of potential years of life lost. Depression is one of the most common causes of work absences.

Since the 1980s the hospital separation rates for psychiatric illness have declined, reflecting a trend to the community management of mental illness. Separation rates in general hospitals fell from 630 per 100,000 in 1982/83 to 598 per 100,000 in 1993/94 (see Chapter Five). This trend was also noted in psychiatric hospitals, where the rates fell from 116 per 100,000 to 94 per 100,000 in the same period. However, during this period, the average length of stay in general hospitals increased from 27 days in 1982/83 to 33 days in 1993/94. In 1994, the leading causes of hospitalization to psychiatric hospitals were affective psychosis for females (26%) and schizophrenia for males (33%). These two diagnoses were also the leading causes of admission to general hospitals (16% for schizophrenia for males and 23% for affective psychosis for females) (56).

Stress

Stress is a ubiquitous feature of modern life. It is part of a larger set of psychological factors that may contribute to illness. Psychological factors include internal factors such as personality and attitudes and reactions to events, and external factors, such as social supports and employment. Stress can be broadly defined as the psychic or physiologic disequilibrium caused by some event. Stress has been linked to increased risk from cardiovascular disease, is considered a predisposing factor for depression, and is linked to decreased work performance.

Twenty-six per cent of Canadians reported high chronic stress. Women are more likely than men to report being stressed (29% versus 23%). Women aged 20 to 24 are most likely to report being highly stressed (39%), compared to men over 75 who are least likely to report being highly stressed (6%). Stress levels decline with age, and well-educated persons tend to report lower stress levels than those with less education (57).

Stress prevention consists in identifying stressors and finding ways of organizing life to reduce demands. Positive guided imagery, relaxation tapes, meditation and exercise have been reported to give benefit. There are no large controlled trials evaluating stress reduction modalities.

3.   INJURIES

Mortality

Injuries are the leading cause of death during the first half of the human life span, and second to cancer as a leading cause of PYLL. In terms of economic burden, they are among the top four, with indirect costs as high as for cardiovascular disease. Injuries are the leading cause of death of children under age five, school-aged children, and young adults. In Canada, six children are killed every day as a result of injury. From the age of 1 to 24, injury is responsible for 63% of all deaths. The causes in younger children are falls at home — particularly in the living room from couches onto coffee tables and "roughhousing" — poisoning, and motor vehicle injuries as a passenger or pedestrian. For school-aged children, bicycle injuries are responsible for 14% of injury-related deaths; three quarters involve head injury. Falls are also an important cause of injury in the elderly, especially fractured neck of femur in elderly women. The leading causes of death in Aboriginals are intentional and non-intentional injury, the latter most frequently due to boating injuries, drowning and poisoning; thirty-five per cent of deaths in Aboriginals are due to violence. Occupational injuries are responsible for 96% of workers' compensation costs. Back complaints represent 15% of these injuries.

Morbidity

In 1993, approximately 18% of the Canadian population over age 15 reported having at least one injury in the previous year. Injuries were second only to cardiovascular diseases in total costs to society in 1993, accounting for $7 billion in direct health care expenditures (58). Pensions and benefits made up over half (57%) of the total direct costs, more than any other category. Motor vehicle injuries accounted for 27% of incidents reported in 1993; 54% resulted in financial loss. Injuries from sports or leisure activities were the next most frequent (26%) and largely occurred among males aged 15 to 34. These were followed by work-related injuries (21%) and injuries in or around the home (14%), frequently falls. Injuries are classified as **non-intentional** (previously termed as accidents), and **intentional** (predominantly homicide and suicide). Injury rates tend to be higher in the western provinces. The injury rate in 1993 was 223 per 1,000 persons. The rate was highest among males aged 15 to 24 (514/1,000), and at all ages men had higher rates than women (58).

An injury surveillance system involving 13 reporting hospitals was established in 1990. The Children's Hospital Injury Research and Prevention Project obtains information on the nature and circumstances related to injuries. Deaths from injury are only the tip of the iceberg in relation to their total impact. It is estimated that for every death there are 45 injuries that involve hospital admission, 1,300 visits to the emergency room, and an unknown number of untreated injuries.

The following sections give specific details on the major causes of non-intentional injury (motor vehicle injuries), followed by intentional injuries.

3.1. NON-INTENTIONAL INJURY

3.1.1. Motor Vehicle Collisions

Mortality

The highest percentage of PYLL arises from fatal motor vehicle injuries, since mortality from this cause occurs primarily in the young. The mortality rate for motor vehicle collisions has steadily declined since the 1960s. Fatality rates are highest in those aged 15 to 24. In 1992, there were 3,792 fatalities associated with motor vehicles: 2,211 (58.3%) were drivers, 1,046 (27.6%) were passengers, and 522 (13.8%) were pedestrians (59).

Risk Factors

Important risk factors for motor vehicle collisions include the mental attitude and condition of the driver, the design and condition of the vehicle, road design and conditions, and seat belt usage. Primary preventive methods therefore include environmental as well as individual measures. Driving while intoxicated is a major factor in collisions. Drinking has been implicated in a large proportion of fatal road injuries. Of 747 automobile drivers killed in road injuries in eight provinces during 1985, 79% had a blood alcohol level of above 80 mg/100 ml (i.e., were legally impaired). By 1992, this percentage of impaired drivers with high blood alcohol levels resulting in fatal injury had declined to 48.1% (59).

Non-Intentional Injury Prevention

It is important to recognize that a major attitudinal change is necessary in order to prevent injuries. That is, injuries just don't happen by chance but in most cases are preventable. There are usually circumstances in which action could be taken in advance to prevent or minimize the extent of damage. A useful framework has been provided by Haddon in which non-intentional injuries are conceptualized as resulting from interactions between host (person), agent or vector (e.g., a car), and environment (see Chapter One). Interventions directed to any factor may reduce the onset or extent of injury sustained. Injury occurs when forces are applied beyond the capability of the organism to withstand. In this model, success of injury prevention depends on the degree of passivity of the measure (therefore requiring minimal effort) and deterrents and incentives. The Haddon matrix concept for public health has been modified to incorporate the concept of behavioural components and health education, affecting predisposing beliefs and attitudes about injuries, safety enabling factors, and reinforcing policies and actions that can be adopted (60).

Preventive injury interventions are visualized as a two-dimensional matrix in which pre-injury, time of impact, and post-injury preventive measures are considered in relation to the person, agent causing injury, or the environment. In the pre-injury phase, attention should be directed to eliminate the source of the energy, reducing exposure to the energy, or reducing the magnitude of resistance to the energy. Attention directed to the injury phase should reduce the magnitude and duration of exposure, and decrease the host's susceptibility to injury. In the post-injury phase, the environment can be altered to reduce the source of the injury in the future and facilitate the rescue and resuscitation of victims in the short term. For example, in relation to motor vehicle injuries, pre-injury strategies include: appropriate use of car seats and seat belts for all children in cars, teaching children road safety, use of bicycle helmets, reduction of vehicular speed especially in areas with schools and in residential areas, and road design. Protection at the time of injury involves the restraining action of the seat belt and helmets' ability to reduce brain damage. Post-injury prevention involves ready access to trauma centres and review of injury sites for future precautions.

The most successful public health measures are also involuntary ones (e.g., those that reduce ejections in crashes or protect vehicle occupants with inflatable air bag cushions in forward deceleration). Recently, daytime running lights have been recommended to increase vehicle visibility. Seat belt legislation enacted in most jurisdictions in Canada has reduced mortality and morbidity due to motor vehicle injuries, with a consequent decrease in the economic burden. Recent work suggests that the Selective Traffic Enforcement Program (STEP) is a useful approach to increase seat belt use; it uses a media and law enforcement blitz for several short periods. The result is a long-term gradual increase in the percentage of vehicle occupants using their seat belts. Risk reduction strategies that require voluntary change in behaviour patterns, such as wearing seat belts, need constant reinforcement (see Chapter Four). Wearing of helmets by motorcyclists is established as a preventive measure, and there is good evidence to support helmet use by bicyclists.

Other strategies against injury that have proven effective are child-proof medicine containers, bars on upper-storey windows, motorcycle helmets and many of which have been demonstrated through case-control study.

3.2. INTENTIONAL INJURY

3.2.1. Suicide

Mortality

Suicide has accounted for about 2% of all deaths in Canada annually since the late 1970s. Suicide rates have increased rapidly since the early 1960s and are currently higher than they were during the Depression 50 years ago. The overall suicide rate per 100,000 Canadians in 1992 was 13. Quebec, Alberta, and Saskatchewan have had the highest rates for the past decade. The male rate for completed suicide is consistently more than double the female rate, and among those aged 15 to 24 the male rate is five times the female rate. In 1992, the mean Canadian suicide rate per 100,000 population for males was 20.6, whereas it was 5.3 for females. There are also distinct gender differences in the most common means of suicide. In 1992, guns and explosives accounted for 35.6% of male suicides, but only 11% of female suicides. Contrarily, poisoning accounted for 40% of female suicides, but less than 10% of male suicides. The PYLL due to suicide is large as it frequently involves young adults. In 1994, there were over 99,700 PYLL for males from suicide, the fourth leading cause of PYLL. These high suicide rates among young adult males only appeared over the last three decades (61).

Risk Factors

People at high risk for suicide include those with AIDS, Inuit, Status Indians, street youth, psychiatric patients (especially schizophrenics and people with affective disorders), prison inmates, people with a past history of attempted suicide, elderly women, both Canadian-born and Asian women, and the bereaved (62). A number of social factors have been associated with suicide, namely mobility, disorganization, and isolation with disruption of family relationships, lack of purpose in life and religious affiliation, and particular cultural attitudes and beliefs. Important contributing medical factors are the lack of adequate community and psychiatric services, since it is apparent that many suicidal persons actually contact such services before committing the act itself (55). The most frequent sets of predisposing circumstances identified in a survey of suicides in a region of Quebec were psychiatric or psychological problems (60%), problematic circumstances (52%) and physical health problem (12%). In 44% of clients there had been suicidal ideation or attempts; alcohol or other drug addiction ranked second to depression-anxiety in terms of risk (63).

Prevention and Health Promotion

There is some evidence that initiation or improvements in community psychiatric services improve the rates of suicide. The four major strategies for primary prevention include public education, reduction in availability and lethality of means, specific education and training programs for health care professionals and gatekeepers, and programs aimed at the high-risk groups. A multifactorial strategy for the prevention of suicide was developed in the Quebec and Chaudiere-Appalaches regions in response to high rates of suicide (23 per 100,000) in this area. The primary prevention recommendations involved increasing professional attention to lifestyle problems, particularly alcohol or drug addictions, and to young people with depression. Education programs should aim at reducing the stigma attached to seeking treatment for mental disorders, alcoholism and drug abuse. Crisis intervention facilities should be available. Strategies to prevent actual attempts may involve confiscation of weapons or limiting medications to those who are depressed or expressing suicidal ideation. The likelihood of successful attempts can be addressed by multiple modalities directed towards the physical environment, and legislation to reduce accessibility to firearms, as well other methods that may be utilized.

The media have a central role in shaping public attitudes and public education. The means for suicide is often related to the availability of lethal substances. Hence, education programs could also aim at discouraging the accumulation of lethal amounts of drugs in household medicine cabinets, for example. Susceptible individuals may attempt suicide if their idol or a prominent person is reported to have committed suicide, thus media coverage of suicides could discourage sensationalism. Professional education should include the early warning signs of persons with suicidal tendencies, knowledge about high-risk populations, commonly used means of suicide, methods of intervention, and available community resources to deal with the underlying problems. Education should be aimed at physicians, clergy, teachers, personnel of correctional facilities, police and others, as well as mental health professionals. There should be specific programs for the high-risk groups. For example, the elderly may benefit from retirement programs, self-help groups, education of family physicians and public education about the typical personality changes in the suicidal elderly person (61).

3.2.2. Homicide

The risk of death from a firearm in Canada by suicide, homicide, or injury is equivalent to the risk of death from a motor vehicle injury. The overall homicide rate in Canada averaged 2.0 to 2.7 per 100,000 in the 1990s. Firearm deaths were the third most common cause of death among Canadians aged 15 to 24 in 1990 (64).

Gun Control

About 1,400 firearm-related deaths occur each year in Canada. Gun control has been highlighted above as an important potential strategy in prevention of both suicides and homicides. Suicides represent 75% of firearm-related deaths in Canada. The number of suicides using firearms has declined since the introduction of gun control legislation in 1978, and no other explanations are plausible to account for this reduction. However, the effects of delay or limitation of access to a firearm until suicidal ideation has passed has not been well investigated. It is estimated that one quarter of Canadian households own a firearm; in 70% of those households it is allegedly for hunting. Over 50% had not used a firearm in the previous 12 months and had no one trained in safe handling. Although protection is often cited as a justification for having a gun, a household member is killed 20 times more often than an intruder (65).

From 1989 to 1992 the mean mortality rate from gunshot wounds ranged from 5.8 per 100,000 in Quebec to 21.2 per 100,000 in the Northwest Territories. A recent cost analysis has estimated that the total costs associated with gunshot wounds approaches $6.6 billion. The vast majority of these costs relate to pain, suffering, and the loss of productive life (66).

Under the newly passed *Firearms Act* (Bill C-68), all owners of firearms must obtain a licence by January 1, 2001. The licence must be renewed every five years and will be required for the purchase of ammunition as well as guns. Firearms are required to be registered by January 1, 2003. The new system will permit the control of who possesses firearms. Those with histories of violence will not be permitted to get a licence. Ownership will now be tied to accountability and education on the proper storage and handling of firearms is possible. As well, more accurate statistics can be kept in order to assess the efficacy of prevention efforts (66).

3.2.3. Domestic Violence

Domestic violence and violence against women and children have become recognized as an important source of morbidity and mortality in the Canadian population: 29% of Canadian women have suffered from violence at the hands of a current or previous partner. It is estimated that 1,435 women and 451 men were killed by their partners between 1974 to 1992 (67). The effects of violence extend beyond the physical harm endured: stress, poor mental health, lack of social connection, and substance abuse can all occur in victims of violence. Children raised in violence-prone homes suffer from depression, post-traumatic stress disorder, peer conflicts, and conduct disorders as well as a host of other behavioural problems.

In 1993, Canada endorsed the United Nations Declaration on the Elimination of Violence Against Women. It is recognized that a multifactorial strategy is necessary for violence prevention. Successful prevention requires first that the problem be acknowledged and addressed by communities and governments. In 1995, the federal government released its Federal Plan for Gender Equality, which clearly recognized violence against women as a crucial area. The following priority issues were identified: supporting community-based actions undertaken by women's organizations, increasing media awareness and involving the media in counteracting violence, supporting shelters for battered women, achieving reform related to criminal justice, addressing violence in Aboriginal on-reserve and Inuit communities, promoting women's safety in the workplace, and undertaking research and analysis on issues related to violence against women.

4. SUMMARY

This chapter summarized the current approaches in disease prevention and health promotion in relation to major non-communicable chronic diseases and injuries in Canada. Many chronic illnesses have *substance abuse* (alcohol and tobacco) and improper diet as major underlying causes. These illnesses are preventable, and hence there has been an increasing emphasis on the role of primary and secondary prevention. Chronic illnesses are the cause of the major burden of illness.

Smoking is the number one preventable cause of death in Canada. In 1993, 33,498 Canadians died of smoking-related deaths. Smoking is associated with lung cancer, chronic obstructive pulmonary disease, cardiovascular illness, and low birth weight. Female smoking-related deaths, while much lower in number than males, have risen proportionately at a greater rate than for males within the last 15 years, parallelling the increase in female smoking. There is good evidence that health care providers, including physicians and non-physicians, can be effective in motivating people to quit smoking using brief interventions by incorporating smoking cessation messages that are repeated on multiple occasions and reinforced. As well, well-designed programs of health promotion with strategies aimed at impressionable and susceptible youth populations to prevent the uptake of smoking, as well as cessation in older smokers, can continue the reversal of smoking prevalence.

There are various diseases and injuries associated with *alcohol* consumption, such as cirrhosis, suicide, breast cancer, respiratory cancer, and motor vehicle and other injuries. Roughly 1.8% of all deaths are directly attributable to alcohol abuse, and an estimated 10.5% of all deaths are alcohol related. The impact of alcohol on the health of Canadians is shown even more strongly in terms of morbidity. There are two defined groups of drinkers: problem drinkers and alcohol-dependent drinkers. There are about 502,700 Canadians who are alcohol dependent.

Physicians are in a good position to identify alcoholism quickly and offer early intervention for those who are drinking at levels that increase their risks for medical and psychosocial consequences of drinking. Many motivated problem drinkers and alcohol-dependent people who want to quit drinking are also being assisted by self-help groups such as Alcoholics Anonymous.

Effective health promotion programs in relation to substance abuse should be comprehensive, coordinated, and participatory. School-based policies on alcohol, drugs and smoking can complement integrated education and prevention programs. In the home setting, parents should be encouraged to discuss alcohol and smoking issues and values with children.

Diet, particularly fat intake, is a major factor in the development of many chronic diseases including cardiovascular disease and cancer. Poor nutrition is also a factor in osteoporosis, chronic liver disease, and dental health. Obesity is a risk factor for diabetes, cardiovascular disease, and endometrial cancer, and increases the risk of breast cancer in postmenopausal women. There is an increasing prevalence of underweight individuals (particularly young women), which makes them susceptible to certain health problems. National guidelines for nutrition have been published by Health and Welfare Canada. For encouraging healthy eating, action should be directed to the community at large, schools, homes, restaurants, grocery stores, workplaces, and health care settings.

Cardiovascular disease (CVD) has been the leading cause of death in Canada, accounting for nearly half of all deaths each year. The most common forms of CVD are ischemic or coronary heart disease (IHD) and cerebrovascular disease (stroke or CBVD). In 1995, IHD and CBVD accounted for over 37% of deaths in Canada, with IHD representing one quarter of all deaths. While CVD is still the leading cause of death, there has been a decline in CVD mortality rates since the mid 1960s, attributed in part to the reduction in the prevalence of smoking, reduced consumption of dietary fat, improved detection, and management of hypertension, as well as improved surgical approaches to the treatment of symptomatic heart disease.

The underlying cause of CVD is atherosclerosis. Factors that contribute to atherosclerosis include smoking, high blood pressure, obesity, lack of physical activity, high levels of dietary fat, and increased LDL fraction. The incidence of CVD increases dramatically with age; 75% of Canadians have at least one of the major cardiovascular risk factors. The rates for women are almost half those of men, except for stroke for which the rates are approximately equal.

Cardiovascular disease is preventable. Community-based population-wide approaches emphasize augmenting community action, reorienting health services, and enhancing prevention. These are believed to reduce the prevalence of risk factors predisposing individuals to CVD.

Cancer ranked second overall as a leading cause of death. More than one in three Canadians will develop some form of cancer in their lifetime. After the age of 55 years, both male and female cancer rates begin to rise at a faster rate; however, the male rate increases more sharply. Despite advances and the better outlook for some cancers, the overall prognosis is still unfavourable and the emphasis must be on prevention and caring.

Environmental factors (such as water and air quality), diet, and lifestyle are considered to be the most important determinants for cancer. Smoking and alcohol are two lifestyle habits that play major roles in a number of non-occupational cancers for which multiple factors may be responsible. Exposures to high concentrations of certain chemicals in the occupational environment are also associated with cancer.

Lung, colon, breast, and prostate are the most common cancers in Canadians. Ninety per cent of lung cancer is caused by smoking. Diets, particularly those high in saturated fat intake, have been linked with increased risk of colorectal cancer. Leukaemia represents the leading cancer in children.

In 1993, *respiratory diseases* ranked the third leading causes of death among men and women. Important factors include smoking, respiratory pathogens, and air pollution. Pollutants interact and their combined effect on a disease may be either additive or multiplicative (e.g., smoking and asbestos combined have a multiplicative effect). Hospitalizations, drug prescriptions, and overall health costs are increasing for asthma.

Congenital anomalies and genetic diseases are now the second leading cause of death in infants. The most common malformations leading to infant death were due to defects of the heart and circulatory system. Aetiological factors for malformations include hereditary or familial tendencies, and non-genetic factors such as maternal diabetes, anticonvulsant drug use during pregnancy, or maternal infection with herpes, syphilis, rubella, toxoplasmosis or cytomegalovirus. Currently, there are 200 known genetic and metabolic disorders. Many of these diseases are preventable with proper counselling in susceptible populations. Selective screening and genetic counselling in susceptible populations are probably the most appropriate form of primary prevention. The advent of new reproductive technologies has raised many ethical issues that were addressed by a major royal commission.

Arthritis and chronic pain conditions are important causes of morbidity in the Canadian population. Although the mortality for these conditions is low, the quality-adjusted life is poorer for those with severe arthritis or chronic pain. These conditions increases in incidence with age and are major causes of health service utilization.

Mental health illnesses such as depression, schizophrenia, and stress cause substantial morbidity. The extent of the problem is not as systematically documented as for other conditions owing to residual stigmatism associated with mental illness.

One in five Canadians had at least one *injury* in 1993, accounting for $7 billion in direct expenditures. The types of injuries included motor vehicle, sports or leisure activity, work-related injuries, and those injuries occurring in and around the home. Injuries are distinguished as either non-intentional (also known as accidents) and intentional (homicide and suicide predominantly). They constitute the leading cause of death during half the human life span and the second leading cause of PYLL. Injuries are the leading cause of death for children under five years, school-aged children, and young adults, due to falling, poisoning, and motor vehicle collisions.

Important risk factors for motor vehicle collisions include the mental attitude and condition of the driver, the design and condition of the vehicle, road design and conditions, and seat belt usage. Primary preventive methods would therefore include environmental measures in addition to those aimed at the individual. Driving while intoxicated is considered a major factor in injuries.

Major attitudinal change is necessary in order to prevent injuries. Pre-injury strategies include appropriate use of car seats and seat belts for all children in cars, teaching children road safety, wearing bicycle helmets, reduction of vehicular speed in specific areas (e.g., near schools), and road signs. Post-injury prevention involves ready access to trauma centres and review of injuries sites for future precautions.

Suicide rates have increased rapidly since the early 1960s. The male rate is consistently more than double the female rate and among those aged 15 to 24, the male rate is five times the female rate. People at high risk for suicide include those with AIDS, Inuit, Status Indians, street youth, psychiatric patients, prison inmates, people with a past history of attempted suicide, the elderly and Canadian-born and Asian-born women.

There is some evidence that initiation or improvements in community psychiatric services produce beneficial effects on the rates of suicide. The four major strategies for primary prevention include public education, reduction in availability and lethality of means, specific education and training programs for health care professionals and gatekeepers, and programs aimed at the high-risk groups.

Violence is an important public health concern. Most homicides are related to firearms. Recent Canadian legislation to make firearm access more difficult should have salutary health effects. Domestic violence is a major cause of morbidity. Recent federal government initiatives should give the issue a higher profile.

5.   REFERENCES

1.   Single E, Robson L, Xie X, Rehm J. The Costs of Substance Abuse in Canada. Ottawa: Canadian Centre on Substance Abuse 1996.
2.   National Cancer Institute of Canada. Canadian Cancer Statistics, 1997. Toronto: National Cancer Institute of Canada, 1997.
3.   Spitzer W, Lawrence V, Dales R, Links between Passive Smoking and Disease: A Best-Evidence Synthesis. Clinical and Investigative Medicine 1990;13(1):17-42.
4.   Ontario Medical Association Committee on Population Health. OMA Position Paper on Second-Hand Smoke. Ontario Medical Review 1996;63(11):29 - 35.
5.   Canadian Council on Smoking and Health. Guide Your Patients to a Smoke-Free Future. A Program of the Canadian Council on Smoking and Health. 1992.

6. Bull S, Pederson L, Ashley M J. Restrictions on Smoking: Growth in Population Support between 1983 and 1991 in Ontario, Canada. Journal of Public Health Policy 1994;15:310-328.
7. Tobacco Control: A Blueprint to Protect the Health of Canadians. Ottawa: Minister of Supply and Services, 1995.
8. Mao Y, Johnson R, Semencins R. Liver Cirrhosis Mortality and Per Capita Alcohol Consumption in Canada. Canadian Journal of Public Health 1992;83(1):80-81.
9. Kahan M. Identifying and Managing Problem Drinkers. Canadian Family Physician 1996;42:661-671.
10. Addiction Research Foundation of Ontario. Alcohol and Your Health. Toronto: 1997.
11. Departments of Preventive Medicine and Biostatistics and Behaviour Sciences, Division of Community Health, Faculty of Medicine, University of Toronto, Addiction Research Foundation. Preventing Alcohol Problems: The Challenge for Medical Education. Proceedings of a National Conference at Niagara-on-the-Lake, Ontario. October 15-17, 1989. Canadian Medical Association Journal 1990;143(10):1041-1042.
12. Selzer ML. The Michigan Alcoholism Screening Test: The Quest for a New Diagnostic Instrument. American Journal of Psychiatry 1971;127(12):1653-1658.
13. Ewing JA. Detecting Alcoholism: The CAGE Questionnaire. Journal of American Medical Association 1984;252(14):1905-1907.
14. Swarbrick M. Model Program for Substance Abuse Prevention. Public Health and Epidemiology Reports Ontario 1991;2(21):320-323.
15. Health and Welfare Canada. Break Free. Directional Paper of the National Program to Reduce Tobacco Use in Canada. Ottawa: Government of Canada, 1987.
16. Health and Welfare Canada. Partners in Canada's Drug Strategy. Health Promotion 1992;30(2):11-12.
17. Rabkin SW, Chen Y, Leiter L, Reeder BA. Risk Factors Correlates of Body Mass Index. Canadian Medical Association Journal 1997;157(1 suppl): S26-S31.
18. Health and Welfare. Nutrition Recommendations: The Report of the Scientific Review Committee. Ottawa: Ministry of Supply and Services, 1990.
19. Miller A, and Health and Welfare Canada. Planning Cancer Control Strategies. Chronic Disease in Canada 1992;13(1):1-40.
20. Joint Steering Committee. Nutrition for Health: An Agenda for Action. 1996.
21. Heart and Stroke Foundation of Canada. Heart Disease and Stroke in Canada. Ottawa: 1997.
22. The Expert Panel. The Canadian Consensus Conference on Cholesterol; Final Report. Canadian Medical Association Journal 1988;139(2):1-8.
23. Greenwood DC, Muir KR, Packham CJ, Madeley RJ. Coronary Heart Disease: A Review of the Role of Psychosocial Stress and Social Support. Journal of Public Health Medicine 1996;18(2):2221-231.
24. Grover S, Coupal L, Gahkry R, Suissa S. Screening for Hypercholesterolaemia among Canadians: How Much Will it Cost? Canadian Medical Association Journal 1991;144(2):161-168.
25. Marshall K. Prevention. How Much Harm? How Much Benefit? The Ethics of Informed Consent for Preventive Screening Programs. Canadian Medical Association Journal 1996;155(4):377-383.
26. Dawber TR. The Framingham Study: The Epidemiology of Atherosclerotic Disease. Cambridge, Ma.: Harvard University Press, 1980.

27. Puska P, Tuomilehto J, et al. The North Karelia Project: Evaluation of a Comprehensive Community Programme for Control of Cardiovascular Disease in 1977-77 in North Karelia, Finland. Copenhagen, Denmark: World Health Organization/EURO Monograph Series, 1981.

28. Shea S, Basch C. A Review of Five Major Community-Based Disease Prevention Programs. Part 2: Intervention Strategies, Evaluation Methods, and Results. American Journal of Health Promotion 1990;4(4):279-287.

29. Shea S, Basch CA. Review of Five Major Community-Based Cardiovascular Disease Prevention Programs. Part 1: Rationale, Design and Theoretical Framework. American Journal of Health Promotion 1990;4(3):203-213.

30. Canada Heart Health Surveys Research Group. The Federal-Provincial Canadian Heart Health Initiative. Canadian Medical Association Journal 1992;146(11):1915-1916.

31. International Heart Health Conference. Victoria Declaration on Heart Health. Bridging the Gap: Science and Policy in Action. Ottawa: Health and Welfare Canada, 1992.

32. Willett W, Hunter DJ, Stampfer MI, et al. Dietary Fat and Fiber in Relation to Risk of Breast Cancer. An 8-Year Follow-up. Journal of American Medical Association 1992;268(15):2037-2044.

33. Miller A, Baines C, To T, Wall C. Canadian National Breast Screening Study. 1. Breast Cancer Detection and Death Rates among Women Aged 40 to 49 Years. 2. Canadian National Breast Screening Study. Breast Cancer Detection and Death Rates among Women Aged 50 to 59 Years. Canadian Medical Association Journal 1992;147(10):1459-1488.

34. Workshop Report. Reducing Deaths from Breast Cancer in Canada. Canadian Medical Association Journal 1989;141(3):199-201.

35. Cole D, Gallinger B, McCready D. Genetic Counselling and Testing for Susceptibility to Breast, Ovarian and Colon Cancer: Where Are We Today? Canadian Medical Association Journal 1996;154(2):149-155.

36. The Steering Committee on Clinical Practice Guidelines for the Care and Treatment of Breast Cancer. Clinical Practice Guidelines for Care and Treatment of Breast Cancer, A Canadian Consensus Document. Canadian Medical Association Journal. Ottawa: Health Canada and Canadian Medical Association, 1998. S1-S83. vol 158 (3 Suppl).

37. Feightner JW, Screening for Prostate Cancer: In the Canadian Guide to Clinical Preventive Health Care. Ed. The Canadian Task Force on the Periodic Health Examination. Minister of Supply and Services Canada, 1994. P. 811-823.

38. Health and Welfare Canada. Proceedings of the Second National Workshop on Cervical Cancer Screening. Chronic Disease in Canada 1992;13(4): Supplement.

39. Parboosingh E, Anderson G, Clarke E. Cervical Cancer Screening: Are the 1989 Recommendations Still Valid? Canadian Medical Association Journal 1996;154(12):1847-1849.

40. Lung Facts. Ontario Lung Association, Toronto, 1995.

41. Krahn M, Berka B, Langlois P, et al. Direct and Indirect Costs of Asthma in Canada, 1990. Canadian Medical Association Journal 1996;154(6):821-831.

42. Ontario Medical Association. Ontario Medical Association Position Paper on Health Effects of Ground-Level Ozone, Acid Aerosols and Particulate Matter. Toronto: 1998.

43. Health Canada. Health and Environment: Partners for Life. Ottawa: Minister of Public Works and Government Services Canada, 1997.

44. Yassi A, Friesen B. Controlling Air Pollution: The Plan to Reduce Nitrogen Oxides (NOx) and Volatile Organic Compounds (VOCs) Emissions in Canada. Canadian Journal of Public Health 1990;81(1):6-9.

45. 1991 Aboriginal People Survey. Ottawa: Statistics Canada, The Daily, 1993.

46. Health Canada, Canadian Society for Exercise Physiology. Canada's Physical Activity Guide to Healthy, Active Living. Ottawa: Health Canada, 1998.

47. Proceed with Care: Final Report of the Royal Commission on New Reproductive Technologies. Ottawa: Royal Commission on New Reproductive Technologies, 1994.

48. Kalter H, Warkang J. Congenital Malformations, Aetiological Factors and Their Role in Prevention Part 1. New England Journal of Medicine 1983;308(8):424-431.

49. Fried P. Marihuana Use by Pregnant Women and Effects on Offspring: An Update. Neurobehaviour Toxicology and Teratology 1982;4(4):451-454.

50. Dick P. Periodic Health Examination, 1996 Update: 1. Prenatal screening for and diagnosis of Down's Syndrome. Canadian Medical Association Journal 1996;154(4):465-480.

51. Update on Folate: Folic Acid Supplementation in the Prevention of Neural Tube Defects. Informed 1996;2:5-6.

52. Badley E. The Impact of Disabling Arthritis. Arthritis Care and Research 1995;8:221-228.

53. The Arthritis Society of Canada. Arthroscope. Toronto: Arthritis Society of Canada, 1995.

54. Millar W. Chronic Pain. Health Reports 1996;7(4):47-53.

55. Canadian Mental Health Association. Depression: An Overview of the Literature. Ottawa: Health Canada, 1995.

56. Beaudet M. Depression. Health Reports 1996;7(4):11-23.

57. Fox B. The Psychological Epidemiology of Cancer Incidence and Prognosis. Chronic Disease in Canada 1995;16(1).

58. Millar W. Accidents in Canada, 1988-1993. Health Reports 1996;7(2):7-16.

59. Mayhew D, Simpson H, Brown S. Alcohol Use among Persons Fatally Injured in Motor Vehicle Accidents. Ottawa: Traffic Injury Research Foundation of Canada, 1994.

60. Gielen A. Health Education and Injury Control: Integrating Approaches. Health Education Quarterly 1992;19(2):203-218.

61. Task Force on Suicide in Canada. Suicide in Canada. Ottawa: Minister of National Health and Welfare, 1994.

62. Mao Y, Hasselback P, Davies J, Nichol R, Wigle D. Suicide in Canada: An Epidemiological Assessment. Canadian Journal of Public Health 1990;81(4):324-328.

63. Bouchard L, Chapdelaine A, Mireault G, Maurice P. Suicides in Quebec and Chaudiere-Appalaches Regions: A Multifactorial Approach for Suicide Prevention. Chronic Disease in Canada 1991;12(6):99-103.

64. Leonard K. Firearm Deaths in Canadian Adolescents and Young Adults. Canadian Journal of Public Health 1994;85(2):128-131.

65. Chapdelaine A, Samson E, Kimberly MD, Viau L. Firearm-Related Injuries in Canada: Issues for Prevention. Canadian Medical Association Journal 1991;145(10):1217-1223.

66. Miller T. Costs Associated with Gunshot Wounds in Canada in 1991. Canadian Medical Association Journal 1995;1553(9):1261-1268.

67. Suderman M, Jaffe P. Summary of Preventing Violence: School and Community-based Strategies. In Health National Forum Health. What Determines Health? Ottawa: Minister of Public Works and Government Services Canada, 1996.

Chapter

8

Communicable Diseases

The turn of this century was characterized by a progressive decline in morbidity and mortality from communicable diseases in the developed world. The last two decades of the 20th century have witnessed the development of emerging and re-emerging infectious diseases: HIV and AIDS, outbreaks of viral haemorrhagia fevers (Ebola), hantavirus, and Cryptosporidium represent examples of the new challenges to public health. Outbreaks of plague in India underscore the failure of health care systems to manage previously controlled diseases. Outbreaks of strains of tuberculosis that resist multiple drugs and vancomycin-resistant enterococci (VRE) have raised the spectre of bacteria not susceptible to antibiotics. This prospect was inconceivable 15 years ago, when the U.S. Surgeon General decreed that the war against infectious agents had been won.

Concern for the dangers posed by communicable diseases have been expressed by high-ranking members of the medical and public health communities. The reasons for the recrudescence of communicable diseases are as broad as the determinants of health. Behavioural intransigence, poverty, war, immigration, environmental desecration, iatrogenesis, and increased international travel figure prominently in the causal underpinnings.

Despite the fears engendered by the extensive publicity given to new communicable diseases, the traditional principles of communicable disease control remain effective. In Canada, immunization programs have nearly eliminated polio and invasive *Haemophilus influenza* type b. Infection control, good hygiene, timely surveillance, and outbreak management remain essential components of the public health response to communicable diseases.

Communicable disease data are collected systematically by provincial and federal authorities in Canada. The information presented below is the most up to date at the time of writing. Interested readers are directed to electronic databases maintained by the Laboratory Centre for Disease Control in Ottawa, the U.S. Centers for Disease Control in Atlanta, and the World Health Organization in Geneva for the most up-to-date Canadian and international data.

1.   BASIC CONCEPTS AND TERMINOLOGY OF COMMUNICABLE DISEASE CONTROL

The investigation and control of communicable diseases (contagious or infectious diseases) requires some knowledge of the spectrum of infectious diseases and the relevant terminology. The spectrum of infectious disease is as follows:

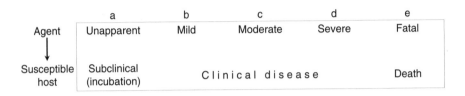

Investigators can characterize the threat of an offending organism by calculating several rates. The **attack rate** is the total number of people who developed clinical disease divided by the population at risk, usually expressed as a percentage. Using the above as an example, the attack rate can be derived by (b+c+d+e)/(population at risk). The **secondary attack rate** is the number of cases among contacts occurring within the incubation period following exposure to a primary case, in relation to the total exposed contacts; the denominator may be restricted to the number of susceptible contacts that can be ascertained. The **pathogenicity rate** describes the power of an organism to produce clinical disease in those who are infected; this is expressed as (b+c+d+e)/ (a+b+c+d+e). **Virulence** describes the severity of disease produced by the organism in a given host and is numerically expressed as a ratio of the number of cases of severe and fatal infection to the total number clinically infected, or (d+e)/(b+c+d+e). **Case-fatality rate** is the proportion of persons contracting a disease who die of that disease, namely e/(b+c+d+e).

A **reservoir of infection** is a person, animal, or inanimate object in which infectious agents can live and multiply for extended periods of time. Transmission of such agents occurs by various means through the environment or from one host (human or animal) to another. **Direct transmission** involves the transfer of infectious agents directly from one host to another. **Indirect transmission** can occur through a vehicle, vector, or the air. In vehicle-borne transmission, organisms are spread via inanimate materials, objects, or media (e.g., toys, clothes, milk, food). Vector-borne transmission may be mechanical (e.g., simple carriage of agents by animals) or biological (e.g., organisms multiplying inside insects). Malaria is an example of biological transmission of parasites from mosquito vectors to human hosts. Air borne transmission may occur via droplet nuclei or dust particles.

A **carrier** is defined as an individual who harbours a specific infectious agent usually without overt clinical disease. A carrier state may be of long or short duration, and it may serve as a potential source of infection.

The **communicable period** is the time during which an infectious agent may be transferred from an infected person or vector to another host. Generation time is the interval between the entry of infection into the host and its maximal infectivity. **Incubation period** is the interval between infection by an agent and the appearance of the first symptom of the disease. Often generation time is equivalent to the incubation period. **Infectiousness** reflects the ease of disease transmission, and is usually measured by the secondary attack rate.

1.1. OUTBREAKS OF INFECTIOUS DISEASES

An **outbreak** of disease is the occurrence of new cases clearly in excess of the baseline, or normally expected, frequency of the disease in a defined community or institutional population over a given time period. An **epidemic** has a synonymous definition, although in common parlance an outbreak usually means an epidemic that is localized, of acute onset, or is relatively short in duration. Notable examples of outbreaks include the cases of lethal meningococcal disease in adolescents and young adults in five provinces of Canada during 1991 and early 1992. Less noticeable are the outbreaks of diseases of moderate morbidity for the general population but of more severe morbidity for those already compromised in health, such as influenza and respiratory syncytial virus among nursing home residents or viral gastroenteritis among infants and children in day care.

There are two other terms worth noting: endemic and panepidemic. **Endemic** refers to the constant presence of a disease or infectious agent within a given geographic area or population sub group. **Pandemic** refers to an epidemic occurring over a wide area, crossing international boundaries, and affecting a large number of people. The investigation of an infectious disease outbreak requires particular epidemiological methods that establish the cause, risk factors, and modes of transmission of the disease (1). The control of the outbreak can then be achieved by removing or neutralizing the agent, strengthening the resistance of the hosts, and interrupting the means of transmission in the environment. Thus, the agent-host-environment triad (mentioned in Chapter One) is utilized. In addition, the outbreak control response must incorporate appropriate communication and sensitivity to public perceptions of risk, which may differ from expert opinions.

1.2. VERIFICATION OF EXISTENCE OF AN OUTBREAK

As mentioned above, defining whether an outbreak exists requires knowledge of the endemic baseline "normally expected" or "usual" frequency of cases of the disease in the specified population. Depending on the type of disease and population, the expected frequency may be a certain number per week or month, or none at all. In addition, in the early stages of an outbreak, the specific diagnosis of the disease or causative agent is usually not yet known, so the most prominent clinical symptoms are used to identify a possible or suspected case. For example, a nursing home might initially define an outbreak as "three or more residents having diarrhea and vomiting within a 72-hour period," since one or two may be considered within the expected frequency.

Once an outbreak is suspected, investigators (usually from local public health departments) must first ascertain the history of symptoms and signs of the affected persons, so that an initial **case definition** can be formulated from the most common symptoms or signs. Included in the case definition is the likely date of onset of illness of the first case (e.g., "any person having onset on or since a specified date, of vomiting, fever higher than 38.5°C and bloody stools"). Laboratory confirmation of the clinical diagnosis is sought as soon as possible — e.g., culture or serology — and results, when available, can define a case more precisely.

After the case definition has been specified, the extent of the outbreak should be determined by **active surveillance** — that is, active efforts to identify all those who may have been exposed to the infectious agent (population at risk) and who may have illness fitting the case definition. In a community outbreak, this may involve contacting hospital emergency rooms, physicians' offices, and local schools. Typical epidemiologic information recorded includes demographics (age, gender, etc.), location (residence, school, or worksite), details about the illness (date and time of onset, prominent symptoms), laboratory tests and treatment (if any), immunization status (if relevant), and close contacts with other persons. A line listing is typically made of all suspected and confirmed cases.

The data from the line listing is used to generate an **epidemic curve**. The epidemic curve is usually constructed as a frequency histogram with the number of cases plotted on the vertical axis and their dates or times of onset along the horizontal axis. The epidemic curve can visually indicate whether the epidemic (outbreak) has a common (or "point") source or whether it is propagated. The location (geographic or institutional) of cases may be depicted as a spot map. Attack rates are often also calculated.

In a **common-source epidemic**, people become ill because of exposure to a single (common) source of infection; the exposure may be of long or short duration. A common-source outbreak is of short duration, with the number of cases rising and falling acutely due to short-term exposure to the infectious source; for example, food poisoning in a group of persons eating the same item at a church picnic. Hence the epidemic curve would show a single, sharp peak. A **propagated epidemic** may begin with only a few exposed persons but is maintained by person-to-person transmission. The epidemic curve will generally show a series of peaks. Hepatitis B provides a good example of a propagated epidemic.

The above information can be used in analytic studies, such as case-control studies, to elucidate further information on hypothesized risk factors and disease transmission patterns as described in Chapter Two.

1.3. IMPLEMENTATION OF INITIAL CONTROL MEASURES

Depending on the symptoms, the suspected agent, the population at risk, and the location, initial control measures will be adopted. These may include isolation of residents in a facility, augmented handwashing and cleaning, cohort nursing (which involves utilizing the same nursing staff in an institution for the duration of the outbreak), exclusion of symptomatic staff, immunization (e.g., for influenza or measles), prophylactic medication for those exposed or at risk (e.g., rifampin for menigococcal disease), or withdrawal of contaminated food from distribution.

Outbreaks of nosocomial infections (i.e., those acquired during stay in a health care facility) require the convening of an outbreak management team to coordinate the efforts of many departments — such as housekeeping, maintenance, dietary, nursing, and medical staff — in implementing investigation and control measures.

1.4. SPECIFIC CONTROL MEASURES

Depending on the cause of the outbreak and the mode of transmission, specific control measures (such as immunization or specific improvements in the processes of food preparation) may be implemented. Readers can refer to standard textbooks of epidemiology and infection control for details regarding the investigation and control of outbreaks (2, 3).

2.   IMMUNIZATION

Immunization remains the most important factor in the prevention of infectious disease. The success of immunization in the reduction of morbidity and mortality from infectious diseases is unrivalled by any other medical intervention both in terms of health benefits and cost effectiveness.

The effectiveness of vaccination in protecting against disease depends not only on the efficacy of individual vaccines, but also on the degree of coverage achieved. These factors rely on administrative aspects of the vaccination program as well as on consumer and provider compliance, and on the maintenance of potency of the vaccine by attention to requirements during transportation and storage. Strategies to improve the effectiveness and efficiency of vaccine-delivery programs have been comprehensively reviewed (4, 5). Table 8.1 indicates a number of steps in vaccine storage and handling that should be undertaken routinely by those involved in vaccine administration (6).

Recommendations concerning immunizations are established by the National Advisory Committee on Immunization (NACI). Each province publishes its own

Table 8.1:	Vaccine Storage and Handling
1. Expiry dates:	Check before each use; discard outdated products.
2. Temperature:	Check temperature routinely; avoid storage of vaccines on refrigerator doors as temperature tends to fluctuate, thus inactivating vaccines.
3. Transport:	Use coolers and cold packs to transport vaccines even over short distances.
4. Protect:	Store light-sensitive products in boxes and allow them to be exposed only briefly to light to avoid inactivation.
5. Dilute:	With diluent provided, consult manufacturer's direction and use as soon as possible.
6. Inspect:	Inspect each vial/ampule before administering for colour change, particles, or precipitation.
7. Discard:	Discard multidose vials that have not been dated at time of first use, and vaccines that have been inadvertently frozen. (Note: Live-virus vaccines with the exception of OPV may be thawed and used more than once, but not repeatedly).

Source: McIntyre L, Shave D. *Update on Immunization Drugs and Therapeutics.* Maritime Practitioners. 1990: 13:(1/2):2. Reproduced with the permission of the authors.

immunization schedule. Interested readers can obtain provincial immunization schedules from each provincial ministry of health. Details on adverse reactions from vaccines are regularly reviewed and published by the Laboratory Centre for Disease Control (LCDC) (7). The recommended schedule for the immunization of infants and children is provided in Table 8.2.

3.   SELECTED VACCINE-PREVENTABLE DISEASES

Although diseases such as tetanus, diphtheria, and polio have been almost eradicated in Canada, sporadic cases and outbreaks of certain diseases that could be prevented by vaccines are still reported. A brief overview of the recent incidence of the major vaccine-preventable diseases in Canada, as well as issues relevant to control, are discussed here. Health Canada publication *Canadian National Report on Immunization, 1996* provides a very good overview of the vaccine preventable diseases in Canada (8).

Pertussis
Periodic outbreaks of pertussis or whooping cough occur in Canada. In 1995, 8,853 cases of pertussis were reported, indicating poor optimal disease control. A small endemic focus exists in Quebec (9). The severity of the disease has decreased due to

widespread vaccination, which affords partial protection. However, the disease has a poorer prognosis in infants under one year of age, in whom the case-fatality rate is 1 in 200. In 1994, the LCDC revised the optimal management of contacts of sporadic cases and outbreaks of pertussis (10).

The development of acellular pertussis vaccines, demonstrated in randomized controlled trials to be safer and more effective than whole-cell preparations, should increase the acceptability, and alleviate parental and physician concerns about safety (11, 12). Increased rates of vaccination against pertussis should result in further reduction in morbidity and mortality.

Measles

A major resurgence of measles occurred in Canada in the late 1980s and early 1990s. The incidence of measles rose from 2 per 100,000 in 1981 to 50 per 100,000 in 1991. After a record low number of 204 cases were reported in 1993, 2,344 cases were reported in 1995. This represented the largest number of cases reported in the Americas (13). The reason for the persistence of measles is that a one-dose vaccine strategy fails to induce protective antibodies in approximately 6% of vaccine recipients. Over a period of years, a pool of susceptible individuals accumulates that allows for periodic outbreaks.

The NACI has recommended a strategy for measles control in Canada that includes a two-dose vaccination program. All provinces embarked on a two-dose strategy by the end of 1996 (14). Recent data indicate that this strategy has been successful at reducing the incidence of measles in Canada (13).

Rubella

There was a marked increase in the number of cases of rubella in British Columbia, Ontario, and other provinces in the late 1980s (15). There were 320 cases reported in the first four months of 1989, affecting people of high school age and those aged 20 to 29 years; 30% of the cases in British Columbia occurred in women of child-bearing age. However, the number of national cases reported went down from 1,384 in 1989 to 402 in 1990. The figure had declined to 286 by 1995 (16). Only two to four cases of congenital rubella syndrome (CRS) were reported annually during the past five years. It is suspected that serious under-reporting of rubella and lack of identification of CRS are responsible for the apparent recent decline in rubella. Female patients should be warned of the dangers associated with rubella infection in pregnancy, if they are not immune.

Influenza

Influenza viruses are a major cause of morbidity, mortality, and lost productivity due to work and school absence in the Canadian population. Influenza A strains (H1N1 and H3N2 variants) and influenza B circulate around the globe annually, usually during the winter months. The overall estimated mortality from influenza and pneumococcal infections, which may arise as a complication of influenza, exceeds that of all vaccine-preventable childhood diseases. In Canada, there are an estimated 6,700 deaths and as many as 75,000 hospitalizations each year from influenza (17). The heaviest toll of morbidity and mortality occurs among those over 65 years of age, although substantial morbidity can occur in young patients who are immunocompromised or have chronic

Table 8.2.   Provincial and Territorial Immunization Schedules for Infants and Children, as of March 1, 1997

Province or territory	DPT (month)	Polio (month)	Hib (month)	DPT-polio (4-6 years)[1]	Td-polio (14-16 years)[2]	Hepatitis B (3 doses) age/grade	MMR 1st dose (months)	MMR/M^R 2nd dose[3]
Newfoundland	2,4,6,18	2,4,6,18 IPV	2,4,6,18	DPT + IPV	Td + IPV	Grade 4	12	18 months MMR
Prince Edward Island	2,4,6,18	2,4,6 IPV 18-OPV	2,4,6,18	DPT + OPV	Td + IPV	Grade 3 (8-9 years) or infants 2,4,15 months	15	4-6 years MMR
Nova Scotia	2,4,6,18	2,4,6,18 IPV	2,4,6,18	DPT + IPV	Td + IPV	Grade 4	12	4-6 years MMR
New Brunswick	2,4,6,18	2,4,6,18 IPV	2,4,6,18	DPT + IPV	Td + IPV	Grade 4 or infants 0,2,12 months	12	18 months MMR
Quebec	2,4,6,18	2,4,6,18 IPV	2,4,6,18	DPT + IPV	Td + IPV	Grade 4	12	18 months MMR
Ontario	2,4,6,18	2,4,6,18 IPV	2,4,6,18	DPT + IPV	Td + IPV	Grade 7	12	4-6 years MMR
Manitoba	2,4,18	2,4,6,18 OPV	2,4,6,18	DPT + OPV	Td	Not planned	12	5 years MMR
Saskatchewan	2,4,6,18	2,4,6,18 IPV	2,4,6,18	DPT + IPV	Td	Grade 6	12	18 months MR
Alberta	2,4,6,18	2,4,6,18 IPV	2,4,6,18	DPT + IPV	Td	Grade 5	12	4-6 years MMR
British Columbia	2,4,6,18	2,4,6,18 IPV	2,4,6,18	DPT + IPV	Td	Grade 6	12	18 months MMR
Yukon Territory	2,4,6,18	2,4,6,18 IPV	2,4,6,18	DPT + IPV	Td + IPV	Grade 4	12	18 months MMR
Northwest Territories	2,4,6,18	2,4,6,18 IPV	2,4,6,18	DPT + IPV	Td + IPV	Grade 4 or infants 0,1,6 months	12	18 months MMR

[1] Ontario, Northwest Territories, Saskatchewan: Diphtheria pertussis-tetanus (DPT)-polio fifth dose is not necessary if the preceding fourth dose was given after the fourth birthday; British Columbia: DPT-polio: DPT-polio fifth dose not necessary if the fourth dose of DPT-inactive polio vaccine (IPV) was given after the first birthday.

[2] New Brunswick: for adolescents of 14 to 16 years of age who received all previous doses as IPV; Quebec: polio vaccine at four to six years and at 14 to 16 years omitted if the oral polio vaccine (OPV) was used for earlier doses; Ontario: polio vaccine at 14 to 16 years not required if the child has completed primary series and received one or more doses of OPV in the past (OPV was used routinely in Ontario from January 1990 to March 1993); Saskatchewan: polio vaccine for 14 to 16 years only if did not receive one dose of OPV; Northwest Territories: polio vaccine at 14 to 16 years not required if the child has completed the primary series and received one or more doses of OPV in the past.

[3] Prince Edward Island: girls in grade 5 who do not have documentation of receiving one dose of measles-mumps rubella (MMR) after their first birthday should be offered a single dose of MMR.

Hib *Haemophilus influenzae* b vaccine; Td Tetanus diphtheria toxoid-adult type.

Source: Laboratory Centre for Disease Control, Health Canada.

diseases such as asthma, chronic obstructive pulmonary disease, ischemic heart disease, or diabetes. Medicare and hospitalization costs for influenza in Canada are approximately $500 million per year.

Influenza immunization programs have been demonstrated to be cost beneficial. It has been shown that if health care providers recommend vaccination, vaccine uptake by individuals in high-risk groups is improved. Increased efforts in organizing influenza programs, particularly in improving provider compliance with national guidelines for immunization, may improve vaccine coverage.

Haemophilus influenza type b

Haemophilus influenza type b (Hib virus) was, until the introduction of an effective vaccine, the leading cause of meningitis in children. The rate of infection in children under age five was 1 in 200. Those with meningitis had a fatality rate of 3-5%, and those who survived had high rates of neurological complications. Since the introduction of the vaccine in 1986, the number of cases of invasive *Haemophilus* disease has declined steadily. In 1985, 485 cases were recorded at tertiary care hospitals in Canada. After the introduction of conjugate vaccines and infant immunization programs, the number of cases in 1995 was 20. This indicates the importance of an effective immunization program (18).

Hepatitis B

The incidence of reported cases in Canada in 1992 was 13 per 100,000, having more than doubled from 5 per 100,000 in 1982. Under-reporting occurs, and Health Canada estimates the overall annual incidence rate for Canada may be as high as 100 infections per 100,000 people. The peak incidence is in males aged 25 to 29 years. There are approximately 2,000 reported cases of hepatitis B per year in Canada. Mortality from this disease has increased from 0.5 to 1.5 per million in Canada in the past decade. The major modes of spread in Canada are sexual transmission and intravenous drug use. Vertical transmission (from mother to newborn) and medical and dental occupational transmission (patient to practitioner and vice versa) account for a small proportion of cases.

Due to the high infectiousness of this virus, the expert consensus in Canada supports universal vaccination against hepatitis B (19). Since 1991, NACI has recommended universal hepatitis B vaccination. There are arguments for immunization in late childhood or early adolescence for maximum protection against sexual transmission of hepatitis B during adolescence and early adulthood (20). In 1996, all provinces except Manitoba have universal pre-adolescent hepatitis B vaccination programs.

3.1. TRENDS IN OTHER SIGNIFICANT INFECTIOUS DISEASES

Tuberculosis (TB)

TB is an important chronic infection, especially in at-risk population such as those with HIV infection, homeless persons, alcoholics, Aboriginal people, and foreign-born individuals from areas where TB is endemic. The incidence of TB in the Aboriginal population is currently 70 per 100,000. The incidence of TB in Canada in 1989 rose for the first time in 30 years to 7.8 per 100,000, representing 2,035 new active and reactivated cases (21). Since then the rate has remained relatively constant varying around 7.4 cases per 100,000. The highest rates are found in Manitoba, Saskatchewan, and the Yukon and Northwest Territories. Apart from the difficulties of control in traditional risk groups and HIV-infected persons, there have been difficulties in preventing transmission by newly arrived immigrants during the period after arrival (22). Most, in fact, are lost to follow-up. Medical practitioners need to be sensitized to the diagnosis management of TB, particularly as it relates to public health hazards and the emergence of multiple-resistant strains in those noncompliant with chemotherapy.

A major obstacle to tuberculosis control is compliance with medication. A course of therapy requires at least three medications for six to nine months. As the acute symptoms rapidly disappear after four to six weeks, it is often difficult to persuade people to remain compliant. As lack of compliance is one of the major determinants of antibiotic resistance, innovative strategies such as Directly Observed Therapy (DOT) have been implemented in populations at high risk for noncompliance. DOT involves giving medications by a health care worker to a patient and making sure the patient takes the medication. This strategy has been effective at reducing the rates of multiple drug-resistant tuberculosis in the United States.

Meningococcal Disease

Bacterial meningitis, a serious inflammation of the coverings of the brain and spinal cord, is usually caused by *Neisseria meningitidis*. Death and permanent neurological impairment are the most severe consequences. Meningococcal disease can also manifest as overwhelming septicemia or arthritis. The incidence of invasive meningococcal disease has varied in Canada from 1 to 3 cases per 100,000 people. In the early 1980s the incidence was low. It rose, however, to a peak in 1989, with an incidence of 2 per 100,000 and then declined in the early 1990s (23). Small clusters (fewer than 10 cases) and unlinked cases of meningococcal disease were reported in at least five provinces in 1991/92: Ontario, Quebec, Prince Edward Island, and British Columbia in 1991 and in Nova Scotia, Labrador, Ontario, Alberta, and Quebec in 1992. There were 250 cases of meningococcal disease reported in 1995. The disease primarily affects children, especially infants. In recent years, however, the proportion of cases occurring in adolescents and adults has been increasing steadily. Group C has emerged as the most frequent *Neisseria* isolate in the 1990s. Despite improved therapeutic management, about 20 people — mostly infants — die from complications every year. The overall case-fatality rate in recent years has been less than 10%, as compared with more than 30% in the 1950s and 1960s.

Hepatitis C

Hepatitis C is now regarded as a serious communicable disease. Most infections are clinically inapparent, but up to 90% of infections become chronic. It is estimated that 300,000 Canadians have been infected with this virus. Over 14,000 cases were reported in 1995, three times the number of cases of hepatitis B. The major modes of transmission are blood transfusions (prior to 1990 when blood screening was introduced) needle sharing, tattooing and body piercing, and needle stick accidents. There is a low but measurable rate of sexual transmission. Currently no vaccine exists. Prevention efforts are focused on screening blood donors and encouraging the use of clean needles (24).

Invasive Group A Streptococcus

Group A *Streptococcus* became prominent when Quebec politician Lucien Bouchard survived a leg amputation from this bacterium. The condition appears to be caused by a heightened immune reaction to the presence of a specific protein in certain strains of Group A *Streptococcus*. The incidence of the disease is low in the population. However, there is compelling evidence that it can be spread from person to person. The disease is reportable to public health authorities in some provinces.

Respiratory Syncytial Virus (RSV)

RSV is a common virus that circulates annually and often precedes the influenza virus. It is an important cause of morbidity and mortality for very young children and for the elderly, and is associated with increased hospitalization for both groups. RSV has increasingly been implicated in nursing home outbreaks of respiratory illness and may be a factor in the increase in winter mortality of the elderly at a magnitude that rivals influenza (25). Although no vaccine exists, basic infection control measures can limit the spread of RSV infections and reduce morbidity and mortality.

3.2. ANTIBIOTIC RESISTANCE

All bacteria are capable of developing resistance to antibiotic medication. The late 1980s witnessed the development of antibiotic resistance of several common bacteria. Hospitals in particular have been troubled by outbreaks of methicillin-resistant Staphylococcus aureus (MRSA) and vancomycin-resistant enterococcus (VRE). *Streptococccus pneumonia*, the most common cause of otitis media in children and community-acquired pneumonia in adults, has shown worldwide resistance to penicillin and other drugs (26).

The determinants of antibiotic resistance are complex. Certainly iatrogenic factors such as the prescription of antibiotics to treat viral infections and personal factors such as non-compliance with full course of treatment with antibiotics have played a role in fostering resistance. The use of antibiotics in feedstocks has also been implicated. Agent factors such as the dissemination of resistance between different bacteria have been documented conclusively (27).

The consequences of antibiotic resistance are sobering: persons with antibiotic-resistant infections suffer higher morbidity and mortality rates and have longer and more expensive hospitalizations. Antibiotic development is expensive and requires considerable time for appropriate testing. Currently there are few promising new antibiotic medications on the development horizon. The prevention of antibiotic resistance requires enhanced epidemiologic and laboratory surveillance, rational prescription practices by physicians, increased compliance by individuals requiring therapy, and scrupulous adherence to hygienic practice in hospitals, nursing homes, and child care facilities.

3.3. VECTOR-BORNE DISEASES AND RABIES

Vectors such as mosquitos and ticks are responsible for a small but important proportion of communicable diseases. Lyme disease is not as prevalent in Canada as in the United States. A small endemic focus of ticks infected with *Borrelia burgdoferii* exists in southern Ontario. Mosquito-borne illnesses such as western equine encephalitis occur in sporadic outbreaks depending on environmental conditions. Vector-borne illnesses such as malaria, dengue fever, and yellow fever are major global causes of morbidity and mortality. There is some evidence linking changes in global climate to the expansion of the range of vector-borne diseases (28).

Rabies is a fatal viral illness. No human deaths have been attributed to rabies in Canada for over two decades. This is likely due to a combination of an effective vaccine available for post-exposure prophylaxis, as well as excellent control of rabies in domesticated animals. Southern Ontario had the highest rates of wildlife rabies in the world, until oral vaccine was given to wild foxes. A raccoon strain of rabies was predicted to cross the United States into Canada in 1995. This prompted an aggressive and successful campaign of vaccinating wild raccoons through bait drops and trap-vaccinate-and-release programs.

3.4. FOOD-BORNE AND WATER-BORNE ILLNESS

Food and water remain important and often unrecognized sources of communicable disease. A massive outbreak of Cryptosporidium infection went largely unrecognized by public health authorities in Milwaukee, Wisconsin. An estimated 500,000 people were infected in the outbreak. There have been recent outbreaks in Collingwood, Ontario, and Kamloops, British Columbia. In 1995 an outbreak of toxoplasmosis in Victoria was linked to reservoir water contaminated by feral or domestic cats (28). These outbreaks underscore the necessity for vigilance and the need to ensure that municipal water supplies are maintained at the highest level of quality.

Food-borne illness is a common cause of morbidity in the population. Common organisms associated with food-borne gastroenteritis are *Salmonella, Staphylococcus aureus*, and *Bacillus cereus*. Reports of food-borne illness to public health authorities is underestimated. This is because the vast majority of food-borne illness occurs at home and does not come to medical attention.

With the increased global nature of the food industry, serious illness and multi-location outbreaks have been associated with contaminated food. Hamburger disease, caused by Escherichia coli 0157:H7, has resulted in severe gastroenteritis and haemolytic uraemic syndrome. A large outbreak in the U.S. was traced to a contaminated shipment of ground beef. A large, geographically dispersed *Salmonella* outbreak in the United States was traced to contaminated ice cream from Minnesota. The recently identified parasite *Cyclospora* was responsible for outbreaks in Canada and the United States.

The Bureau of Infectious Diseases, Laboratory Centre for Disease Control, and the Health Protection Branch convened the 1996 National Consensus Conference on Food-borne, Water-borne and Enteric Disease Surveillance to develop a plan to better control human illness from these sources (29).

4. SEXUALLY TRANSMITTED DISEASES

4.1. INCIDENCE

In general, socioeconomic conditions and changes in lifestyle in North America are likely to have contributed to the observed increase in sexually transmitted diseases (STDs) in Canada. The 1960s brought new affluence, and with it more leisure time, social mobility, and changes in sexual behaviour. In addition, the ready availability of birth control methods decreased the probability of unwanted pregnancy. The emergence of AIDS as a major cause of death in homosexual males in the 1980s and early 1990s was also related to these changes in social norms. Subsequently, however, HIV infection in users of intravenous drugs, in new immigrants from AIDS-endemic countries, and in the sexual partners of these groups, has established the disease in the socioeconomically disadvantaged and their next generation.

Genital chlamydia, gonorrhea, and AIDS now account for more than half of the reported cases of all notifiable diseases combined. Infection with genital *Chlamydia trachomatis* has emerged as the most frequent STD in recent years in Canada, occurring three to five times more frequently than gonorrheal infections and responsible for over 40,000 reported cases of STD during 1994 (30). The rise in the number of reported cases is in part related to an increase in awareness of the disease and better diagnostic techniques, resulting in increased reporting. Chlamydial infection became nationally notifiable only in 1990. The disease is most prevalent among sexually active adolescents, particularly females aged 15 to 19 years. Rates of infection for women in that group range from 1,400 to 1,600 per 100,000 females compared to rates of 200 per 100,000 in women aged 20 to 44 years. Serious long-term consequences for females are pelvic inflammatory disease, ectopic pregnancy, and infertility.

The incidence of gonorrhea and syphilis has declined steadily over the past decade. Gonorrhea reports fell from 12,457 in 1991 to 4,443 in 1994; syphilis reports fell from 1,429 in 1991 to 194 in 1994 (16). Gonorrhea is more common in men than women and accounted for 27% of STD reports in men in 1994, compared to 7.6% in women. Syphilis accounted for 0.1% of reports in women and 0.7% of reports in men (31). The incidence of congenital syphilis is related to young maternal age, ethnicity (Aboriginal peoples), lack of prenatal care, and failure of health care professionals to repeat nontreponemal tests (VDRL/RPR) in the third trimester.

AIDS was first identified in Canada in 1979, and its incidence has increased since then. It became a reportable disease in Canada in 1982. As of October 1996, 14,185 cases of AIDS had been reported (32). Epidemiological evidence indicates that about 50% of HIV carriers will develop AIDS within 10 to 11 years after infection, and it is estimated that 30,000 Canadians have been infected so far. Most AIDS cases were reported from Ontario (40.2%), Quebec (32.8%), and British Columbia (16.3%). Men who have sex with men account for 79% of AIDS cases. Intravenous drug use accounts for the fastest growing segment of AIDS and HIV incidence. After a rapid rise through the 1980s, the annual incidence of new cases in Canada appears to have levelled off or declined slightly. Behaviour changes among gay men are a likely reason for this stabilizing effect. Globally, the HIV pandemic continues unabated. In sub-Saharan Africa, the prevalence of AIDS is estimated at 1,814 per 100,000.

AIDS is caused by the human immunodeficiency virus (HIV), which is transmitted by four routes: sexual contact with an infected partner, via infected blood and blood products, from an infected mother to her unborn child perinatally, and through needles and syringes shared among intravenous drug abusers. Sexual contact is the most frequent route, both homosexual and heterosexual. Unprotected anal and vaginal intercourse pose the greatest risk. Not all individuals exposed to HIV are at risk of HIV infection; the factors influencing this are poorly understood. With rare exceptions, most patients have seroconverted (that is, antibodies have developed in the blood as a result of infection) by six months after exposure, the majority seroconverting within two to six weeks. Evidence from virus isolation studies indicates that the majority of individuals who are HIV-antibody positive have the virus in their lymphocytes. All people with reactive HIV serology must be considered infectious. However, since some infected individuals may not develop the HIV antibody or may be in the incubation period, any person who has been exposed or belongs to a high-risk group should be considered potentially infectious regardless of serologic status.

In women, HIV infection occurs mainly among those of reproductive age and results from heterosexual activity with a person at risk (31%) or with a person from an AIDS endemic country (28%). The number of cases has grown from 13 in 1983 to 866 in 1996 (32). Studies of HIV seroprevalence in child-bearing women in Canada show rates of 3.2 per 10,000. There were 150 cases of AIDS diagnosed in children under age 15 by October 1996, with 80% being the result of perinatal transmission. AIDS is associated with increases in tuberculosis morbidity. Between 2% and 5% of all AIDS cases have tuberculosis as well. AIDS has a very high mortality rate (72% of all persons diagnosed with AIDS in Canada have died), with the median length of time between onset of AIDS and death estimated at 10 months.

4.2. TRADITIONAL STD PREVENTION

The mainstay of STD services has attempted to control syphilis, gonorrhea, and other sexually transmitted diseases by secondary prevention involving diagnosis and treatment, and primary or secondary prevention for contacts. AIDS marks a departure from this model as curative treatment is not available. People with gonorrhea, syphilis, and chlamydia may be asymptomatic, making it difficult to control infections and trace contacts. The other problems associated with control are difficulties in the follow-up of contacts, poor compliance with treatment regimens by patients, and the lack of physician reporting of cases. Contact tracing provided by public health staff is often more effective than that provided by medical practitioners. Current treatment schedules for STDs are established by Health Canada (33). Each province establishes and circulates specific guidelines for the treatment of STDs.

It is important to note that effective prevention for one sexually transmitted disease is likely to have an effect on others. Condom use is successful for not only the prevention of HIV, but also reduces the rates of syphilis, gonorrhea, and chlamydia. HIV prevention programs in the developing world have shown consistent reductions in these diseases and unplanned pregnancies as a benefit of the promotion of condom use.

4.3. HEALTH PROMOTION IN SEXUAL HEALTH

More recently the concept of healthy sexuality has been introduced as a modality of primary prevention (34). Healthy sexuality is comfort with one's own sexuality, body characteristics, and self-efficacy in making decisions related to sexuality, such as contraception, pregnancy, and prevention of sexually transmitted disease. Developing positive sexual health involves a multifaceted approach of health education, self-esteem, and decision-making skills for behavioural change, as well as communication of specific knowledge such as methods of birth control (oral contraception and barrier methods) and STD prevention (safer sex techniques).

Education and communication in this area must be innovative and sustain the interest of youth. For example, it has been recognized in a number of surveys on sexual attitudes of Canadian youth that barriers exist to behaviour change allowing the adoption of safer sex practices. Although young people appear to have adequate knowledge about STDs, they are unlikely to interpret risks personally and will take the view that "it cannot happen to me" (35). Approaches that personalize the information on AIDS, for example a speaker with the disease, may be more successful. Public health units have developed rap videos on safer sex in an attempt to reach youth. Practising putting a condom on a model may also enhance personal skill development.

Efforts to provide better communication about sexual health and services with high-risk groups are also being developed. These include more accessible clinics (such as locating clinics in high schools (36) and providing other user-friendly types of facilities in shopping malls), reaching homeless youth in the community through outreach workers, and community development. Health promotion strategies are multifaceted. For example, a healthy public policy approach would encourage schools to provide condom machines in washrooms. Community development, as exemplified by gay communities, can result in widespread behaviour change. The continued incidence of HIV infection in the 1990s — especially in groups previously largely unaffected — remains a major concern, as is the chlamydia epidemic.

5.   AIDS

Strategies to control AIDS have focused on preventing the spread of HIV infection and providing multi-drug therapy early. Strategies to control sexual transmission of the virus include the promotion of behavioural change to encourage the use of condoms for safer sex. To prevent transmission by infected blood and blood products, the Canadian Red Cross Society has initiated a policy of requesting members of high-risk groups to refrain from donating blood. Since the fall of 1985, all blood collected by the Red Cross has been screened for HIV antibodies, and further transmission through blood products is one in a million. Similarly, all factor VIII concentrate now used by haemophiliacs is heat-treated to inactivate the virus. However, AIDS may still develop in some individuals infected by this route before 1985. Sperm and organ donors are screened for the presence of HIV antibody. The Krever Commission of Inquiry on the Blood System in Canada has comprehensively reviewed the issues of the transmission of HIV through blood and blood products (37).

Strategies for preventing the spread of HIV among drug users involve the use of harm reduction techniques (see Chapter One) such as the establishment of needle exchanges (where clean equipment can be obtained) and the training of intravenous drug users in disinfecting their equipment using bleach kits (38). Finally, recommendations have been made for health care personnel to adopt universal precautions for handling body fluids (see Chapter Ten). The administration of the antiviral agent AZT is successful in reducing the rate of maternal transmission of HIV infection to newborns (39). Newly developed protease inhibitors have given rise to the hope that HIV can become a manageable chronic disease. A vaccine for HIV remains a remote hope. Primary prevention should still be regarded as the best possible way to prevent the spread of HIV.

Testing those at risk for HIV has assumed importance largely as a means of reinforcing the need for adopting safer sex behaviour as well as allowing early HIV treatment. Guidelines for HIV testing that involve pre- and post-test counselling have been established and disseminated because it is important that people being tested understand the disease and the implications of the test. Although public health has never been responsible for a breech of confidentiality regarding HIV/AIDS, this pathogen is unique in that anonymous testing is available to individuals. All other lab testing for communicable diseases requires a doctor's order.

The components of health promotion (as established in the Ottawa Charter) have been applied to AIDS in terms of a comprehensive and integrated basis for action in the 1990s (40). The implementation of healthy public policy, interpreted as minimizing structural discrimination against those who are HIV infected, reduces the alienation of those needing health and social services. A social environment supportive of safer sex practices, such as the use of condoms (and safer intravenous drug use), can utilize the principles of social marketing. Development of personal skills in safer sexual behaviour can be achieved by applying the communication-education theory, particularly by developing infrastructures for communication to at-risk groups, such as outreach programs and small group sessions. Promotion of the strengthening of communities has resulted in action to enhance behaviour change and behavioural norms in at-risk groups. Strategies for the last component of the Ottawa Charter approach, reorientation of the health system emphasizing a community approach, have been indicated throughout the above section.

Global experience in AIDS prevention indicates that population-based strategies need to be supplemented with messages adapted to the specific culture and practices of those at risk. Peer-led education models and the use of influential celebrities can bring health messages tailored to the particular concerns of those who perceive themselves to exist outside the mainstream. A recent review of AIDS prevention has emphasized the effectiveness of community-based strategies in the prevention of AIDS (41).

6.   SUMMARY

Despite the widespread availability of most vaccines, outbreaks of communicable diseases such as measles, meningitis, and tuberculosis continue to occur in Canada and are associated with significant mortality and morbidity.

Although vaccine-preventable diseases have declined, sporadic cases and outbreaks of a number of infectious diseases are being reported. These include:

In 1989 and 1990, there were *pertussis*, or whooping cough, outbreaks. The virulence of this bacteria has decreased due to widespread vaccination which affords partial protection.

A major resurgence of vaccine-preventable cases of *measles* occurred in Canada in the late 1980s and early 1990s. The cases have largely been among those aged 10 to 14, most of whom had been previously vaccinated. The resurgence of measles incidence in Canada is largely due to primary vaccine failure. A two-dose immunization strategy should eliminate measles in Canada.

There was a marked increase in the number of cases of *rubella* in the late 1980s. Cases have been occurring in those of high school age and among those aged 20 to 29.

Influenza is of special significance in the winter months. The mortality from influenza (particularly in the elderly) and pneumococcal infections (which may arise as a complication of influenza infection) now exceeds that of all vaccine-preventable childhood disease.

Meningococcal disease, a bacterial meningitis, is an inflammation of the covering of the brain and spinal cord. Its incidence was low in the early 1980s; however, it peaked in 1989 and then declined in the 1990s. The disease primarily affects children, especially infants. In recent years, the proportion of cases occurring in adolescents and adults has been increasing steadily.

Haemophilus influenza type b prior to 1987, occurred in 1 in 200 under the age of five. However, in the early 1990s the incidence was reduced to 27 from 54 per 100,000. The decrease was largely due to new conjugate vaccines given to infants.

Hepatitis B is one of the most important communicable diseases. From 1982 to 1992, the incidence has almost doubled, with the peak incidence in those aged 25 to 29. Hepatitis B is a sexually transmitted disease, particularly among young adults. Universal immunization of school-aged children should eventually reduce the incidence of hepatitis B.

Tuberculosis is a significant chronic infection in a number of at-risk population (e.g., alcoholics, persons with HIV, immigrants, and Aboriginal peoples).

Vector-borne diseases, although rare in Canada, are an important cause of morbidity and mortality worldwide. Food-borne disease contributes significantly to the burden of morbidity from communicable disease in Canada. Food-borne and water-borne diseases can be caused by bacteria, viruses, and rare parasites.

It is important to realize that the effectiveness of vaccination in protecting individuals depends on both the efficacy, or performance of the vaccine under ideal conditions, and on the degree of coverage achieved. Primary immunization for infants and children against diphtheria, whooping cough, tetanus, poliomyelitis, and Hib disease started at the age of two months and is given at four and six months, with booster doses at 18 months and at four to six years of age. Measles, mumps, and rubella vaccine is given after the first birthday and before school starts.

Genital chlamydia, gonorrhea, and AIDS now account for more than half of the reported cases of all notifiable diseases combined. Infection with genital chlamydia has emerged as an epidemic STD in recent years in Canada. The disease is most prevalent among sexually active young women aged 15 to 19. Despite effective antibiotic therapy, there has been a rise in the incidence of gonorrhea in the past two decades and a persistence of syphilis.

AIDS incidence appears to have levelled off, but continues to rise among intravenous drug users. Carriers of HIV will develop AIDS within 10 to 11 years after infection. Most Canadian AIDS cases have been reported in Ontario, Quebec, and British Columbia. AIDS is caused by HIV, which is transmitted by four routes: sexual contact with an infected partner, via infected blood and blood products, from an infected mother to her unborn child perinatally, and through the use of needles by intravenous drug abusers. AIDS is one of the major causes of death among males between 30 and 39 in Canada. Strategies to control

AIDS have focused on preventing the spread of HIV infection. Strategies to control the sexual transmission of the virus include promoting behavioural change to limit the number of sexual partners and the use of condoms for safer sex. As well, the Canadian Red Cross Society has initiated a policy of requesting that anyone belonging to a high-risk group refrain from donating blood.

7. REFERENCES

1. Last JM. A Dictionary of Epidemiology (third edition). Toronto: Oxford University Press, 1995.
2. Benenson AS. Control of Communicable Diseases in Man (16th edition). Washington, DC: American Public Health Association, 1995.
3. Giesecke J. Modern Infectious Disease Epidemiology. Boston: Little, Brown and Company, 1994.
4. Gyorkos T, Tannenbaum T, Abrahamowicz M, et al. Evaluation of the Effectiveness of Immunization Delivery Methods. Canadian Journal of Public Health 1994; 85(S1):S14-S29.
5. Tannenbaum T, Gyorkos T, Abrahamowicz M. Immunization Delivery Methods: Practice Recommendations. Canadian Journal of Public Health 1994; 85(S1):S37-S47.
6. National Guidelines for Vaccine Storage and Transportation. Canada Communicable Disease Report 1995;21(11):93-97.
7. Pless R, Duclos P. Reinforcing Surveillance for Vaccine-Associated Adverse Events: The Advisory Committee on Causality Assessment. Canadian Journal of Infectious Disease 1996;7:98-99.
8. Health Canada. Canadian National Report on Immunization, 1996. Ottawa: Division of Immunization, Laboratory Centre for Disease Control, 1997.
9. Resurgence of Pertussis in Montergie, Quebec, 1990-1994. Canada Communicable Disease Report 1995;20(22):41-45.
10. Statement on Management of Persons Exposed to Pertussis and Pertussis Outbreak Control. Canada Communicable Disease Report 1994;20(22):193-199.
11. Greco D, Salmuso S, Mastrantonio P, et al. A Controlled Trial of Two Acellular Vaccines and One Whole-Cell Vaccine against Pertussis. New England Journal of Medicine 1996;334:341-348.
12. Gustafson L, Hallander H, Olin P, et al. A Controlled Trial of Two Component Acellular and a Whole-Cell Pertussis Vaccine. New England Journal of Medicine 1996;334:349-355.
13. Furesz J. Elimination of Measles in the Americas. Canadian Medical Association Journal 1996;155(1):1423-1426.
14. Supplementary Statement on Measles Elimination in Canada. Canada Communicable Disease Report 1996;22(2):9-15.
15. Arbuckle T, Sherman G. Is Congenital Rubella Syndrome a Vanishing Disease? Chronic Disease in Canada 1992;13(2):24-28.
16. Statistics Canada. Catalogue no. 82-221-XDE. 1995.
17. Canadian Consensus Conference on Influenza. Canada Communicable Disease Report 1993;19(17):136-146.

18. Department of Paediatrics, British Columbia Children's Hospital. Recent Trends in Paediatric Haemophilus Influenza Type B Infections in Canada. Canadian Medical Association Journal 1996;154(7):1041-1047.
19. Hepatitis B in Canada: The Case for Universal Vaccination. Position Statement. Canadian Medical Association Journal 1992;146(1):25-27.
20. Gold R. Hepatitis B Vaccine: Revisited. Paediatric Child Health 1996;1:95-96.
21. Wilkins K. Tuberculosis, 1994. Health Reports 1996;8(1):33-39.
22. Statistics Canada. Tuberculosis Incidence in Canada, 1989. Health Reports 1990;2(4):303.
23. Guidelines for Controlling Meningococcal Disease. Epidemiologic Report. Canadian Medical Association Journal 1992;146(6):939-942.
24. Prevention and Control of Hepatitis C, Guidelines and Recommendations. Canada Communicable Disease Report 1995; 21(S2).
25. Nicholson K. Impact of Influenza and RSV on Mortality in England from January 1975 to December 1990. Epidemiology and Infection 1996;116:51-63.
26. Friedland I, McCracken G. Management of Infections Caused by Antibiotic-Resistant Streptococcus Pneumonia. New England Journal of Medicine 1994;331(6):377-382.
27. Travis J. Reviving the Antibiotic Miracle. Science 1994;264:360-362.
28. Epstein P, Rogers D, Sloof R. Satellite Imaging and Vector-Borne Disease. Lancet 1993;341:1404-1406.
29. Summary of the National Consensus Conference on Foodborne, Waterborne and Enteric Disease Surveillance. Canada Communicable Disease Report 1996;22(11):81-84.
30. Davies H, Wang E, et al. Periodic Health Examination, 1996 Update: 2. Screening for Chlamydial Infections. Canadian Medical Association Journal 1996;154(11):1631-1642.
31. Public Health Intelligence Reinvestment Twelve-Month Progress Report 1996. 1996.
32. Health Protection Branch. Quarterly Surveillance Update: AIDS in Canada, October 1996. Ottawa: Laboratory Centre for Disease Control, 1996.
33. Gully P. Canadian Guidelines for the Prevention, Diagnosis, Management and Treatment of Sexually Transmitted Diseases in Neonates, Children, Adolescents, and Adults. Ottawa: Laboratory Centre for Disease Control, Health and Welfare Canada, 1992.
34. Ministry of Health Ontario. Mandatory Health Programs and Services and Guidelines. Program Standard, Sexual Health. Toronto: Ministry of Health Ontario, 1989.
35. Bowie W, Warren WK, Fisher WA, et al. Implications of the Canada Youth and AIDS Study for Health Care Providers. Canadian Medical Association Journal 1990;143(8):713-716.
36. Rafuse J. MD's, Nurses Play Major Role in Success of "Sexuality Clinics" at Ottawa High Schools. Canadian Medical Association Journal 1992;146(4):593-596.
37. Krever H, Health Canada. The Commission of Inquiry on the Blood System in Canada (Krever Commission Report). Ottawa: Canada Communication Group, 1997.
38. Des Jarlais D. Harm Reduction: A Framework for Incorporating Science into Drug Policy. American Journal of Public Health 1995;85(1):10-11.
39. Connor E, Sperling R, Gelber R, et al. Reduction of Maternal-Infant Transmission of Human Immunodeficiency Virus Type 1 with Zidovudine. New England Journal of Medicine 1994;331(18):1173-1180.
40. Nutbeam D, Blakey V. The Concept of Health Promotion and AIDS Prevention. A Comprehensive and Integrated Basis for Action in the 1990s. Health Promotion International 1990;5(3):233-242.
41. Coates T, Aggleton P, Gutzwiller F. HIV Prevention in Developed Countries. Lancet 1996;348:1143-1148.

9

Environmental Health

1. GENERAL FRAMEWORK

In recent years, there has been increasing recognition of the interdependence of human health and the health of the global ecosystem, with its many life forms. Much of this awareness has been generated by community-based environmental advocacy groups such as Greenpeace and Pollution Probe, as well as Aboriginal peoples, who have all highlighted the importance of the environment. Historically, the field of environmental health has usually dealt with food and water safety, and with inspection and investigation of environmental hazards that may arise from inadequate sanitation. In most of Canada (apart from areas such as Aboriginal reserves where physical facilities may be grossly inadequate), provision of sanitation, potable water supply, and food free from gross contamination have been largely achieved. There is, however, growing concern over the status of the environment and the consequences of environmental pollution, particularly of chemical contamination. This concern is not only limited to the effects on human health but also to the viability of ecosystems in general and many species in particular.

Public attention has been captured by recent reports detailing the effects of acid rain on forest and aquatic ecosystems, climatic changes resulting from the "greenhouse effect", the depletion of the ozone layer, and the effects of marine pollution on aquatic life. Public interest has also been heightened as a result of numerous reports linking environmental exposure to adverse human health outcomes. Environmental factors may contribute to the development of breast cancer, and the reported decrease in the sperm count of men in some developed nations has led to increased research of the role of chemical contamination on human reproductive capacity (1).

There is a growing awareness of possible links between illness and many features of industrialized society (2). Indoor air quality has been investigated in many modern buildings, following reports of symptoms in employees or residents, resulting in a newly identified illness pattern: the "sick building syndrome." The evacuation of St-Basile-le-Grand near Montreal in August 1988, following the fire-related release of polychlorinated biphenyls (PCBs), and the 1997 Hamilton (Ontario) fire of a warehouse containing plastic are examples of events that focused public attention on emergency response measures and the control aspects of environmental health.

Environmental health may be defined as the study of conditions in the natural and built (physical) environment that influence human health and well-being. As the impact of the environment on human population is widespread, environmental health is generally categorized as a discipline of public health. While other disciplines assess the impact of environmental agents or hazards on the individual patient, the focus of study in environmental health is the impact of these agents on the health of the population.

The environment (as it affects health) can be divided into working and non-working categories. The workplace environment is often associated with high-level exposure of a population predominantly of adult age and in good health. In contrast, non-workplace environmental exposures are generally low level and may be chronic. The population at risk consists of persons at the extremes of age, developing fetuses, and the ill or immunocompromised. Thus, while many of the pathogenic agents are similar, there is an arbitrary distinction between working and non-working environmental health. The specific concerns relating to the working environment (occupational health) are addressed in Chapter Ten. An overview of environmental health in Canada is given in the publications by Health Canada entitled *A Vital Link: Health and the Environment in Canada: (3)* and *Health and Environment: Partner for Life (2)*.

Despite the uncertainty associated with many environmental health problems, health care providers are considered to be the most credible source of information regarding the health effects of environmental exposures. Consequently, it is important for every health care provider to be familiar with the concepts employed and the issues involved in environmental health.

2.   STUDY OF ENVIRONMENTAL HEALTH

The study of environmental health issues relies on two primary disciplines, toxicology and epidemiology. **Toxicology**, the science of "poisons" (toxins), attempts to identify adverse effects of substances on health and to predict harmful dosages. One of the fundamental tenets of toxicology is that any substance can be a poison if given in a large enough dose. By contrast, a carcinogen may have no "threshold" dose below which it no longer causes cancer. The other discipline, **epidemiology**, as has been previously defined in Chapter Two, is the study of the distribution and determinants of health and disease in human population. Although these disciplines provide a vast amount of information on specific environmental health hazards, the interpretation of these data and subsequent regulatory decisions is often difficult. This section addresses some of these difficulties.

There are a variety of problems in the measurement of a specific toxic agent. The levels are often difficult to determine, both in the human body and in the ambient (surrounding) environment. As technology progresses, the detection of minute quantities of chemicals is enhanced, but the interpretation of their significance to human health may remain difficult. When a level is measurable, it often does not reflect the concentration in the target organ of interest; rather, it represents a crude attempt to assess dose by measuring tissue fluid levels (usually blood). Often the agent itself is not toxic but is metabolized to toxic endproducts within the body. When ambient levels can be defined, the dose-response relationship at low levels is often difficult to predict because most toxicological or epidemiological data are obtained from high-dose animal experimentation or occupational exposure. Extrapolation to low doses is uncertain, and there are several models to choose from. Often an arbitrary safety factor is applied to the threshold dose to derive an acceptable intake (exposure) level for humans. This safety factor attempts to account for both inter- and intra-species variation.

The study of other adverse health outcomes, particularly mutagenic or carcinogenic effects, is complicated by the long latency period following exposure. During the latency period for most cancers, exposures to causal agents may be terminated or periodic. Adverse outcomes may manifest only in a small fraction of the exposed population. This again makes epidemiologic analysis difficult (4). Furthermore, the effects of a specific agent are often masked by the confounding effects of multiple exposures. The relationship between agents grows even more complex when one accounts for synergistic, promoting, or attenuating interrelationships of chemical mixtures. The study of environmental health is also complicated by the fact that many adverse outcomes are nonspecific and subjective. The upper respiratory and conjunctival symptoms of the sick building syndrome, for example, are difficult to quantify objectively. Analysis becomes more difficult when one considers that such nonspecific and ill-defined psychosomatic symptoms have also been induced by fear of ill effects from the environment. Frank et al. (5) reviewed the strengths and weaknesses of a number of epidemiologic studies related to environmental concerns and summarized these as lack of certainty of exposure to putative agents, large potentially exposed population, and relatively common adverse health effects.

Recent research has extended the domain of concern about persistent chemicals in the environment to include reproductive and neuro-behavioural outcomes. There is an emerging body of literature that examines the effects of chemicals on the hormone systems of humans and animals. Consequently, the focus of research will expand beyond concerns about carcinogenesis and look at a broader range of outcomes (6).

2.1. ASSESSMENT AND MANAGEMENT OF HEALTH RISKS

Each of us is exposed to a variety of risks, environmental and behavioural, every day. Health Canada, Environment Canada, provincial ministries of health and environment, municipal departments of health, and various consumer groups are among the leading authorities responsible for identifying and assessing the risks to human health posed by the environment. Evaluation of the political, economic, societal, and technological implications of the risk is undertaken. Options for managing risks are identified according to the best available evidence. Decisions are then made for the development of policy, regulations, and other measures for protection of the public.

Risk assessment is the first approach to assessing health risks posed by contaminants. Two closely associated concepts, risk management and risk communication, deal with actions taken to reduce risk and to communicate with the public about the environmental hazards which people perceive. Another method, outlined in Chapter Two, deals with the investigation of clusters of non-communicable diseases, such as congenital defects or cancer in the community due to putative environmental agents.

2.1.1. Risk Assessment

There are four major steps in the risk assessment of any environmental contaminant: hazard identification, exposure assessment and monitoring, dose-response assessment, and risk determination.

Hazard Identification

Does the substance have potentially adverse effects and what are they? What organ systems do they affect? Information is obtained from laboratory, genetic, animal, and human epidemiological studies.

Exposure Assessment and Monitoring

Exposure can be defined as any contact between a substance and an individual. An exposure pathway has five components:
- The source of contamination;
- The environmental media;
- The point of exposure;
- The receptor person or population;
- The route of exposure.

With this general framework in mind, it is possible to develop a model of the variety of possible exposures and their potential impact on humans. The principal environmental media for the exposure to contaminants are water, food, soil, and air. The major routes of exposure for humans are inhalation, ingestion, and dermal contact. Once these factors are characterized, it is possible to calculate an estimated daily intake (EDI), which sums the estimated dose from all possible exposure routes. As data are often not available for all routes of exposure or on the toxicology of all contaminants, it is often necessary to make assumptions about the estimated dose that a person may have achieved. The averaging process that occurs may not take into account variability with respect to differences in body weight or duration of exposure, and may not precisely calculate consumption rates for food and water.

Exposure must be estimated in order to characterize safe levels of exposure to potentially hazardous substances. Toxicological studies are used to determine the dose response relationship between a substance and its potential health effects. An essential component of a health risk assessment is the concept of a threshold. Animal data from toxicological studies and data derived from epidemiologic data on humans are used to determine the level of exposure at which no observable adverse effects occur (NOAEL) or the lowest dose at which a measurable adverse effect occurs (LOAEL). Once the LOAEL or NOAEL has been estimated, it is possible to estimate a likely safe exposure level to a contaminant. This is called the tolerable daily intake (TDI).

These estimates are always uncertain, however, so the TDI usually includes a safety factor. Depending on the extent of the laboratory studies and the adverse effects that the substance can cause, the safety factor may range from 100 to several thousand or more.

The estimated daily intake from the various exposure routes can be compared to the tolerable daily intake in order to determine whether an individual or population is exposed to greater than acceptable exposures. If this occurs, then risk management strategies, as outlined below, can be implemented.

There are a large number of potentially harmful exposures from environmental sources, and monitoring the levels of selected potential exposures is necessary. However, it is not feasible to monitor all potential exposures, so selected indicators are usually chosen for surveillance purposes.

Identification of potential contamination of nutritional sources includes the monitoring of breast milk for contaminants such as dioxins and PCBs and the levels of these contaminants in fish and animals in local environments where subsistence fishing and hunting is practised by Aboriginal peoples.

In Canada, water quality should conform to accepted guidelines, such as the Guidelines for Canadian Drinking Water Quality (7). These are designed to ensure that the water is free from pathogenic organisms, harmful chemicals, radioactive matter and should be palatable. Maximum acceptable concentrations (MACs) for a wide range of chemicals, esthetic objectives, and microbiologic characteristics for water have been defined. The microbiologic assessment of drinking water generally involves assessment for coliform organisms as a marker of faecal contamination. More recently, in recreational water, the presence of *Escherichia coli* at specified levels is regarded as an indicator of faecal contamination (8). Although viruses have been implicated in waterborne disease outbreaks, no specific virologic standard applies. The turbidity of water is assessed for esthetic purposes. Turbidity can also interfere with the detection methods for bacteriologic quality and with the disinfection process.

MACs are also applicable in assessing individual air contaminants. The Air Quality Index described in Chapter Two only addresses six important pollutants that are related particularly to acute health effects. Evidence of long-range transport and deposition of airborne contaminants such as mercury and organochlorine pesticides indicate the need for the measurement and surveillance of other air-borne pollutants (9).

Dose-Response Assessment

Dose-response analysis uses data from toxicological and epidemiological studies to determine how much exposure to a potential contaminant is associated with adverse health outcome. Dose-response models are either threshold or non-threshold in nature. A threshold model indicates that there is a level of exposure below which no adverse effect is likely. Non-threshold models indicate that any exposure is likely to result in some adverse effect. The concept of dose response is particularly important for carcinogenic chemicals for which it may be necessary to specify exposures with an acceptable degree of risk: less than one chance in a million for an individual to develop cancer over a lifetime (if exposure cannot be eliminated entirely).

Risk Determination

Given the potential toxicity of the substance, the actual or estimated exposure and the dose-response relationship, what are the likely effects on human health? What is the measure of uncertainty inherent in this calculation? Options for minimizing the risk are then developed and analysed to complete the "risk assessment cycle".

2.1.2. Risk Management

Risk management is the next series of steps following risk assessment. It involves decision making and implementation of options for management of the identified risk. For example, when considering food contaminants, if a potential daily intake exceeds the tolerable daily intake, certain risk management options are considered. The options include:

- establishing guidelines or promulgating specific regulations controlling the toxic substance or substances;
- restricting the sale or distribution of food produced in an area that may have been identified as the source of the contamination; recommending changes in dietary habits.

Before initiating any specific action, however, the federal Health Protection Branch must assess its advantages and disadvantages. For example, removal of certain foods from the market or recommendations to change dietary habits could deny the people at risk of an essential source of nutrition, which might cause a more serious health problem than that associated with the chemical contaminant.

2.1.3. Risk Communication

The communication of risk in relation to environmental hazards, and public health hazards in general, depends on an important concept: the perception of risk by the lay public often differs from that of "experts". Experts tend to express risk in terms of the actual numbers affected and numerical probabilities. The lay public tends to perceive risk according to the degree of "unfamiliarity" of the threat and whether there is a threat of a catastrophe involving serious adverse events (particularly death) for many people at one time. The model for this concept of risk perception is the factorial model, the two factors being fear of the unknown and dread. These factors can be quantified on two-dimensional axes. For example, in Canada, nuclear installations score very highly on both of these factors (both x and y axes), and public reaction to any possibility of an environmental threat is likely to be high. Another principle of risk communication is that the potential risk of an environmental health hazard should be expressed in readily understandable terms. For example, expressing the risk of cancer from a contaminant in drinking water as less than one chance in a million of a lifetime for an individual is more useful than using scientific language.

In general, however, the public has difficulty with the expression of risk as a probability; it prefers to know whether the agent does or does not pose a risk to health (the "risk dichotomy" concept). Since it is usually impossible to dichotomize risk so absolutely, effective risk communication may involve informing the public that the measured level of the agent is either above or below a certain guideline or regulated safe level. It is essential, however, to have an accurate understanding of the perception of risk in the community and an accurate understanding of the range of risk acceptable to the community. Otherwise, reassurance may be perceived as false and not truly addressing the degree of concern and stress in the community. The relevant aspects of risk perception and communication have been well summarized by Covelho (10).

3.   ENVIRONMENTAL HEALTH ISSUES

In the following section, some environmental agents that have been incriminated as causing ill health are described. The sources of the agents, routes of human exposure, adverse effects, and approaches to control are included in the discussion.

3.1. OUTDOOR AND INDOOR ENVIRONMENTS

3.1.1. Ionizing Radiation
There are two types of radiation: ionizing and non-ionizing. Ionizing radiation is emitted from radioactive substances and is capable of producing ions in matter, including cellular matter, causing altered cell physiology. More than 80% of the radiation to which humans are exposed are produced from natural sources, whether from the radioactive elements in the earth's crust, cosmic radiation, or ingested or inhaled isotopes. With one major exception, non-background radiation exposure is primarily an occupational hazard for certain categories of workers and are discussed in greater detail in Chapter Ten.

Radon
Radon is a naturally occurring radioactive gas that forms as a decay product of uranium 238. Uranium is a trace element found in all soils. As part of the radioactive decay process, radon produces four progeny that emit alpha radiation. Human skin acts as a barrier, but inhaled radon progeny deposit alpha particles internally in the localized

area of the bronchial epithelium, which eventually leads to lung cancer. Due to its accumulation indoors it is more of a concern for indoor air pollution, although it is present in the natural environment as well. Radon gas passes from porous soil into buildings through cracks in basement floors and walls. Given that the majority of an individual's time is spent indoors, there is a potential health risk from natural sources of radon. Health Canada has recommended that the Canadian guideline for existing homes for radon should be 20 picocuries per litre, and for newly constructed homes, 4 picocuries per litre. When the level of radon is in doubt, houses must be individually tested for radon levels; extrapolation from neighbouring homes is not appropriate.

Estimates of the lung cancer risk following household radon exposure have been extrapolated from studies of lung cancer incidence in uranium miners. The relative risk for exposed households has been estimated to range between 1.1 and 1.5. It has also been estimated that up to 15% of lung cancer deaths may be attributable to domestic radon exposure. Occupational standards have been set for exposure to radon for uranium miners and for dwellings in uranium mining communities. In dwellings with high levels, measures such as increased basement ventilation and sealing cracks and holes in the foundation are simple and effective methods for decreasing radon concentrations. Tobacco smoking increases an individual's chance of getting lung cancer with radon exposure.

3.1.2. Living Near Nuclear Facilities

Nuclear accidents at Chernobyl and Three Mile Island have raised public anxiety and affected perceptions of the safety of living in close proximity to nuclear facilities. The major issue is better communication between the public and health care providers and authorities, based on an expanded knowledge base about radiation effects and the realistic potential for exposure (which is minimal) (11). Many factors can influence the health effects of radiation, including the type of radiation, the rate at which energy is deposited in tissues, the dose of radiation administered and received by tissues, and the radiation sensitivity of the affected tissue. The total dose is also important. The effects of high-dose radiation are well documented and are described in Chapter Ten. Less is known about low-dose exposure. A study of the rates of childhood leukaemia in the vicinity of nuclear facilities in Ontario (Chalk River, Port Hope, Elliot Lake, Pickering, and Bruce) demonstrated only a slightly increased number of observed leukaemia deaths. In the United Kingdom, the higher incidence of childhood leukaemia has raised the issue of paternal exposure to possible workplace hazards. A study in Ontario has not provided support for this hypothesis (12).

Electromagnetic Fields

The use of electricity creates two kinds of invisible fields: electric and magnetic. Electric fields are produced by voltage, magnetic fields by current. Together they are referred to as "electromagnetic fields," a form of non-ionizing radiation. In Canada, the strongest electric field normally encountered by the public is about 10 kilovolts per metre and is found under high-voltage transmission lines. Other sources of exposure to electric fields are electric blankets, computers, fluorescent lighting, household appliances, and wiring. From most of these sources the electric field strength seldom exceeds one kilovolt per metre. The strongest domestic magnetic fields are those produced by hair dryers.

Considerable research has been carried out on the health effects of exposure to electromagnetic fields. The results of this research are conflicting, and therefore it is not clear whether a health hazard exists. For example, some studies have linked exposure to electromagnetic fields with increased cancer rates, particularly leukaemia and brain cancer (13). A recent Canadian study demonstrated excess of cancer only for a small subset of workers employed in very high exposure settings. In general, the research failed to indicate an excess of cancer for those exposed at lower levels (14).

3.1.3. Outdoor Air Pollution, Acid Rain, and Their Control

Air pollution exists when certain substances are present in the atmosphere in sufficient concentrations to cause adverse affects. Natural sources include volcanoes and forest fires. In Canada, air pollution results primarily from the incomplete combustion of fossil fuels, particularly by cars, with release into the atmosphere of various oxides of sulphur, nitrogen, and carbon. In addition, a variety of toxic trace elements (lead, cadmium, beryllium, asbestos) have also been detected. Air pollution also consists of aerosols, which reduce visibility, particulate matter, such as lead or asbestos particles, and organic and inorganic gases.

Recent Canadian research indicates that the exposure to a high level of ozone for one hour a day or to a high level of average sulphate level on a given day are associated with increased hospital admissions for respiratory admissions. Furthermore, there seems to be an association between mortality and increased levels of air pollution (15). The range of effects of air pollution measured in these studies represents only the most severe end of the spectrum. As a consequence of these studies, air pollution control has assumed a higher priority on the environmental health agenda at all levels of government.

Ozone Depletion and Pollution

Ozone (O_3) is a gas in the stratosphere, forming a layer that protects the earth from harmful ultraviolet radiation. Recently, there has been growing concern about the depletion of ozone in the stratosphere causing an increased incidence of skin cancer of all types including melanoma, as well as expected increases in other health effects, such as cataracts and other ophthalmic conditions, and depressed immune function, which may increase susceptibility to cancers. The mechanism for the destruction of the ozone layer is that some synthetic chemicals such as chlorofluorocarbons (CFCs) and halons are released into the atmosphere during the production, use, and disposal of products such as air conditioners, plastic foams, and solvents. In the presence of sunlight in the atmosphere, these molecules are split and the chlorine reacts with the ozone, breaking it down. CFCs, along with carbon dioxide and methane, also trap heat close to the earth's surface causing global warming ("greenhouse effect") (16).

A number of strategies have been introduced to address these concerns. In 1987, a major conference of industrial nations in Montreal agreed to stop production of CFCs by the year 2000 in a document known as the "Montreal Protocol" (17). Under the influence of the Montreal Protocol, new supply of ozone-depleting substances in Canada fell from a high point of 27.8 kilotonnes in 1987 to 5.8 kilotonnes in 1995 and fell to less then 1.6 kilotonnes in 1996 (18). Other initiatives are the conservation, recovery, and recycling of ozone-depleting chemicals. A recent awareness-raising campaign about the health effects of ozone depletion ("Ozone Watch Program") has been introduced by Environment Canada (18). A weekly ozone index is published along with the recommendations appropriate to the level, such as limiting the amount of time spent in direct sunlight to avoid sunburn in persons with fair skin. In addition, skin-protection precautions are being promoted, such as the wearing of hats, sun screens, and protective clothing.

Ozone pollution in the troposphere or ambient air, however, can cause a variety of health problems such as irritation of the upper and lower respiratory tract (2). Ozone is not directly released into the atmosphere in significant amounts, but forms when nitrogen oxides and hydrocarbons react in the presence of sunlight or electrical discharges such as lightning storms. Nitrogen oxides are produced when fossil fuels are burned in motor vehicles, power plants, furnaces, and turbines. In Ontario, for example, vehicle emissions account for about 60% of total nitrogen oxide emissions. Hydrocarbon emissions result from incomplete combustion of gasoline and from evaporation of petroleum fuels, industrial solvents, paints, and dry-cleaning fluids. Ozone in the troposphere may result in decreased functional capacity of the lungs. Ozone may be related to increased hospital admissions for respiratory ailments. Adverse health effects may be exacerbated in those suffering from respiratory diseases and those engaging in heavy exercise when the air quality is poor. Children may also be particularly vulnerable to the effects of ozone.

Smog

The word "smog" was coined several decades ago, derived from the combination of the words "smoke" and "fog", to describe the brownish yellow haze that sometimes hangs over urban areas. A complex product of motor vehicle exhaust and industrial pollution, smog is a chemical ozone-laden soup that most often occurs over large cities, although suburban and rural communities are not always spared. Smog tends to form under conditions of bright sunlight, high temperature and a stationary air mass. Therefore, the afternoons and early evenings of hot summer days are peak smog periods; by late in the day, the sun's rays have "baked" the exhaust from motor vehicles and industries into smog (2).

Ground-level ozone is the principal ingredient of smog. Smog may also contain acidic air pollutants, peroxyacetyl nitrate, particulates, nitrogen oxides, sulphates and carbon monoxide. The health effects of smog resemble those of ozone. However, because smog is a mixture of pollutants, its effects can vary, and the impact of one pollutant may be intensified when the pollutant is combined with another. More research is required to identify and understand fully the health effects of various chemical combinations and of long-term exposure to low levels of smog (2).

Acid Rain

Acid rain refers to the oxidation of the sulphur and nitrogen precursors to acidic compounds. Consequently, nitrogen oxides are transformed into nitric acid and sulphur oxides become sulphuric acid. These compounds can remain suspended in the atmosphere (pre-depositional) or can fall to earth as precipitation (depositional). The chief sources of sulphur dioxide (SO_2) are industrial emissions, although motor vehicle exhaust also plays a role. The negative impact on plant and aquatic ecosystems has been widely studied, but only recently have human health hazards been investigated (19).

Air Pollution and Adverse Health Effects

Increases in mortality and morbidity have been temporally associated with periods of high atmospheric concentrations of pollutants in ecological studies. The Great London Fog of 1952 demonstrated an association between cardiorespiratory mortality and SO_2 concentrations. Particulate matter of smaller than 10 microns (PM-10s) that are easily deposited in the lung are also implicated in contributing to respiratory morbidity. Analysis of hospital admissions in Ontario and in different Canadian cities have revealed an association between admissions for respiratory illness and levels of atmospheric pollutants (20, 21). Animal studies have confirmed decreased pulmonary function and impaired clearance mechanisms, although human volunteer studies have yielded conflicting results. An estimated 4,000 deaths per year occur in Canada as a result of atmospheric pollution, primarily in heavily industrialized urban centres. Outdoor air quality varies considerably in Canadian cities. In Toronto and Vancouver, over 70% of days in 1994 were reported to be fair to poor for outdoor air quality. By contrast, Halifax reported only 6% fair to poor air-quality days (22).

Control of Outdoor Air Pollution

A number of strategies have been developed to minimize air pollution. The air-pollution index implemented in some provinces, based on the continuous measurement of levels of sulphur dioxide and suspended particulate matter, gives warnings of air pollution build-ups; these can then be aborted by closing down polluting industries if necessary. Monitoring air quality is undertaken on a national basis, and recent trends have been encouraging. The establishment of emission standards for all sources has contributed to control of air pollution, including those for cars (for which catalytic converters have been introduced), ferrous foundries, and asphalt paving producers. Pollution abatement technology has been developed and adopted, such as tall stacks to disperse pollutants over wider areas (if they cannot be eliminated entirely), and high-temperature incinerators. Optimal use of road and transit systems are objectives to be achieved and are being addressed, such as the Healthy Cities approach as a part of healthy public policy in Toronto (see Chapter One). Healthy public policy in the environmental context has great potential in involving major stakeholders vital to the development and implementation of workable solutions to pollution. Many proposed solutions have enormous cost implications. Round-table conferences of industry and government, for example, have been held in Ontario on environmental issues and illustrate a collaborative approach. However, enforcement of legislation has led to penalties for non-observance of regulations regarding environmental pollution, and although these are not considered severe enough by some interest groups, enforcement could still have a deterrent effect.

3.1.4. Indoor Air Pollution

Indoor air quality has recently been scrutinized, following complaints of adverse health effects and discomfort in occupants of sealed buildings. A variety of non-specific health effects have been identified, including eye and upper respiratory tract irritation, as well as headache, fatigue, and nausea. Other building-associated illnesses include Pontiac fever (an influenza-like illness) and Legionnaires' disease. A variety of indoor pollutants can be measured, originating from building materials, furnishings, heating, and human activities. Indoor pollutants also originate from the external environment. The most frequent pollutants include tobacco smoke, volatile organic compounds, formaldehyde, and other gases. The degree of ventilation and entry rate of fresh air, as well as the reaction rate between chemicals, determines the concentration of indoor pollutants. Other factors such as temperature and humidity are important for comfort. Psychological factors also play a role.

There is a correlation between levels of carbon dioxide in indoor air, a measurable surrogate marker, and the prevalence of complaints about indoor air quality. At levels of CO_2 less than 500 parts per million (ppm) there are usually no complaints; from 500 to 1,000 ppm, occasional complaints, and over 1,000 ppm, many complaints. Increasing the ventilation should be the first response to complaints of poor indoor air quality. There is a tendency to avoid precise measurement of actual contaminants, as these have not proved helpful in reducing adverse health effects to date. The proposed 1995 National Building Code is intended to set standards for residential mechanical ventilation systems and to ensure adequate ventilation. Exposure guidelines have been published for indoor air (23).

Associated with indoor air quality is the recent identification of the health hazards of passive smoke exposure. These are discussed in Chapter Seven.

3.2. WATER QUALITY

Ensuring a safe potable water supply has long been a prerequisite for public health. Recently, people have become concerned about chemical contamination of water. There are more than 70,000 industrial chemicals, and hundreds of new chemicals are developed each year. Many of these chemicals, including household detergents, fail to biodegrade, resulting in their accumulation in soil and water. The major chemical contaminants in water that affect health are PCBs, dioxins, furans, mercury, lead, and pesticides (these are discussed below). Of the combined pollutants that endanger health in the modern world, experts estimate that only about 6% come from drinking water, about 90% come from food, and 1% to 2% from air (24).

In response to the public's increasing use of bottled water and devices to treat municipal water, the City of Toronto Department of Public Health undertook a risk assessment of drinking water in 1990 (25). Comparing municipal tap water with bottled and device-treated water, the study's results reinforced confidence in tap water. Bacterial contamination was not found in tap water, but was found in both device-treated and bottled water. Trace chemical contaminants were found in all three types of water; however, tap water was considered superior overall due to the variability of the chemical contaminants in the other water sources and the lack of guidelines for acceptable levels. Four groups of chemicals caused some concern in tap water. Lead usually enters drinking water while standing in water pipes and can be avoided if recommendations are followed (see page 229). Aluminum levels are largely present as a result of added alum, for which alternative technologies can be adopted. Trihalomethanes are produced when chlorine is added to the water for disinfection; alternatives are available such as the use of pre-ozonation for disinfection to reduce the need for chlorine. A number of other organic, potentially carcinogenic compounds were also detected in trace levels for which further investigation is required.

Interest in water quality and its possible human health effects has also been centred, on the Great Lakes, due to the known persistence of toxic chemicals arising from industrial and commercial production and use. Current knowledge of the level of contamination in open waters and in aquatic biota has come from the findings of a study undertaken by Environment Canada, Health Canada, and the Department of Fisheries and Oceans (26). Although this is a polluted ecosystem, the levels of toxic chemicals in open waters were well below Canadian and international drinking water standards. Sediment studies demonstrated that pollution by synthetic organic chemicals and heavy metals peaked in the 1960s and early 1970s, declining in the 1980s. Levels of contaminants in Great Lakes aquatic birds and fish have decreased since the 1970s; however, sub-lethal effects on enzyme systems and reproductive effects and congenital defects in a number of species have been attributed to chemical contaminants.

3.3. TOXIC CHEMICALS

Only a minute fraction of the total number of chemicals in use today have had adequate toxicological testing prior to their introduction. Less than 1% have an established threshold limit value to regulate occupational exposure. Furthermore, toxicity testing is limited to tests for acute large-dose toxicity and mutagenicity. A review of the adverse health outcomes of the differing classes of chemicals is beyond the scope of this chapter. Instead, this section will examine a small number of the most prominent chemical classes in relation to environmental health.

3.3.1. Metals

Many metals are essential human micronutrients. At higher doses, however, these elements can have serious toxic effects (these are discussed in detail in Chapter Ten).

Environmental exposures to metals have also been documented as a cause of disease in human population. Best known are the neurological and teratogenic consequences following contamination of Minamata Bay in Japan with organic mercury. In northwestern Ontario, consumption of fish obtained from rivers contaminated by industrial effluent has also led to mercury poisoning in the Aboriginal population.

Lead

Source and Exposure. Lead is a naturally occurring metal present in rocks, soil, water, and air. It has been mined, smelted, and used in making tools and ornamental objects since prehistoric times, and concentrations of lead in the environment have increased steadily since the Industrial Revolution. The most dramatic increase has occurred since the 1920s, following the introduction of lead additives into automobile gasoline to prevent engine knocking. Lead is released into the air through industrial emissions and the combustion of leaded gasoline. While industrial emissions (i.e., from smelters and refineries) can cause high concentrations of lead near the source, most of the lead in the air is a byproduct of the combustion of leaded gasoline. Concentrations of air-borne lead are therefore generally higher in cities than in rural areas. Regardless of their source, lead can be inhaled or ingested by humans and may circulate in the blood and be deposited in bone and other tissues. Either long-term exposure to low levels or short-term exposure to high levels can seriously affect human health. Measures taken in recent years have significantly reduced human exposure to lead.

Concentrations of lead in the air have declined significantly since the introduction of unleaded gasoline in Canada in 1975. In fact, studies indicate that between 1973 and 1985, air-borne lead concentrations fell by 76%, a change that matches almost exactly the increased use of unleaded gasoline. The most recent data available show that levels of lead in the air of large cities in eastern Canada and the Maritimes have declined even further and are now close to levels observed in rural areas.

All Canadians are exposed to lead in the air, dirt, household dust, food, drinking water and various consumer products. For the general population, food is the largest source of exposure to lead, accounting for up to 80% exposure in adults and 90% in children. Lead is in virtually all of the food we eat. In addition to naturally occurring lead, food can become contaminated from several sources: air-borne lead can be deposited directly onto crops and can also seep into soil and be absorbed into plants; the use of lead soldering in the manufacture of cans results in lead dust, which can directly contaminate food; and the lead in the solder itself can leach from the container into the food.

Intake of lead from this latter source is declining as the use of cans without lead solder becomes more common in food-processing industries. In addition, Canadian food processors have improved quality control in order to reduce lead levels in food. These and other initiatives have contributed to a dramatic decrease in the intake of lead from food.

In most areas of Canada, the concentration of lead in natural water supplies is very low. However, the use of lead solder in plumbing in newer homes, lead service connections to the main water supply, or lead pipes in very old homes can all contribute to significant levels of lead in domestic water. These problems are more evident in areas with very soft or acidic drinking water (low pH). Lead levels in domestic water increase with the length of time water is left standing in the plumbing system. It is a good idea for people living in areas that have soft water to flush domestic plumbing systems by letting water run through the taps for a few minutes prior to first use for drinking each day. As well, only water from the cold tap should be used for drinking and cooking and, in particular, for making baby formula.

Air-borne lead particles are often deposited in household dust. This source of lead appears to be especially important to young children who ingest a significant amount of soil and dust through their common habit of putting things in their mouths (pica). Paint manufactured prior to the current regulations may contain lead, and ingested paint chips can pose a threat to children. Also, stripping or sanding old paint during home renovations can produce lead particles that may be inhaled or ingested by the occupants.

Health Effects and Control. Lead is absorbed into the bloodstream and deposited in bone and other tissues. Results of long-term exposure to lead may be less noticeable but are nevertheless serious. While the most obvious manifestation is anaemia, exposure to lead has also been linked to impairment of mental function, visual-motor performance, memory, and attention span, as well as lack of appetite, abdominal pain and constipation, fatigue, sleeplessness, irritability, and headache. It has also been determined that chronic exposure to lead may affect kidney function (27, 28).

In the general population, two groups — the unborn child and children up to six years of age — are at a greater risk of the adverse health effects of lead. During pregnancy, lead can cross the placenta and reach the unborn child. Researchers believe that the last trimester of pregnancy may be the most critical time for this to occur. In the past when workers were exposed to high levels of lead, increased spontaneous abortions and stillbirth rates were noted in female workers in the lead industry. Young children are a high-risk group for several reasons: they take in more lead per unit of body weight than adults; they develop at a rapid rate; and are more susceptible to the adverse effects of lead. Children also absorb a higher proportion of lead from food sources (about 50% absorption, compared to about 10% by adults). Over the past decade, some researchers have found that exposure to even low levels of lead prior to birth or during infancy and early childhood can cause impaired intellectual development, behavioural disturbances, decreased physical growth, and hearing impairment. Although scientific evidence is so far insufficient, the impact of lead on young children is an ongoing concern in Canada.

Elevated blood lead levels can be detected by a simple fingerprick blood test. There are guidelines that dictate the safe level of lead for individuals and the community, and these are recommended by the joint Federal/Provincial Advisory Committee on Environmental and Occupational Health. When the recommended levels are exceeded then intervention is appropriate: identification of the source of exposure, control of the source, or removal of individuals from further exposure. The proposed Canadian guidelines for lead in drinking water is a maximum acceptable level of 0.01 milligrams per litres, or 10 parts per billion. Municipal water treatment removes lead effectively and the alkalization of water can reduce leaching from corroded pipes. To avoid post-treatment exposure, taps should be flushed for two minutes if water is left standing for more than eight hours, and replacement of lead pipes and lead solder by municipalities and home-owners may be necessary if lead levels at point-of-use exceed recommended levels (27).

Mercury

Source and Exposure. Elemental mercury is either a vapour or liquid and is used in electrical equipment and the tanning industry. The major source is natural degassing of the earth's crust. Industrial releases may also be deposited in the environment, both close to industry and at great distances (for example, in the far North). Acidic environments favour mercury deposition. Organic mercury (predominantly methyl mercury) is more toxic to humans, and it may be formed by the action of micro-organisms on elemental mercury deposited in the flooding of land or by their action in the human body after elemental mercury has been ingested.

Fish bioconcentrate mercury in their muscle tissue by a factor of 10 to 100,000 times the ambient (surrounding) levels. Most exposure to mercury today occurs through the eating of fish.

Canadians who are at risk for organic mercury poisoning are those who rely on subsistence fishing and do not heed guidelines. In particular, the fetus of a fish-eating mother is at risk if maternal levels are elevated. Surveys of mercury levels (in hair and blood) undertaken in 350 Aboriginal communities revealed a disturbing prevalence of elevated mercury levels in 2.5% of communities (3). Neurological effects in adults were not detected in these population.

Health Effects and Control. Methyl mercury is rapidly absorbed when elemental mercury is converted into this organic form. Acute intoxication can cause paraesthesia, ataxia, impairment of vision, hearing, psychosis, and kidney damage. This level of poisoning has not been reported in Canada. Chronic low-dose poisoning of up to 300 milligrams per day results in an asymptomatic period (of some months), during which time the mercury penetrates cell membranes and binds with proteins and sulphhydryl groups. Liver and kidney damage can occur, as can central nervous system impairment of sensory, coordinating, and visual functions.

The brain of the developing fetus is particularly at risk if exposed to high levels of circulating maternal organic mercury. Possible effects include retarded physical growth and coordination, cerebral palsy and more subtle effects on coordination, behaviour, and intelligence quotient (29).

The MAC for mercury, as recommended by the Guidelines for Drinking Water Quality, is two parts per billion (ppb). Advisories are issued if the concentration in fish is greater than 0.05 parts per million (50 ppb). It is recommended in certain areas that white fish be preferred over lake trout for consumption. Pregnant women living in certain areas should not consume large amounts of fish.

Conventional water treatment removes up to 80% of inorganic mercury in turbid waters and less in clear water. Organic mercury is not affected by conventional water treatment but is effectively removed by activated carbon filtration.

Cadmium

Source and Exposure. Cadmium is a relatively rare element in the earth's crust; however, as a result of industrial and municipal wastes it is accumulating in the soil at a rate of 1% increase per year. Cadmium is used in the process of electroplating metals, as a stabilizer for plastics, in batteries, and high-technology industries (e.g., the manufacture of television tubes and nuclear reactor shields). It is also released in the burning of fossil fuels, incinerator discharges, and cigarettes. It is one of the five most common leachates in water near hazardous waste sites.

Plants taking up cadmium from contaminated soil, and the use of sewage sludge as fertilizers for feed crops, result in bioconcentration of cadmium in vegetables, poultry, and beef. The settling of incinerator deposits on crops augments the levels found in plants. Fish also bioconcentrate cadmium. Most exposure to cadmium therefore occurs by food intake. Cigarette smokers who smoke a pack a day double their usual intake of cadmium.

Health Effects and Control. Cadmium is a known animal carcinogen and a "probable human carcinogen". Acute high-dose inhalation exposure causes severe lung irritation, nausea, vomiting, diarrhea, and chills. Long-term low-dosage exposure in humans leads to kidney damage and multiple system effects including emphysema, liver damage, testicular, immune system, and central nervous system damage. Unlike lead and mercury, there does not appear to be transplacental transfer of cadmium.

The World Health Organization has set the provisional tolerable daily intake of cadmium at 1 to 1.2 micrograms per kilogram. The MAC for cadmium in drinking water is 5 ppb. Activated carbon filtration removes cadmium from water. Control measures in the future will likely involve regulation of the use of sewage sludge as a fertilizer and of incinerator discharges. Occupational measures are discussed in Chapter Ten.

Aluminum

Source and Exposure. Aluminum is one of the most common elements in the earth's crust. Food ingestion is responsible for 96% of the usual human aluminum intake, drinking water for 3.5%, and antacids and other consumer products for the remainder. The concentration of aluminum in drinking water varies according to geological factors, soil acidity, and acid rain. It may also be added in the form of alum (aluminum sulphate) during the treatment of municipal water in the coagulation-flocculation stage. This process causes the formation of larger particles, which then settle out water impurities.

Health Effects and Control. The potential health effects of aluminum in drinking water are the cause of ongoing controversy, particularly in relation to its putative role in Alzheimer's disease (AD), the most common cause of dementia. Animal toxicological studies have demonstrated that cats and rabbits whose brains were injected with aluminum developed neurofibrillary tangles similar to those found in patients with AD. A disorder known as dialysis encephalopathy, a rapidly fatal neurologic syndrome, has been observed in dialysis patients, who were also found to have high levels of aluminum in their brains. The characteristic pathological changes of AD, however, were absent. Many researchers have found elevated levels of aluminum in the brains of AD patients who have died, although this evidence is not consistent. At this point the role of aluminum in causation of AD has not been established, according to the criteria described in Chapter Two (30, 31).

3.3.2. Polychlorinated Biphenyls and Dioxins

Polychlorinated Biphenyls (PCBs)

Source and Exposure. PCBs are a class of highly stable, non-corroding, and relatively non-flammable chemicals first manufactured on a commercial scale in 1929. For several decades, they were used extensively in a wide range of industrial applications, especially the manufacture of electrical and heat exchange equipment. In the past, PCBs have also been used in such products as ink, oil, sealant, caulking compound, and carbonless copy paper. In the 1970s, concerns over health and the environmental impact of PCBs led to their substitution by other compounds and eventually to a North American ban in 1977 on the manufacture, importation, and most non-electrical uses of PCBs. Electrical uses of PCBs are now being phased out, with stringent requirements for handling and disposal.

Studies have found trace levels of PCBs everywhere in the environment. This is thought to be due primarily to improper disposal practices and accidental releases from the 1930s to 1970s, followed by long-range transport of PCBs by air currents. PCBs do not readily break down in the environment. This persistence, coupled with their tendency to accumulate in the fat of living organisms, means that they are often present and biomagnified in the food chain. Although PCBs are no longer being manufactured, significant amounts remain in certain types of equipment. As well, public concern over how to dispose of PCBs properly has led to stockpiling of these substances at sites across Canada. Despite stringent safeguards on storage of PCBs and PCB-contaminated wastes, releases into the environment remain a potential risk.

Humans are regularly exposed to minute amounts of PCBs through food, air, and water. As a result, all humans have a detectable level of PCBs in their body fat and blood. These levels are not likely to cause adverse health effects. Ingestion is the most common route of entry. The average Canadian intake of PCBs for adults from all routes has been estimated at less than 10 micrograms per day. Uncontrolled fires involving PCBs can pose a significant threat to human health. When PCBs are heated, they are transformed into an array of dangerous chemicals, including furans and occasionally dioxin. Following a fire, particles containing these toxic chemicals may settle on a variety of surfaces, including the ground and water, thereby resulting in a potential for human exposure.

Health Effects and Control. Sustained, high-level exposure to PCBs has been associated with adverse health effects. These include a severe form of acne (chloracne), eye discharge, swelling of the upper eyelids, hyperpigmentation of the nails and skin, numbness of limbs, weakness, muscle spasms, chronic bronchitis, and decreased birth weight and head circumference in newborns. These health effects were identified following an incident in Japan in 1968 involving the accidental mixing of PCBs with cooking oil. Scientists generally agree that short-term, low-level exposure to PCBs is unlikely to have a significant health impact. However, there is potential cause for concern over long-term exposure to low concentrations (29).

The International Agency for Research on Cancer recently concluded that there is some evidence to link long-term, high-level PCB exposure with an increased incidence of cancer, particularly liver cancer. This is based on studies of humans exposed to high concentrations of furan-contaminated PCBs. Laboratory rats exposed for a lifetime to high levels of a PCB mixture also developed liver cancer.

Associations have been found between prenatal exposure to PCBs and slight reductions in mental development in children. Transplacental transfer has been documented and was predictive of low birth weight, smaller dimensions of the infant, neonatal hypotonia and hyporeflexia, and cognitive, motor, and behavioural development deficits. There is no evidence of any harmful effects from the small amounts of PCBs found in breast milk. Health care professionals advise that the known benefits of breast-feeding outweigh any potential risks that may be associated with PCBs in human milk.

PCBs bioconcentrate in fish, and those who eat fish on a regular basis are thus at risk of health effects associated with PCBs. Aboriginal people who survive on subsistence fishing are at risk as they may not heed guidelines. The guideline for avoidance of eating fish is 2 ppm.

As mentioned previously, PCBs are being phased out following legislation banning their production. However, transport and storage of existing wastes containing PCBs (more than 50 ppb) pending destruction are also regulated under the *Transportation of Dangerous Goods Act* and *Canada's Environmental Protection Act,* respectively, as well as under provincial legislation. Suitable disposal facilities for the destruction of PCBs are not widely available in Canada but are planned, including mobile facilities for on-site high temperature incineration. Chemical processes for decontaminating PCB contaminated oil are currently used predominantly.

Dioxins and Furans

Source and Exposure. Dioxins are a family of toxic substances called polychlorinated dibenzo-para-dioxin. A second family of closely related toxic substances known as polychlorinated dibenzofurans is very often present with dioxin. Recent research has indicated that elevated doses of dioxins and furans can significantly damage the health of laboratory animals. The impact of these substances on humans and wildlife is less certain. Dioxins and furans are therefore the subject of considerable controversy, both in the public realm and within the scientific community. Dioxins and furans have never been purposely manufactured, but are rather byproducts of the production of certain chemicals (such as some pesticides and wood preservatives) of the chlorine-bleaching process used in some pulp and paper mills, and of the incomplete combustion of materials that contain both chlorine atoms and organic matter. Although they are most often human-made, some natural occurrences, such as forest fires, are believed to contribute to the presence of dioxins and furans in the environment.

Dioxins and furans originate from a variety of sources and can be transported in the atmosphere over long distances. As a result, they are found at very minute levels throughout the environment. High concentrations can generally be linked to specific polluting sources, such as chemical dumps, obsolete municipal incinerators, or pulp and paper mills using chlorine in the bleaching process. Polychlorinated biphenyls used to be an important source of furans, which are contaminants in commercial PCB mixtures. As indicated above, today most PCBs are contained in secure facilities, and are a source of furan releases to the environment only in the event of accidental leakage or fires.

People living in industrialized nations are constantly being exposed to minute amounts of dioxins and furans through their presence in food, air, water, soil, or some consumer products. Scientists have shown that food is the major source of dioxins and furans for humans.

Health Effects and Control. As dioxins and furans are soluble in fat they can accumulate in the bodies of all animals, including humans. No long-term effects have been found in fish, wildlife, or domestic animals that can be definitively linked to exposure to the low levels of dioxins and furans typically found in the environment. However, the remarkable loss of reproductive capability in fish-catching birds in the Great Lakes area in the 1970s may have been associated with dioxins and furans. The toxic effects of dioxins and furans on vegetation are not known.

On the other hand, recent scientific studies do indicate that high levels of dioxins and furans can significantly damage the health of laboratory animals, including weight loss, skin disorders, effects on their immune system, impaired liver function, induction of liver enzymes, impaired reproduction (including birth defects), and increased numbers of tumours. While dioxin has been shown to have a range of long-term effects on laboratory animals, effects on humans are equivocal. In studies of humans who have been exposed to high levels of dioxins and furans through their work or accidentally, the health effect that has been most consistently observed is a chloracne, which is not exclusive to dioxins and furans and usually disappears several months after the affected person ceases to be in contact with the contaminant. Some of the people exposed to chemicals contaminated with dioxins and furans have also displayed other adverse effects on the skin, liver, immune system, sensory organs, or behaviour. No conclusive link has been established between human exposure to dioxins and furans and effects such as cancer or abnormal reproduction.

Recent developments in research have enabled scientists to measure dioxins and furans at levels as low as several parts per trillion or even parts per quadrillion (a part per quadrillion is equivalent to one cent in $10 trillion). Establishing levels of exposure to dioxins and furans that might be considered acceptable for the general population is controversial.

Despite the lack of direct evidence that current exposures to dioxins and furans in Canada contribute to health problems in humans, the government of Canada recognizes that these compounds are undesirable environmental contaminants and that, where possible, their unintentional production should be limited. Investigations by both government and industry is continuing on several fronts. These include sampling and analysis of air, sediments, wildlife, fish, industrial effluent and sludge, and pulp from pulp and paper mills using chlorine bleaching. The Health Protection Branch of Health Canada monitors dioxin levels in a variety of foods, human breast milk, water, and some paper products. The federal government no longer permits the sale and use of pesticides containing 2,3,7,8-TCDD (a form of dioxin) and has regulated the content of other dioxins in pesticides remaining on the market. Monitoring programs indicate that 2,3,7,8-TCDD is not found in currently marketed pest control products. The government of Canada, in conjunction with the provinces, has also established codes of practice to reduce contamination by the wood preservation industries. These efforts to control sources of dioxins and furans have had a positive impact. One indicator of this is that levels of dioxins and furans in Great Lakes fish-eating birds have declined (32).

Pesticides

Pesticides are toxic chemicals unique as a class of environmental agents as they are deliberately added to the environment for the express purpose of killing some form of life. They have been categorized as "economic poisons" as they have important beneficial effects on food supply and on health. For example, the use of insecticides has eliminated or controlled vector-borne disease in many parts of the world.

Both acute and chronic human health effects related to pesticide exposure have been identified. The acute effects are primarily occupational in origin. Among the variety of delayed health effects associated with pesticides, none has been more prominent than the carcinogenic effects of "Agent Orange". This compound containing the herbicide 2,4,5-T and combined with the potent carcinogen 2,3,7,8-TCDD (a dioxin), was sprayed over many of the Vietnam field camps, jungles, and roadways during the Vietnam war. Studies of exposed Vietnam veterans have revealed an excess of soft-tissue sarcomas and lymphomas. Studies of the teratogenic consequences of Agent Orange exposure have produced inconclusive results. In 1980, the International Agency for Research on Cancer (IARC) published a review of the carcinogenicity of compounds (33). It concluded that the pesticides chlordane-heptachlor, DDT, diedrin, and HCH-lindane could not be classified as carcinogens but require further investigation.

In general, pesticide residues contaminate food products and can concentrate in the ecological food chain. Every human body is born with measurable pesticide levels, related to widespread use of pesticides. The delayed effects of pesticide exposure are difficult to investigate as exposures are universal and not easily measured, a latency period applies to all carcinogenic outcomes, and there are no unexposed control groups. Given these difficulties, the delayed health risks of pesticide exposure are often below the power of detection of epidemiological studies.

4.   CREATING A SAFE ENVIRONMENT

With increasing recognition of the importance of the ecosystem has come respect for the maintenance of the integrity of the environment for its intrinsic value, as well as for human needs. A number of strategies have been developed and are discussed below. They include the broad framework of healthy public policy in relation to the environment, sustainable development, the management of waste, and response to environmental emergencies. Strategies to protect human health in relation to the environment include both direct and indirect approaches. Establishing guidelines for human exposure to toxic substances are direct strategies. It is anticipated that reduction of the production of chlorofluorocarbons to sustain the atmosphere's integrity will also have beneficial effects on human health. This is an example of an indirect environmental health approach. In the restoration and maintenance of a safe environment, the responsibility and role of individual commitment and action, as well as of government, is fundamental to the success of environmental measures.

4.1. HEALTHY PUBLIC POLICY

Healthy public policy aims at mobilizing many segments of the community to reduce the adverse health effects on humans that may result from deleterious environmental exposures. The measures utilized include intersectoral and interdepartmental action, legislation, regulations and guidelines, community organization, education, and advocacy (see Chapter One). A unifying approach to public policy in environmental protection has developed in the form of the sustainable development concept. Specific strategies are discussed below. First, however, it is instructive to review the population-based theoretical position that provides the rationale for healthy public policy approaches in relation to the environment, as articulated by Rose (34). He proposed that in a continuous distribution of exposures, large numbers exposed to small risk from environmental exposure generate the bulk of the resulting disease. In comparison, far fewer cases occur in those at high risk due to extreme exposure, as may occur, for example, in an occupational setting. As well as paying attention to those at high risk, Rose recommended mass measures as part of the solution to reducing exposures of the substances in the total population that have the potential to generate most of the illness.

4.1.1. Regulations and Guidelines

Federal
Jurisdictional responsibility for environmental issues are shared between the federal and provincial governments and areas of overlap are usually resolved through close cooperation. The *Canadian Environmental Protection Act* is the cornerstone of federal environmental legislation, providing the framework for protection from pollution, especially hazardous substances. Under the Act, a list of priority toxic substances is to be developed. Substances identified as toxic are transferred to the Toxic Substances List and subject to regulations that may be applied to their entire life cycle. Environment Canada enforces the Act, and Health Canada contributes to the development of regulations and guidelines. Other pieces of federal legislation relevant to environment

and health are the *Food and Drugs Act and Regulations* (Health Canada); the *Pest Control Products Act* (Agriculture Canada), and the *Hazardous Products Act and Regulations* (Consumer and Corporate Affairs Canada). There is, however, fragmentation at this level of government with the federal government's role in the control of hazardous substances partitioned between 24 departments administering 58 Acts of Parliament. The federal government is also entirely responsible for setting national policy with regard to environmental pollutants that can travel across provincial or international boundaries. Examples of such pollutants are atmospheric sulphur and nitrogen dioxides that cause acid rain.

A new area of federal legislative development is the environmental assessment and review process, which is intended to be formalized into the *Canada Environmental Assessment Act*. This process is used to identify and review the implications to multiple sectors, including health, of all projects, with both public and professional input being obtained. The issue of the siting of dams and nuclear facilities is a major one in Canada, and environmental assessments are a means of identifying implications for the whole ecosystem as well as for human health. Provinces have also developed environmental assessment processes and regulations.

Federal government departments also make health-based guidelines for air, drinking and recreational water. These are not enforceable but are used by many jurisdictions as guidelines for development of their own regulations. Guidelines have the advantage of a capacity for greater responsiveness in comparison to legislation but the disadvantage of unenforceability.

Provincial

The provinces have primary responsibility for the quality of local air and water, the quantity and types of emissions allowed to industries, the disposal of toxic waste products and the identification and management of environmental health hazards. For example, Ontario's *Environmental Protection Act* and *Amendments* requires control of pollutants below any level known to produce a hazard or discomfort to humans, livestock, damage vegetation, or cause corrosion or soiling of buildings. Provinces are also responsible for setting soil contamination guidelines. Provincial ministries of the environment play a primary role in this field, but share responsibilities with the ministries of labour, natural resources, and health, among others. Responsibilities in relation to environment and health are fragmented at the provincial level as well as at the federal level as previously indicated.

Municipal

Local municipalities are responsible for garbage disposal. Some municipalities have taken initiatives such as recycling programs and are at the forefront of cleaning up the environment to improve health. Local government can request the province to pass enabling legislation to allow local regulations regarding environmental hazards to be developed and implemented.

Role of Public Health

Public health departments usually have municipal and provincial mandates for the enforcement of regulations regarding safe food and water, sanitation, and other environmental hazards such as restriction of smoking in public places. In addition, the role of public health in environmental issues is frequently that of an "honest broker" (getting the stakeholders to the table, providing information on health effects, legitimizing concerns and issues by encouraging expression of these by stakeholders, and then negotiation of solutions that address the concerns of all parties to the extent possible). A stakeholder is a party affected in some way, frequently economic, by a decision or issue, or who has a mandate or responsibility for involvement; the community is a major stakeholder. The role of public health is described in more detail in Chapter 15.

Intersectoral Initiatives

Recently in Canada there have been a number of initiatives undertaken in relation to the environment that have included many departments of government and other sectors. For example, the Great Lakes Action Plan, a five-year plan initiated in 1989, involves six federal departments: Agriculture Canada, Environment Canada, Fisheries and Oceans, Public Works Canada, Transport Canada, and Health Canada. The three distinct components of the plan are the Great Lakes Cleanup Fund, the Great Lakes Health Effects Program, and the Preservation Program for environmental quality and assessment. The significant findings of a study on toxic chemicals in the Great Lakes undertaken under the program's auspices were highlighted earlier in this chapter.

Canada's Green Plan, published in 1990, incorporates community involvement and education, legislation, and participation by stakeholders in partnerships to improve the environment. The environment is likely to be placed on the agenda of many sectors, both private and government. Canada's Green Plan is an excellent example of healthy public policy related to the environment. The federal government and provinces have made a commitment in this plan: to clean the air, water, and land, to eliminate dumping of toxic substances into the environment, to sustain forestry, agriculture, and fisheries development, to protect 12% of Canada as park space, to preserve the integrity of the Arctic and the global environment, including a reduction of greenhouse gases, to develop partnerships in environmental literacy, and to prepare for environmental emergencies.

4.1.3. Sustainable Development

This is the concept of productive economic activity that leaves resources in the natural environment intact. Human development and the achievement of human potential require a form of economic activity that is socially as well as environmentally sustainable, for present and future generations. Certain widely held human values, such as support for growth in population, need for material production, increasing material expectations and belief in technology, have caused specific ecological phenomena that threaten human health. The major issues are global warming and climatic change with possible consequent food shortages and change in distribution of vector-borne diseases, ozone depletion, ecosystem contamination, and resource depletion. Sustainable development is a conceptual model incorporating a number of generic approaches to reverse the deterioration of the earth, prevention of pollution beyond the point where natural systems cannot cope, conservation of natural resources by sparing or reduced use, recycling and reuse, with municipal recycling programs a positive indication of action in this area, and sustained yield, whereby renewable resources are utilized at a rate that does not exceed their continued replenishment. Earlier sections in this chapter describe relevant control strategies.

Waste Management

Waste management involves the disposal, destruction or storage of solid waste and sewage (and industrial discharges and nuclear waste). More recently, it has begun to include other waste management practices, such as recovery from the waste stream and the adoption of a sustainable environment framework, to reduce the volumes of waste produced. Canadians produce over 30 million tons of solid waste per year: garbage and refuse, sludge from waste treatment plants, water supply treatment plants, or air pollution control facilities, other discarded material, including solid, liquid, semisolid, or contained gaseous material from commercial, mining, and agricultural operations and from community activities. Hazardous waste, a major component of this solid waste (comprising eight million tons per year), refers to radioactive or biomedical material, material produced during particular industrial processes, and waste containing one or more particular potentially hazardous substances at certain concentrations or containing corrosive, ignitable, or otherwise hazardous material.

There are three main approaches currently to solid waste disposal in Canada: burial, ideally in modern sanitary landfills that satisfy criteria relating to aesthetics, health, and prevention/monitoring of leaching (diffusion of substances into ground water from the landfill site), incineration (in which controlled combustion is used to stabilize and eliminate hazardous material, convert organic into inorganic matter, and kill pathogens), and transformation, for example, anaerobic digestion by microorganism or pyrolysis (chemical decomposition caused by combustion in an oxygen-starved environment), which can reduce waste volume by 91%. Sewage (apart from areas where septic tanks are used) is treated in Canada in municipal sewage treatment plants. After a process of screening and settling, the sludge produced is digested and dewatered to form sludge cakes that are then incinerated. Effluent liquids are chlorinated and discharged into bodies of water, causing concerns as to the possible effects of chlorinated organic compounds (such as trihalomethanes and chloramines) on the aquatic life.

Canada's Green Plan 1990 indicates a federal commitment to a 50% reduction of wastes in Canada by the year 2000. Packaging, which accounts for 36% of waste, has been targeted in particular. The best way to manage waste is for society — including government, industry, and individuals — to produce less, by following the "4 Rs": reduce, reuse, recycle, and recover (2). Reducing consumption of goods is the most effective waste management strategy, because it results in less waste and consumes less energy. Reusing products is the next best option. Examples of this strategy include returnable beer and soft drink bottles, garage sales and second hand furniture and clothing outlets operated by commercial businesses and charitable organizations.

Recycling involves using material from old products to make new products. Commonly recycled materials include newspapers, metal cans, glass bottles, plastics, cardboard, and used auto parts. Recovery involves the harvesting of energy or economically worthwhile components from waste materials. Industrial-scale examples include heat energy generated from the incineration of solid wastes and methane gas recovered from composting organic wastes. It is estimated that backyard composting could reduce the volume of residential waste in Canada by up to 60%.

Special provision is made for disposal of hazardous waste with support for household hazardous waste drop-off programs and location of new hazardous waste destruction facilities (e.g., for PCBs) and supporting technology. The Green Plan acknowledges the need for consultation, discussion, and involvement of stakeholders, such as industry, in developing and implementing environmental policies.

4.2. MANAGING ENVIRONMENTAL ACCIDENTS

The management of life-threatening incidents involving exposure to toxic chemicals (such as in Bhopal) or radiation exposure (such as in Chernobyl) is difficult. It requires collaboration from several levels of government and at times from international experts. Most of these incidents are not so dramatic but are nonetheless serious. Guidotti (35) has outlined the necessary steps to evaluate unknown health effects. The first step is to evaluate the problem, documenting evidence and obtaining accurate information on the nature and magnitude of the hazard. The second step is to contain the problem, coordinating efforts with responsible public and private agencies. The third step is to evaluate health effects, focusing on specific outcomes, when the exposure is known, and on the primary organ systems of concern (dermal, respiratory, hepatic, neurological, and renal) and carcinogenic and fetotoxic effects when the exposure is not known.

5. SUMMARY

Environmental health may be defined as the study of conditions in the natural and human-made environment that can influence health and well-being. The focus of study in environmental health is the impact of environmental or hazardous agents on the health of the population. The environment as it affects health can be divided into workplace and non-workplace categories. The workplace environment (occupational health) is often associated with high-level exposure, with the exposed population being predominantly of adult age and in good health. In contrast, non-workplace environmental exposures are generally low level and often chronic. The population at risk contains the extremes of age, developing fetuses, and the ill or immunocompromised persons.

The study of environmental health relies on epidemiology and toxicology. *Epidemiology* is the study of the distribution and determinants of health and disease in human population. *Toxicology*, the science of poisons, attempts to identify adverse effects and predict harmful dosages. One of the fundamental tenets of toxicology is that any substance can be a poison if given in a large enough doses.

Canadians are exposed to toxic substances through a variety of sources, including food, water, air, soil, and consumer products. *Risk assessment, management, and communication* are strategies for dealing with health risks posed by the environmental contaminants. There are four major steps in the risk assessment of any environmental contaminant. These are *hazard identification, exposure determination and monitoring, dose-response determination*, and *risk determination*. Risk management follows risk assessment and involves decision making and implementation of options for managing the identified risk. The communication of risk in relation to environmental hazards depends on the perception of risk by the public versus the perception of risk by the "experts".

Environmental health issues focus on the outdoor and indoor environment, water quality, and toxic chemicals. Factors in the *outdoor and indoor environment* that affect health consist of ionizing radiation, electromagnetic fields, air pollution, and acid rain. Ionizing radiation, emitted from radioactive substances and the natural background, leads to altered cell physiology. Due to conflicting research results, it is not clear whether or not electromagnetic fields are a health hazard. The main sources of exposure to these fields are high-voltage transmission lines, computers, electric blankets, fluorescent lighting, and household appliances. Air pollution results primarily from the incomplete combustion of fossil fuels, particularly by cars. Recently, there has been a depletion of ozone in the stratosphere, causing an increased incidence of skin cancer of all types including melanoma, cataracts, and depressed immune function. Acid rain refers to the oxidation of the sulphur and nitrogen precursors to acidic compounds. Increases in mortality and morbidity have been temporarily associated with periods of high atmospheric concentrations of pollutant.

With respect to *water quality*, the major chemical contaminants in water are PCBs, dioxins, furans, mercury, lead, and pesticides.

Toxic chemicals include metals (such as lead, mercury, aluminum), polychlorinated biphenyls, and dioxins. Although metals are essential micronutrients, at higher doses these elements can have serious toxic effects. For example, excessive exposure to lead results in its deposition in bone and other tissues. The most obvious clinical manifestation of lead toxicity is anaemia, but impaired mental function, visual-motor performance, memory, and attention span have also been cited. PCBs do not readily break down and hence remain in the environment. This persistence, coupled with their tendency to accumulate in the fat of living organisms, means that PCBs are often present in the food chain. Some of the health effects attributed to PCBs include a severe form of acne, swelling of the upper eye lid, muscle spasm, chronic bronchitis, and decreased birth weight and head circumference in newborns. Thus, the major substances posing environmental threats to human health are ozone pollution, tobacco smoke, acid rain, pesticides, PCBs, and lead.

A number of strategies have been proposed in order to create a safer environment. These strategies consists of healthy public policy, waste management, and managing environmental accidents. *Healthy public policy* aims at mobilizing many segments of the community to reduce the adverse health effects on humans that may result from deleterious environmental exposures. The measures utilized include regulations and guidelines, education and advocacy, legislation, and community organization. Sustainable development is also a form of healthy public policy. It is the concept of productive economic activity that leaves resources in the natural environment intact. Sustainable development is a conceptual model incorporating a number of generic approaches to reversing the deterioration of the earth: prevention of pollution, conservation, and sustained yield. *Waste management* involves the disposal, destruction or storage of solid waste, and sewage. There are three main approaches currently to solid waste disposal in Canada. These are burial, incineration, and transformation. The best way to manage waste is for society — including government, industry, and individuals — to produce less, by following the "4 Rs": reduce, reuse, recycle, and recover. The *management of life-threatening exposures* to toxic chemicals requires collaboration from several levels of government. The steps in management are evaluating the problem, containing the problem, and evaluating the health effects.

6. REFERENCES

1.   de Krester D. Declining Sperm Counts. British Medical Journal 1996;312(7029):457-458.
2.   Health Canada. Health and Environment: Partners for Life. Ottawa: Minister of Public Works and Government Services Canada, 1997.
3.   A Vital Link. Health and the Environment in Canada. Ottawa: Health and Welfare Canada, 1992.
4.   Morgenstern H, Thomas D. Principles of Study Design in Environmental Epidemiology. Environmental Health Perspectives Supplements 1993;101(4):23-37.
5.   Frank JW, Gibson B, McPherson M. Information Needs in Epidemiology: Detecting the Health Effects of Environmental Chemical Exposure Environment. In Fowler CD, Grim AP, Munn RE, eds. Information Needs for Risk Management. Monograph No. 8 ed. Toronto: Institute of Environmental Studies, University of Toronto, 1988:129-144.
6.   Colburn T, vom Saal F, Soto A. Developmental Effects of Endocrine Disrupting Chemicals in Wildlife and Humans. Environmental Health Perspectives 1993;101:378-384.
7.   Federal-Provincial Subcommittee on Drinking Water of the Federal-Provincial Committee on Environmental and Occupational Health. Guidelines for Canadian Drinking Water Quality. Ottawa: Minister of Supplies and Services, 1996.
8.   Federal-Provincial Working Group on Recreational Water Quality of the Federal-Provincial Advisory Committee on Environmental and Occupational Health. Guidelines for Canadian Recreational Water Quality. Ottawa: Minister of Supplies and Services, 1992.
9.   Barrie L, Gregor D, et al. Arctic Contaminants: Sources, Occurrence and Pathways. Science of Total Environment 1992;122:1-74.
10. Covelho V. Risk Perception and Communication. Canadian Journal of Public Health. 1995;86(2):78-9.

11. Klich B. Medical Symposium Explores Radiation Risks and Public Concern. Ontario Medical Review 1992;59(10):23-30.

12. McLaughlin J, Anderson T, Clarke EA, King W. Occupational Exposure of Fathers to Ionizing Radon and the Risk of Leukaemia in Offsprings: A Case Control Study. Ottawa: Atomic Energy Control Board, 1992.

13. Savitz D. Epidemiologic Studies of Electric and Magnetic Fields and Cancer: Strategies for Extending Knowledge. Environmental Health Perspectives 1993; 101(s4):83-100.

14. Miller A, To T, Agnew D, et al. Leukaemia following Occupational Exposure to 60-Hz Electric and Magnetic Fields among Ontario Electric Utility Workers. American Journal of Epidemiology 1996;144:150 -160.

15. Great Lakes Health Effects Program. Outdoor Air and Your Health. Ottawa: Health Canada, 1996.

16. Maskell K, Mintzer I, Callander B. Basic Science of Climate Change. Lancet 1993;342:1027 -1031.

17. Gindi M. Ultraviolet Radiation: A Public Health Perspective. Ontario Ministry of Health. Public Health and Epidemiology Reports Ontario 1992;3(9):136-140.

18. Environment Canada. Canada's Ozone Layer Protection Program: A Summary (3rd ed.). Ottawa: Government of Canada, 1996.

19. Naus M. Health Effects of Acid Rain Exposure. Ontario Disease Surveillance Report 1988;9(17):296-298.

20. Bates D, Sizto R. Relationship between Air Pollution Levels and Hospital Admissions in Southern Ontario: Acid Summer Haze Effect. Environmental Research 1987;47:317-331.

21. Burnett RT, Brook JR, Yung WT, et al. Association between Ozone and Hospitalization for Respiratory Diseases in 16 Canadian Cities. Environment Research 1997;72:24-31.

22. Canadian Council on Social Development. Growing Up in Canada. Ottawa: 1995.

23. Federal-Provincial Advisory Committee on Environmental and Occupational Health. Exposure Guidelines for Residential Indoor Air Quality. Ottawa: Ministry of Supply and Services, Government of Canada, 1995.

24. University of Toronto. Is Our Drinking Water Safe? Health News 1989;7(4):1-6.

25. Department of Public Health. The Quality of Drinking Water in Toronto: A Review of Tap Water, Bottled Water and Water Treated by a Point-of-Use Device. Toronto: City of Toronto, 1990.

26. Environment Canada, Health and Welfare Canada, Department of Fisheries and Oceans. Toxic Chemicals in the Great Lakes and Associated Effects: Synopsis. Ottawa: Ministry of Supply and Services, 1991.

27. Metropolitan Toronto Teaching Health Units and South Riverdale Community Health Centre. Why Barns are Red: Health Risks from Lead and Prevention. A Resource Manual to Promote Public Awareness. Toronto: City of Toronto Public Health Department, 1995.

28. Rice D. The Neurotoxicity of Lead, Methyl Mercury, and PCBs in relation to the Great Lakes. Environmental Health Perspectives 1995;103 (Supplement 9):71-87.

29. Rice D. Neurotoxicity of Lead, Methylmercury, and PCB's in Relation to the Great Lakes. Environmental Health Perspectives 1995;103 (Suppl 9):71-87.

30. Nieboer E, Gibson B, Oxman A, et al. Health Effects of Aluminum: A Critical Review with Emphasis on Aluminum in Drinking Water. Environmental Reviews 1995;6(277-286).

31. Smith L. Public Health Role, Aluminum and Alzheimer's Disease. Envirometrics 1995;6:277-286.

32. Harrison K. Between Science and Politics: Assessing the Risks of Dioxin in Canada and the United States. Policy Sciences 1991;24:367-88.

33. International Agency for Research in Cancer Working Group. An Evaluation of Chemicals and Industrial Processes Associated with Cancer in Humans Based on Human and Animal Data. Cancer Research 1980;40(1):1-12.

34. Rose G. Environmental Factors and Disease: The Man Made Environment. British Medical Journal 1987;294(6577):963-965.

35. Guidotti T. Managing Incidents Involving Hazardous Substances. American Journal of Preventative Medicine 1986;2(3):148-154.

Chapter

10

Occupational Health
and Disease

Most adults spend a considerable amount of time at their workplace and are exposed to a variety of situations. Some of these situations are pleasant, but others expose the workers to stressful situations, and also to physical, chemical, mechanical, ergonomic, and biological hazards. The effects of these hazards are not always immediate and some of them have a long latency period. This chapter deals with the impact of the workplace environment as it relates to Canadian workers.

1.   OCCUPATIONAL HEALTH

Occupational health is defined as the maintenance and promotion of health in the work environment. The delivery of occupational health services involves not only physicians and nurses but also hygienists, engineers and safety officers, ergonomists, chiropractors, physicists, and technicians. The jurisdiction for enforcement of occupational health legislation lies with the provinces. Exceptions to this are 16 federally regulated industries covered under the Canada Labour Code, such as the grain industry and the transportation industry. Because of this provincial jurisdiction, there are variations in legislation and regulations governing occupational health across Canada. However, the principles of the worker's right to know, the worker's right to refuse dangerous work, and the need for workers and management to participate in joint safety and health committees exist across most of the country. The joint safety and health committee is an important bipartite forum where employees and employers can manage issues of concern.

The work environment contains a wide range of potential environmental exposure grouped as chemical (solvents, poisons), physical (radiation, noise), biological (blood products, viruses), mechanical and ergonomic (repetitive strains, awkward posture), and psychosocial (stress, isolation). Protecting the worker from exposure to these factors requires a commitment on the part of management to ensure that activities are carried out in the areas of health promotion (worker education and work design), health protection and disease prevention (protecting workers from hazards and monitoring the health of the worker), and rehabilitation (returning the worker to safe, meaningful, productive work).

1.1. CANADIAN WORKFORCE

Although Canada is a country born from the wealth of its natural resources, it is today a modern country with most of its workers employed in the service sector. As of July 1996 there were approximately 15.6 million people in the workforce, 10.8 million of whom are employed in the service industry. It is noteworthy that although men outnumber women in the total workforce — 8.6 to 7.0 million — there is a slightly higher representation of women in the service industry (5.7 million women to 5.1 million men). The reason for this is the fact that men are to a greater extent over-represented in the goods-producing industry, 3.3 million to 1.0 million. The goods-producing industry is defined by Statistics Canada as including manufacturing, construction, utilities, agriculture, and the other primary industries (fishing, trapping, logging, mining, quarrying). All other sectors of industry, including government, are considered service. The gender distribution of workers in the following employment sectors is as follows: manufacturing, 2.3 million total, of whom 69.6% are male; construction, of whom 0.9 million (88.9%) are male; and agriculture, of whom 0.5 million (60.0%) are male. The sex distribution suggests that gender is a determinant with respect to type of workplace injury encountered (1).

1.2. HEALTH INDICATORS AMONG CANADIAN WORKERS

Preliminary data collected under the auspices of the National Work Injuries Statistics Program (NWISP), a program coordinated by Statistics Canada to collect information from the provincial and territorial workers compensation boards, suggest that in 1994 there were 818,687 injuries related to activity in the workplace; 387,287 (47.3%) of these did not result in lost time, 430,630 (52.6%) resulted in lost time (worker absence from the workplace), and 770 resulted in fatalities (0.09%). This amounts to an incidence rate of workplace injuries of 6.9 per 100 workers, with 3.6 involving lost time. The incidence of workplace fatality rate was 6.0 per 100,000 workers.

The 818,687 injuries reported in 1994 represents a decline of more than 30% from the high of 1.2 million injuries in 1980. Many factors apart from safety issues may have contributed to this apparent decrease, including the level and nature of economic activity and the employment rate. Considering injuries and fatalities on an absolute basis, of the total 430,630 lost-time injuries, 119,083 (27.7%) occurred in manufacturing, 102,078 (23.7%) in service industry, 72,963 (16.9%) in wholesale and retail trade, and 38,816

(9.0%) in the transport, communication, and utilities sector. Of the 770 fatalities, 145 (20%) occurred in construction, 137 (19.3%) in manufacturing, 108 (15.2%) in transportation, and 84 (11.9%) in mining (2). The highest annual incidence of occupational fatality rates in Canada for 1993/94 per 10,000 workers employed were as follows: mining, 6.2; logging and forestry, 5.6; fishing and trapping, 4.0; construction, 2.0; transportation, 1.3; and manufacturing, 0.7 (3, 4).

Compensation payments to workers by workers' compensation boards (WCBs) for 1994 totalled approximately $5 billion; as indirect costs generally equal compensation claims, the estimated cost to the Canadian economy for 1994 is at least $10 billion. Injuries account for 97% of all compensated cases by WCBs; the remainder are occupational diseases.

Depending on the nature and severity of the injury or disease, the result may be a temporary or permanent disability that may require either modified work or time off work (a lost-time injury) during the period of disability. The percentages of work injuries that result in temporary or permanent disability are 45% and 5% respectively, with 50% suffering no sequelae. The pattern of occupational injuries and disease causing temporary disability is shown in Figure 5.5 in Chapter Five, with back injuries being the most common type of injury.

Common occupational injuries and diseases that cause permanent disability in Ontario are hearing loss, diseases affecting joints and tendons, and dermatitis; permanent disabilities secondary to injuries are related to strains and sprains, contusions, fractures, cuts, wounds, amputation, and multiple injuries. The economic impact results in both direct and indirect costs. In 1994, approximately $5 billion was paid to workers for occupational injuries of which $2.3 billion was paid out by Ontario's WCB, the most of any of the provinces or territories (3).

1.3. ISSUES RELATED TO OCCUPATIONAL HEALTH DATA

Injury and illness prevention is considered one of the most important issues in occupational health. The lack of coordinated collection of data in Canada has long been recognized as a major hindrance to the prevention of occupational injury and illness (5-7). One of the problems is deciding who should be responsible for collecting this information — a difficult problem as occupational health falls under federal, provincial, and territorial jurisdictions as well as potential occupational exposure data collected by hospitals, primary care physicians, emergency room visits, medical examiner reports, health surveys, death certificates, occupational medicine specialists, industry, cancer registries, health insurance firms, and WCBs. In fact, WCBs provide the bulk of the information, with cancer registries and health insurance firms collecting most of the rest of the information. Unfortunately, these sources of information remain largely unrealized. WCB data tend to be imperfect; the data focus mostly on the illness of the worker with little information on any substances to which all workers were exposed in the same work situation, i.e., pooled exposure data. Information is collected from the WCBs through Statistics Canada's NWISP, but the inconsistency of the type of data is a problem.

What are needed for epidemiological studies are unique patient-identifying data, accurate medical diagnosis, acceptable causes of disease, and defined industry and occupation coding — none of which is accepted as the standard today.

An additional problem exists with the interpretation of epidemiological data, even if data collection is satisfactory, as there is the confounding effect of nonoccupational disease. For example, when trying to determine the causation between coal mining and lung cancer, smoking becomes an extremely powerful confounding factor. This makes for challenging study design as well as problematic WCB compensation claims in miners who smoke.

In addition to lifestyle, there is also the issue of genetic, or inherent, disease. For example, it is important to identify the confounding effect of the "natural" occurrence of asthma in the worker population studied when trying to determine the association between diisocyanate and workplace asthma. It is the realization of the confounding effect of nonoccupational disease that presents a special problem in occupational epidemiology. As the stakes are high from the worker's perspective with respect to compensation for illness, it is very important for both worker and the employer that the employer perform the proper preplacement and periodic health screening exams.

2.   OCCUPATIONAL HEALTH RESOURCES

Occupational health resources are based in government, industry, educational institutions, union-based centres, and hospitals. The federal government relies on two ministries to set standards and provide appropriate health services: Labour Canada and Health Canada. At the provincial level, responsibility for regulation lies with one or more departments or ministries (e.g., ministry of labour, ministry of mining, ministry of health) and service provision to the civil service lies with another (ministry of government services). Major industries have corporate medical departments where company-hired health care professionals are responsible for the surveillance and monitoring of workers as prescribed by law and corporate policy. The range of health care professionals hired depends on the size and complexity of the industry or corporation and may include a physician, nurse, industrial hygienist, psychologist, chiropractors, and physiotherapists. Educational institutions, hospitals, union-based centres, and consultants provide some, if not all, occupational health services either on a fee-for-service basis or other payment mechanisms. The occupational health services provide health promotion and health protection (**primary prevention**), disease (**secondary prevention**), and rehabilitation services (**tertiary prevention**).

There are no legislated requirements for specific health and safety expertise in the workforce. Consequently, there is a wide variation in the skill set available for ensuring a safe and healthy work environment. In the smaller companies there may be no one assigned the role of a health and safety professional. In the larger companies there may be a large health care staff, often led by a physician, that includes industrial hygienists, nurses, and technicians. Generally, at a particular site it is often an occupational health nurse or safety professional who provides the day-to-day functioning of the health and safety function. A physician may be called upon to provided diagnostic information or act as a consultant with respect to return-to-work programs or health surveillance. The industrial hygienist is usually concerned with monitoring the environment for workplace hazards and protecting the worker from these hazards. Engineers play a role in designing any process with safety in mind, substituting dangerous materials, and implementing changes to the work environment to protect the worker with engineering controls where necessary. Clearly, however, these are generalizations and, except where mandated by professional requirements (e.g., diagnosing disease by physicians and designing equipment by professional engineers), there is a great deal of variability in what various degrees of training can bring to the workforce.

The specifics of corporate responsibility to workers' safety is determined to a large part by the provincial legislation; however, there are three aspects that are universal across the country. The first is the concept of due diligence. That is, the employer must demonstrate that he or she took reasonable steps to become familiar with the inherent dangers in the workplace and that action was taken to ensure that the workplace was safe. Ignorance is no excuse for an unsafe workplace if it can be demonstrated that no effort was made to understand the hazards of the workplace.

Secondly, the federally legislated Workplace Hazardous Materials Information System (WHMIS) applies across Canada. The intent of WHMIS is to ensure that workers are protected from hazards in the workplace by keeping a centralized record of all hazards in the workplace on Material Safety Data Sheets (MSDSs), which detail important information on handling hazardous substances and cleaning up spills properly, labelling all chemical substances in the workplace, and educating all workers at the work site with respect to the WHMIS program.

Thirdly, provincial occupational health and safety acts mandate the existence of joint health and safety committees. These committees are composed of representatives drawn from the management and workers. Their purpose is to identify workplace health and safety hazards and to communicate their concerns to management in writing. Workers must be granted time, with pay, to prepare for and attend committee meetings and to participate in inspections of the workplace.

2.1. HEALTH PROMOTION AND HEALTH PROTECTION

As already explained, the prevention of injury and illness is very important for maintaining the physical, mental, and social well-being of employees in the workplace. The goal of primary prevention is to take action in the workplace so that the worker is protected from injury and illness. These interventions can take place at the source, along the path, or at the worker level. Ideally, of course, this is the preferred level of prevention and includes such activities as identifying hazards in the workplace (**hazard identification**), assessing the actual level of risk associated with the identified hazards (**risk assessment**), and reducing exposure to environmental stressors in the workplace (through risk control and risk communication), similar to those described in Chapter Nine. **Risk control** is achieved through the reduction of exposure, which can be achieved in a variety of ways, such as engineering practices; an example is substitution — the replacement of a hazardous substance with one less so, e.g., replacement of silica powder with a silica-free inert powder in the moulding trade. Other engineering practices include enclosure — the physical containment of hazards — and exhausting (or ventilation). Enclosure and exhausting are sometimes referred to collectively as segregation methods to reduce worker exposure.

Industrial engineers use several methods for setting standards for the exposure limits to hazardous substances in the work environment. When legislation recognizes these limits, they constitute legal standards. Where levels are not defined, the acceptable code of practice is usually set on a 40-hour work week (i.e., eight hours a day). They rely on threshold limit values (TLVs). TLVs place a limit on exposure as measured by time-weighted averages (TWAs). Guidelines are set by the American Conference of Governmental Industrial Hygienists for these values. They are based on the assumption that a small percentage of workers will suffer adverse effects as a result of exposure at the TLV-TWA set. These values are published annually (8). The values are revised if the scientific literature provides justification. All provinces have lists of designated substances that provide regulations for employers, employees, and joint health and occupational safety committees, which cover the control of worker exposure to toxic substances.

Administrative strategies for controlling exposure include job rotation, or rotating employees through jobs that have exposure to hazardous materials. Work practice strategies include clean working procedures and wetting of surfaces contaminated with dust. Personal protection equipment is the control strategy of last resort, because it is expensive to purchase and maintain, training is generally required of the worker, and equipment must be individually fitted. Nonetheless, personal protection equipment can be very effective provided the worker wears the equipment. Noncompliance is commonly a problem in the workplace, as personal protection equipment is often uncomfortable to wear and the long-term benefits of improved health are often not perceived as desirable as the relief afforded in removing the equipment.

2.1.1. Healthy Lifestyle Promotion

Health promotion in the workplace has emerged as an effective approach, enabling access to the substantial numbers of persons in the workplace not only for prevention of work-associated health problems, but also for wellness programs that incorporate attention to lifestyle and other health determinants (9, 10). These determinants include the broad, systemic work, and social conditions or environments that influence employee health. Specific work practices, job design, work process, and lifestyle may need change. A comprehensive approach beyond lifestyle, based on community development and healthy public policy strategies, as discussed in Chapter One, is relevant. For example, provision of a day care centre on-site and flexible work hours facilitate the health of women employees of child-rearing age. Worker empowerment can be enhanced by small group development and community organizing. Joint collaboration of employers and workers, beyond the collective bargaining process, help fulfil employee needs as well as organizational goals.

The federal government has introduced the Corporate Model of a Workplace Health System, which has been piloted throughout the country (11). Employers can request a survey of workers' health and health concerns to determine the health needs of employees. The survey is then analysed and recommendations made, in conjunction with management, through a workplace health committee for the introduction of prevention programs for prevalent problems or risk factors. Recently, the emphasis has moved away from provision of expensive gymnasiums and equipment, which were part of the initial response to health promotion in the workplace by larger companies. Programs now often include dietary advice, including attention to the type of items offered by the cafeteria (if one is provided), stress management, and smoking cessation counselling, as well as opportunities for enhancing fitness and broader changes to the work environment as discussed above (10).

Smoking cessation programs have been extensively studied and are one of the few lifestyle programs that are justifiable to the company based on cost effectiveness alone, as the investment in the program is less than the savings achieved through a reduction in absenteeism from smoking-related illnesses. Other healthy lifestyle programs include blood pressure reduction, weight loss, alcohol and caffeine moderation, and cholesterol reduction.

Employee assistance programs (EAPs) help employees deal with stress. They provide for a third party to be available for counselling services to help employees deal with workplace and home problems (which may include stress of relationships, financial issues, or drug or alcohol abuse).

2.2. DISEASE PREVENTION

The goal of disease prevention (secondary prevention) is to monitor workers' health to prevent the development of disease. Secondary prevention in occupational health involves the use of preplacement and periodic examinations. The preplacement examination findings help in establishing an individual's baseline characteristics. Periodic examinations facilitate early, and often presymptomatic, diagnosis and may also serve as an early indicator of the effectiveness of plant hygiene controls.

It must be emphasized that the periodic exams are not the "regular check-ups" performed by the family physician, but are highly selective examinations that focus on the organ systems at risk due to specific hazards in the work environment. This includes directed histories (with respect to specific symptoms), directed physicals, and appropriate physiological, biochemical, and imaging studies.

Another aspect of secondary prevention in the workplace is the issue of employee screening for substance abuse. Mandatory pre-employment and random testing have been introduced in many industries in the United States. The Canadian Medical Association (CMA) has issued a statement advising that employee testing for substance abuse is not warranted, except as an adjunct, if performance impairment is suspected on other grounds in employees in safety-sensitive jobs (12). Although a great many drugs can be detected in urine, the test characteristics are very poor with regard to sensitivity, specificity, and predictive value (see Chapter Two), nor do the tests indicate when the substance was used, as levels may persist for weeks. There is also little correlation between levels detected and extent of impairment of work performance, which is the most germane issue. The most commonly abused substance, alcohol, is generally not tested for as the emphasis has been on detecting illicit drugs. The issue generates much concern with regard to civil liberties.

If substance abuse is detected, whether by organized screening or observation of impaired performance, such as may occur with alcoholism, an organizational response is warranted. This includes provision of counselling and cessation programs, and many employers provide employee assistance programs for those with alcohol problems.

2.3. REHABILITATION

Tertiary prevention in occupational health refers to the treatment of injury or illness with the safe return to the workforce in the most timely and appropriate manner. A rapid return to the workplace reflects the employer's desire to reduce costs associated with a worker off work convalescing and the employee's desire to be a functioning and productive member of society. The cornerstones of a successful rapid return-to-work philosophy include the provision of treatment and rehabilitation as soon as possible and the return to the workplace as soon as possible, utilizing a modified program where appropriate. A modified program is work that has been selected to accommodate any limitations that the worker may have while recovering. The CMA has released a policy summary describing the physician's role in helping the worker to a safe return to meaningful work following injury or illness. These guidelines focus on the physician's role in diagnosing and treating injury or illness, advising the patient, communicating, and working with the patient and the employer to facilitate the patient's return to productive employment (13).

Following a work-related injury or illness, the individual may be temporarily or permanently disabled. If these individuals are covered under their provincial workers' compensation act, financial compensation is available for rehabilitation services.

2.3.1. Workers' Compensation Board

The injury and disease related to work are compensable in all provinces and territories. The agency that deals with compensation in most provinces is called the Workers' Compensation Board; in Ontario it is called Workplace Safety and Insurance Board. Workers' compensation falls within the jurisdiction of provincial statutes, although the general principles are uniform. The main features of workers' compensation are as follows: the WCB is autonomous; employers pay for costs; the WCB decides benefits; negligence is not a factor; first aid, medical treatment, lost time, and rehabilitation are covered for most workers; a no-fault insurance system; and workers abdicate their right to sue the employer. The employer must notify the WCB within a specified time (ascribed in legislation) of an employee becoming injured, and is responsible for first aid to the worker and transport to hospital. The treating physician should submit a report to the WCB (in Quebec the legislation requires mandatory reporting). In addition to treatment, the WCB offers rehabilitation consisting of physiotherapy, occupational therapy, counselling, social work, and chiropractic services for accepted claims.

3.   COMMON OCCUPATIONAL EXPOSURES

The balance of this chapter provides a brief overview of the clinical aspects of common occupational exposures and diseases. More detailed clinical reviews are available in textbooks on occupational medicine, some of which are included in the bibliography (14-16).

The occupational health history must be a routine component of any health history. When occupational disease is suspected, the history should be suitably detailed. Generally speaking, there are two main parts: a work history, which includes exposure and controls, and a health history, which reviews the symptoms in order to determine any relationship to work. While this history is being elicited, other significant environmental exposures (such as hobbies or travel history) should also be ascertained. While occupational diseases have their origin in the working environment, it should be noted that similar diseases may be caused by nonoccupational exposures, the distinction being the location of the exposure.

The agents causing occupational disease may be divided into five broad groups: chemical, physical, biological, mechanical and ergonomic, and psychosocial. It is essential to note that at the time of diagnosis some conditions must be fulfilled before attributing causality to the workplace as described in Chapter Two. These conditions, where applicable, include adequate concentration and duration of exposure, absorption by the body, appropriate temporal sequence, and consistency of ill-health effects with the putative exposure. The list of occupational diseases may be endless. However, this chapter focuses on those deemed significant because of their frequency of occurrence in Canada or the severity of the disability produced. Known or highly suspected carcinogens in the workplace are listed in Table 10.1.

3.1.   CHEMICAL AGENTS

3.1.1. Organic Dusts

Organic dusts contain carbon and are largely derived from substances of animal or plant origin. Common examples are dusts and fibres arising from the handling or manufacture of wood, bone, shell, fur, skins, hides, leather, brooms, straw, flour, grain, tobacco, jute, flax (linen), hemp, cotton, wool, felt, carpets, rag, paper, or sweepings.

Table 10.1: Known Carcinogens in the Workplace

Aluminum Production	Iron and steel founding
Arsenic and arsenic compounds	Isopropyl alcohol manufacture, strong acid-process
Asbestos	Magenta, manufacture of
Auramine, manufacture of	Mineral oils, untreated and mildly-treated
Benzene	Mustard gas
Benzidine	Nickel and nickel compounds
Boot and shoe manufacture and repair	The rubber industry
Coal gasification	Shale-oils
Coar-tar pitches	Soots
Coke production	Talc containing asbestiform fibre
Furniture and cabinet making	Vinyl Chloride
Haematite mining, underground, with exposure to radon	

Source: WHO, International Agency for Research in Cancer. *IARC Mongraphs on the Evaluation of Caricinogenic Risks to Humans.* Supplement 7: 40-42, 1987, Lyon, Paris

Most organic dusts do not cause lung disease of a specific disabling nature. Many are irritants to the upper respiratory passages and to the conjunctivas and skin, causing bronchitis, conjunctivitis, and dermatitis. Many organic dusts may elicit allergic reactions in sensitized persons, with production of asthma and urticaria (hives). Workers may exhibit no outward symptoms until they are exposed to a dust to which they are sensitized, when they develop an allergic reaction characterized by a decrease in the vital capacity of lung from a normal level of about 5 litres to 2.5 or 3 litres and by a decrease in the timed forced expiratory ventilation fractions (FEV_1, FEV_2, FEV_3) indicating bronchiolar spasm, wheezing, and dyspnoea (shortness of breath). Such adverse effects are usually relieved by cessation of the exposure, and tend to recur when the person returns to the job. A typical history includes symptoms of cough, wheeze, or shortness of breath, worsening during the work week with improvement on weekends and holidays.

3.1.2. Mineral Dusts

No dust can be regarded as entirely harmless; however, for practical purposes mineral dusts can be divided into two classes: active and inert. The majority of dusts encountered, industrially or otherwise, are relatively inert. Some of the inert dusts may cause radiological pulmonary shadowing from the deposition of radio-opaque material in the lungs, without initiating fibrosis or loss of pulmonary function. Their main importance lies in the problem they present in differential diagnosis. Siderosis, which is due to the deposition of iron dust in the lung, is probably the most frequently encountered non-disabling pneumoconiosis.

Among the active dusts, silica, asbestos (a silicate), and the fume from processing of bauxite ore are the chief offenders in producing disabling pulmonary disease in this country. It has been conclusively established that the vast majority (over 90%) of the particles that reach the alveoli are less than 3 microns (3/1000 mm) in diameter. Most particles larger than 3 microns either settle out of the air before it is breathed, or are trapped in the secretions of the nose and throat and are eliminated or swallowed. As a rule, dusts vary greatly in size, depending to some extent upon the mechanical processes involved in their production, for example, wet versus dry drilling of hard rock.

Silica

With regard to the numbers of people exposed and cases of disability produced, "free" silica (silicon dioxide, SiO_2) is the chief cause of pulmonary dust disease; in contrast, "combined" silica (silicate, SiO_3) is probably inert. Silica is the main constituent of sand, sandstone, and granite, and is present in iron ore and coal. Exposure to crystalline silica occurs in several occupations (such as hard rock mining, sandblasting, granite cutting). The approximate average duration of exposure required for the development of silicosis varies widely for different occupations from five years in unprotected sandblasting to 30 years in moulders and granite cutters. The prolonged inhalation of dusts containing free silica may result in the development of a disabling pulmonary fibrosis known as silicosis. The Committee on Pneumoconiosis of the American Public Health Association defines silicosis as "a disease due to the breathing of air containing silica (SiO_2)". It is characterized by generalized fibrotic changes and the development of miliary nodules in both lungs, and clinically by shortness of breath, decreased chest expansion, lessened capacity for work, absence of fever, increased susceptibility to tuberculosis (some or all of which symptoms may be present), and characteristic x-ray findings that show rounded opacities, localized initially to upper lung fields, and "egg shell" calcification of hilar lymph nodes in a minority of cases.

A controversy emerging in occupational medicine is the relationship between silicosis and lung cancer. Numerous studies have been reported in the literature. The additive effects of silica and carcinogens such as benzopyrene have been proven without a doubt. However, whether silica by itself is a carcinogen has not been clearly established.

In diagnosing silicosis, it is essential to ascertain whether the worker was exposed to silica and, if so, whether sufficient exposure to cause the disease occurred.

The x-ray on its own is of little value in determining disability and in fact may be misleading.

Asbestos

Canada is one of the principal asbestos-producing countries. There are three forms of asbestos, namely chrysolite, amosite, and crocidolite. Canada produces mainly chrysolite, which is chiefly hydrated magnesium silicate that occurs as a white fibrous ore. The fibres, when separated, may be spun into yarn and woven in much the same manner as ordinary textiles, or they may be ground and mixed with other materials to form insulating boards or sheets. Exposure to the dust occurs in the crushing, carding, spinning, and weaving of the material, and in the manufacture of brake linings and insulating products.

The essential lesion in asbestosis is a diffuse fibrosis, which probably begins as a "collar" around the terminal bronchioles. Usually, at least four to seven years of exposure are required before a serious degree of fibrosis occurs. Apparently there is less predisposition to tuberculosis than is the case with silicosis. Lung cancer was reported in 15% to 23% of men who died with asbestosis and had autopsies. Thus there is evidence for accepting lung cancer as an occupational disease in those who have asbestos fibrosis of the lungs. The sentinel carcinoma for asbestos is mesothelioma.

Coal

Graphite is a crystalline form of carbon; ash-free anthracite coal is an amorphous form of the same element. In their pure state, these dusts cause no fibrosis of the lung. As they occur in nature, however, graphite and anthracite frequently contain considerable amounts of free silica, and exposed workers may develop a modified form of silicosis or coal worker's pneumoconiosis characterized by diffusely scattered, small stellate patches of fibrosis, each surrounded by an area of focal emphysema. Like true silicosis, coal worker's pneumoconiosis may be disabling. The incidence of the disease has been shown to be related to the concentration of silica dust in the air and to the length of exposure.

3.1.3. Metallic Dusts and Fumes
Lead

Of the metallic dusts and fumes, lead and its compounds are probably the most important, not only because of their widespread use in industry, but also because of the serious disability that may result from poisoning. The environmental aspects of lead contamination are described in Chapter Nine. The occupations that expose workers to the highest levels of lead are the manufacture of storage batteries and the reclamation of scrap metal. Exposure also occurs in soldering operations and lead burning, in the manufacture of paints containing lead, and in the sanding of surfaces coated with lead paints. Other exposures occur in the printing trade, the breaking up of ships coated with lead paints, the glazing of pottery, the manufacture and use of certain insecticides, and the blending of tetraethyl lead gasoline additive.

The toxicity of the various lead compounds appears to depend upon several factors: the solubility of the compound in the body fluids, the size of the particles (solubility is greater, of course, in proportion to the smallness of the particles), and conditions under which the compound is used. Where a lead compound is used as a powder, atmospheric contamination is reduced if the powder is kept damp. Of the various lead compounds, the carbonate, the monoxide, and the sulphate are considered to be more toxic than metallic lead or other lead compounds. Lead arsenate is very toxic, due to the presence of the arsenic radical. The toxicity of lead chromate or chrome yellow is less than would be expected due to its low solubility.

To study the effects of lead exposure in workers, two separate entities must be kept in mind: lead absorption and lead poisoning. Lead absorption is that condition in which workers experience absorption but do not have clinical evidence of lead poisoning. There is an increased lead urinary excretion rate, perhaps an increased blood lead level, a reduced or falling haemoglobin, perhaps an increased basophilic stippling of red blood cells, and, on rare occasions, a lead line along the gum margin (although the lead line occurs after very prolonged exposure and rarely without other, more prominent symptoms). Despite this evidence of increased lead absorption, these workers feel well and have no complaints about their health.

Lead poisoning (or lead intoxication) may be acute or chronic. Acute lead poisoning results from a single exposure to a large dose and is rarely encountered in industry. Accidental ingestion of lead acetate or lead subacetate is the main source of lead. Signs and symptoms of acute lead poisoning include metallic taste, vomiting, colic, and constipation or bloody diarrhea. Central nervous system symptoms predominate when exposure is from organic lead compounds (such as tetraethyl or tetramethyl lead).

Chronic lead poisoning is a classic example of a cumulative poison. It occurs from the inhalation or ingestion of small amounts of lead dust, fumes, or vapours over a relatively long period of time. The diagnosis of early lead poisoning is often difficult since the presenting symptoms are very general (such as headache, weakness, and pallor; see also Chapter Nine). To make a diagnosis of occupational lead poisoning, the following criteria must be met: there must be a history of significant exposure to lead at work, there must be clinical signs and symptoms compatible with lead poisoning, and there must be supportive laboratory evidence (i.e., increased urinary or blood lead levels, increased erythroprotoporphyrin, low haemoglobin). It also requires the medical professional to be cognizant of the possibility of the occupational hazard of lead in order to consider the diagnosis.

Ideally, prevention of lead poisoning consists of avoiding exposure to lead. Minimum requirements for examining workers exposed to lead consists of a complete medical examination periodically and periodic inquiry into general health, together with urine or blood lead measurements. If blood lead is above 0.08 micrograms per 100 millilitres that individual is at a high risk for developing lead poisoning.

Mercury

Mercury and mercury compounds are used widely in many industries. For example, they are used in the manufacture of scientific instruments and industrial chemicals, in the photographic industry, in the pharmaceutical industry, in the manufacture of amalgams with copper, tin, silver, and gold, in dentistry, and in power generators. The effects of environmental exposure to mercury are described in Chapter Nine.

Acute exposure to mercury is fairly rare, particularly in industry. Ingestion produces severe corrosion of the upper alimentary tract. Chronic exposure usually results in any or all of the following: erethism (a form of anxiety neurosis, illustrated by the "Mad Hatter" in Lewis Carroll's Alice in Wonderland, an unfortunate victim of chronic mercury exposure secondary to the mercury that was used at one time in hat manufacturing), vasomotor disturbances, renal damage, depression, central and peripheral nerve disorders, lesions in the mouth and teeth, and nausea and vomiting.

There are some clinical differences between organic and inorganic mercury poisoning. Erethism, stomatitis, and salivation are less marked with organic compounds, whereas motor and sensory disturbances are greater. Urinary excretion of mercury of more than 300 micrograms per day is associated with a chronic condition.

Cadmium

Today the largest use of cadmium is the electroplating industry. Almost all industrial exposures are due to the inhalation of fumes emitted in smelting impure zinc, in distilling cadmium sponge, or in welding or burning cadmium-plated metal. The occurrence of cadmium poisoning is increasing due to its increased use. The effects of acute and chronic cadmium toxicity are described in Chapter Nine.

Nickel

It is used in the manufacture of alloys of iron, chromium, and tungsten. Its salts are also used widely. In industry, exposure occurs through the inhalation of the dusts and fumes that are by-products of the production of the metal. Nickel and its salts are not considered to cause systemic poisoning. Recently, cases of lung and sinus cancer have been found in greater than normal numbers among men employed in the calcining and sintering operations. However, the most common effect resulting from exposure to nickel compounds is the development of nickel-itch seen most commonly in people doing nickel plating.

3.1.4. Volatile Solvents and Organic Materials
Aromatic Hydrocarbons

Benzene is perhaps the most dangerous of solvents used commercially. In acute poisoning, the worker becomes confused or dizzy, complains of tightening of the leg muscles and pressure over the forehead, then passes into a stage of excitement. A worker who continues to be exposed may lapse into a coma. In non-fatal cases, recovery is usually complete. In chronic poisoning, the onset is slow with vague symptoms (e.g., fatigue, headache, nausea). With continued exposure, aplastic anaemia or leukaemia may develop. Toluene and xylene are closely related chemically to benzene but are less toxic and do not produce the same effects.

Chlorinated Hydrocarbons

Chlorinated hydrocarbons are used widely in oils, greases, and waxes. They are generally nonflammable, and their toxicity to the liver and kidney ranges from very high to very low. Carbon tetrachloride is the most toxic of this group. Following exposures to high concentrations, the worker may become unconscious and, if exposure is not terminated, death can follow from respiratory failure. Exposure to lower concentrations, insufficient to produce unconsciousness, usually results in severe gastro-intestinal upset and may progress to serious kidney and hepatic damage.

Alcohol, Esters, and Ketones

These categories include methyl, propyl, and butyl alcohol, and methyl and ethyl acetate, as well as acetone.

Methyl Alcohol

It is used as a solvent in the manufacture of lacquers, varnishes, shellac, and cleaning and polishing materials. In industry, exposure occurs mainly through inhalation of the vapour, but also via absorption through the skin. Severe exposure leads to dizziness, unconsciousness, cardiac depression, and, eventually, death. In mild to moderate exposure, blurring of vision, photo phobia, and conjunctivitis, followed by blindness, may occur secondary to the metabolism of methyl alcohol to toxic formic acid. If the level of methyl alcohol in the blood, or of formic acid in the urine, exceeds 150 micrograms per day, there is absorption of methyl alcohol.

3.1.5. Gases

Industrial gases may be divided into three groups: those irritating to the upper respiratory tract (e.g., ammonia, sulphur dioxide), those that are toxic (e.g., carbon monoxide, arsine), and those that are asphyxiants and displace oxygen (e.g., methane, nitrogen).

Sulphur Dioxide

This gas occurs widely in industry. Higher concentrations (20 parts per million, or ppm) produce immediate irritation of the eyes and coughing. Concentrations above this level cannot be tolerated, and continued exposure may result in oedema of the larynx and lungs, and bronchopneumonia. Repeated exposure to the gas results in nasopharyngitis, bronchitis, shortness of breath on exertion, increased fatigue, and alteration of the sense of taste and smell. Brief exposures, lasting up to half an hour, to concentrations up to 100 ppm do not produce disability, but concentrations of 400 to 500 ppm are dangerous, even for short exposures.

Carbon Monoxide

Carbon monoxide is produced by the incomplete combustion of carbon-containing materials and is nearly always present in the gases given off from burning substances. Poisoning is most common from automobile exhaust gas, and from poorly designed or unvented gas burners in stoves or heaters.

Carbon monoxide combines with haemoglobin in blood to form carboxyhemoglobin, which negates the ability of haemoglobin to carry oxygen to the body's tissues. With concentrations up to 10% of carboxyhemoglobin in the blood, there are rarely any symptoms. Concentrations of 20% to 30% cause shortness of breath on moderate exertion and slight headache. Concentrations from 30% to 50% cause severe headache, mental confusion and dizziness, impairment of vision and hearing, and collapse and fainting on exertion. With concentrations of 50% to 60%, unconsciousness results, and death may follow if exposure is long. Concentrations of 80% result in almost immediate death. There is usually no cyanosis (blue skin, as one might expect from the presence of deoxygenated haemoglobin); since carboxyhemoglobin is a bright red compound, the lips may take on a "healthy" red appearance. Acute cases of poisoning, resulting from brief exposures to high concentrations, seldom result in any permanent disability if recovery takes place. The possibility of chronic effects as the result of repeated exposure to lower concentrations is controversial.

Hydrogen Sulphide (Sour Gas)

Hydrogen sulphide is a colourless gas that has an offensive, rotten-egg odour. However, the gas rapidly paralyses the olfactory nerve endings, so that heavy exposure may occur without the patient being aware of it (which is perhaps the biggest danger of hydrogen sulphide at the workplace). It presents as a by-product in industry (such as the petroleum industry where sulphur-rich crude is processed). Additionally, it is a hazard in sewers, mines, wells, and tunnels. Hydrogen sulphide causes asphyxiation due to paralysis of the respiratory centre. High concentrations may cause rhinitis, bronchitis, and, occasionally, pulmonary oedema. Exposure to very high concentrations causes immediate death. Chronic poisoning results in headache, inflammation of the conjunctiva and eyelids, digestive disturbances, loss of weight, and general debility.

Silo Filler's Disease

Silo filler's disease is due to poisoning by oxides of nitrogen. A silo is an airtight structure in which green crops such as corn and clover are pressed and kept for fodder. The decomposition of organic material produces oxides of nitrogen, which can cause pulmonary oedema; this may clear or result in the development of a condition known as bronchiolitis fibrosa cystica. There is haemorrhage in lung, edema, hypertrophy of alveolar epithelium, and the formation of hyaline membranes. X-rays show a diffuse fine nodular infiltrate in the lungs, concentrated in the suprahilar area.

3.2. PHYSICAL AGENTS

3.2.1. Excessive Noise

The effects produced by excessive noise may include impaired hearing, fatigue, increased blood pressure, decreased efficiency, and emotional disturbances. Noise can be measured by a sound level meter, which determines the intensity of a sound in the immediate environment in terms of decibels. Ordinary conversation varies from 35 to 65 decibels. The normal threshold of audibility is 0 decibels. Intensity above 80 decibels are annoying and noise levels of 100 to 130 decibels have been found to cause temporary and permanent deafness. Levels above 130 decibels are painful to the ear.

Although industrial noise is usually a combination of sounds at different frequencies, it is still possible to establish the main source of a noise and take appropriate steps to eliminate or reduce it. Initial loss in acuity occurs for sounds with high frequencies, particularly those around 4,000 cycles per second (Hz). Brief exposures to high noise levels results in temporary hearing loss, with recovery occurring over several days to weeks. On the other hand, exposure during the work day to sustained noise levels of 85 decibels or higher for several months may result in permanent partial impairment of hearing. In general, the greater the loss in acuity for conversation, the more seriously the person is handicapped. Often the first time that someone may notice a hearing problem is during a telephone conversation.

In assessing the importance of noise in producing deafness, a careful search must be made to rule out other conditions that are also recognized as causing deafness. There is considerable individual susceptibility to the effects of noise. Preplacement and periodic audiograms are essential for employees working in high noise levels. It is necessary also to distinguish between occupational impairment and the normal deterioration in hearing that occurs with advancing age (presbycusis). Noise may be prevented or eliminated by one or more of the following methods: elimination of noise at its source, isolation of noisy operations, reduction of noise by sound insulation, and use of personal protective devices against noise.

3.2.2. Temperature and Humidity

Excessively high temperature and humidity occur in many industries, principally as a result of the heat and moisture produced by industrial processes. This may be accentuated during the summer months by a high external temperature. Very high temperatures may bring about heat cramps, heat exhaustion, or heat stroke.

Heat Cramps

Heat cramps may occur in people who sweat profusely as a result of heavy physical work performed in hot environments, and are due to sodium chloride depletion. The characteristic symptoms consist of spasmodic contractions of the muscles of the extremities and abdominal wall. The body temperature is usually normal or slightly elevated, the pulse rate slightly increased, the blood pressure normal, and the skin moist. Nausea and vomiting may occur. The cramps disappear completely and rapidly following intravenous injection of physiological saline and can be prevented by oral administration of salt and water.

Heat Exhaustion

This usually occurs in hot weather, with the initial symptoms being fatigue, headache, and dizziness. These may proceed to a state of unconsciousness or collapse. The body temperature may be low or elevated (although not exceeding 102°F or 126°C), the skin may be moist, the pulse is rapid and weak, and the blood pressure is usually low. The clinical picture is the same as shock.

Heat Stroke

This is often called sunstroke when the cause is the radiant heat from the sun. In industrial workers, heat stroke occurs most frequently during prolonged heat waves. The condition is due to failure of the temperature-controlling centre of the hypothalamus. The onset may be sudden, with the outstanding symptom being a high body temperature falling between 107°F and 110°F (135°C and 140°C). The pulse is rapid (except in the late stages) and the blood pressure is elevated. Other characteristics include laboured respiration, hot and dry skin, flushed face, depressed nervous system, incontinence, and vomiting. The state of coma may last for hours or days.

Cold

Exposure of extremities to the cold can cause chilblains or precipitate attacks of Raynaud's disease. Raynaud's disease is an idiopathic, paroxysmal, bilateral, asymmetrical cyanosis of digits, due to arterial or arteriolar contractions, brought on by cold or emotions. Re-warming the affected part reverses the temporary damage. Frostbite is a more severe and largely irreversible form of local cell injury. Upon thawing, hyperaemia and increased capillary permeability cause edema, swelling and thrombosis, followed by ischemia and gangrene in the digits.

3.2.3. Abnormalities of Air Pressure

Exposure to abnormally high atmospheric pressures occurs in diving operations and in occupations where compressed air shafts and caissons are used, as in construction of tunnels, bridge piers, and building foundations. Workers are exposed to air pressures exceeding the hydrostatic pressure of water at the depths in which they work.

Decompression Sickness

Most frequently encountered by industrial workers, symptoms usually appear within the first few hours following too-rapid decompression. This rapid decompression leads to the formation of bubbles of nitrogen gas that block off the blood supply to various parts of the body, including the spinal cord. The most common symptom is severe pain in the muscles and joints of the arms and legs. Other symptoms include epigastric pain, dyspnoea, paralysis of skeletal muscle, and shock. Death may occur rapidly or may follow secondary complications. Prevention consists of limiting the lengths of time a worker may stay in compressed air at specified pressures, and requiring adequate periods for decompression after each work period.

Barotrauma

Occurs as the result of too sudden increases or decreases in atmospheric pressures. A sudden increase with a blocked eustachian tube may result in otic barotrauma (rupture of the tympanic membrane), whereas a sudden decrease, with blocked nasal sinuses, may cause sinus barotrauma. A similar effect can occur in other gas containing cavities (e.g., intestines), if the external air pressure is suddenly decreased.

3.2.4. Radiation

Radiation exposure occurs from X-rays (medical and dental) primarily but also from radon progeny, radioactive minerals in building materials, phosphate fertilizers, smoke detectors, and nuclear power plants. There are two types of radiation: ionizing and non-ionizing.

Ionizing Radiation

Ionizing radiation consists of X-rays, gamma rays, alpha particles, beta particles, and neutrons. X-rays are streams of photons that have great penetrability and move at high speed. Gamma rays are higher energy photons that have greater penetrability. Beta particles are electrons that can penetrate several centimetres of body tissue. Alpha particles are positively charged helium nuclei and have poor penetration. They can be easily impeded but deposit a lot of energy in a short track. Neutrons are uncharged particles that exist independently only for a fraction of a second.

Exposure from x-rays and gamma radiation is measured in grays (1 Gy = 100 rads, or radiation absorbed dose) while the unit sievert (1 Sv = 100 rem, or roentgen equivalent man) expresses a dose equivalent. The exposure of radiation workers is limited to 2 mSv (2 rem) per year averaged over a five-year period (the background radiation exposure varies by geographical location but is about 0.03 rems per year in North America). This exposure limit is determined pursuant to the Atomic Energy Control Board of Canada, which is responsible for most regulations in the radiation field.

As a result of these regulations, all atomic radiation workers must wear dosimeter film badges to measure exposure. These are periodically measured to determine the exposure dose. The effects of alpha and beta particles, neutrons, X-rays, and gamma rays on the body are believed to be due to the process of ionization. The ultimate effect of ionization is damage to, or death of, the cells. The ability of the body to repair the damage varies with the total energy absorbed (the sievert), the frequency of exposure, and the period of time over which the exposure is spread. Greater doses can be tolerated if fractionated than if given as a single exposure.

The type and severity of the injury depend on the extent of the tissue exposed and on the particular tissue that absorbs the radiation. The lymphoid tissue, including bone marrow, lymphocytes, and Peyer's patches, appears to be the most sensitive to radiation, followed by, in decreasing order of susceptibility, polymorphonuclear leucocytes, epithelial cells (including the hair), gonads, endothelial cells (including blood vessels and peritoneum), connective tissue, muscle cells, and the nerve cells.

The effects of ionizing radiation may be subdivided into somatic and genetic. The somatic effects, in turn, may be acute or delayed. The acute somatic effects are known as radiation sickness; this varies in severity from mild skin erythema (redness), to severe illness with death occurring within a week of exposure. The latter follows exposures of greater than 50 Sv. Nausea and vomiting develop within an hour of such exposures; these may subside for a few days, only to be followed by the return of nausea, vomiting, diarrhea, fever, bleeding, and ulceration of the mucous membranes. The blood lymphocyte count declines and secondary infection may occur. Death is usually the result of intestinal or haemopoietic injury. Treatment of acute radiation sickness is so far only palliative.

The delayed somatic effects of ionizing radiation include leucopenia, anaemia, sterility, fetal injury, bone necrosis, and sarcomata (as occurred among dial painters who ingested radium paint during World War I), lung cancer (reported among uranium miners in Czechoslovakia and the Colorado plateau), chronic atrophic dermatitis, hyperkeratoses, epitheliomata, leukaemia, breast and thyroid cancer (reported among survivors of Hiroshima and Nagasaki), and production of cataracts by neutron exposure. Except for leukaemia, a long latency period of 15 to 25 years is characteristic of malignancies secondary to radiation exposure.

With respect to the genetic effects of ionizing radiation, there are few human data. The majority of both natural and radiation mutations is of recessive inheritance, and the probability of their becoming manifest in future generations is small. In follow-up studies on the survivors of the Japanese bombings, so far there has been little evidence of a deleterious effect on succeeding generations.

Protecting workers who are exposed to ionizing radiation requires a combination of engineering controls, environmental monitoring, and employee monitoring. This includes distancing the worker from the radiation source as far as possible (exposure to radiation varies inversely with the square of the distance from the source), shielding the worker (lead walls or lead impregnated clothing), and hygiene measures (exhausting, proper clean clothing, and environmental cleaning). Dosimeters (radiation dose registering devices worn by the worker) are changed at regular intervals (typically every two weeks) and records of the dose received are kept. Workers are temporarily removed from the environment if they are receiving levels too high. Preplacement investigations include blood work and regular employee blood work may be taken depending on dose of radiation received.

Non-Ionizing Radiation

Non-ionizing radiation refers to emission from those parts of the electromagnetic spectrum where emitted photons generally have insufficient energy to produce ionization of atoms. These forms of radiation include microwave, television and radio waves, visible light, and infrared and ultraviolet radiation, among others. Important workplace forms of non-ionizing radiation are ultraviolet and infrared radiation.

Ultraviolet (UV) Radiation. Occupational exposure to ultraviolet rays occurs chiefly from sunlight in such workers as farmers and construction workers. The risks are acute (sunburn) or delayed (skin cancer or cataract). Welding is a source of ultraviolet radiation exposure. The intensity of the ultraviolet radiation increases with the temperature of the welding process. Exposure may also occur in the use of ultraviolet rays for inspecting razor blades, blue prints, and golf balls, and in the examination of bedding for the presence of used materials. Ultraviolet rays are also used in the diagnosis and treatment of skin diseases.

UV radiation primarily affects the eyes, skin and superficial blood vessels. Symptoms appear 4 to 12 hours after exposure, with skin developing an erythema, followed by freckling and pigmentation. The eyes may react by developing ophthalmia with acute conjunctivitis, lacrimation, photo phobia, and burning. In severe cases, corneal ulceration, iritis, and cataracts may develop.

Infrared Radiation. Infrared radiation (heat radiation) is given off by everything with a temperature of greater than absolute zero but is of a concern in high temperature processes such as welding, glass-blowing, foundry work, and other occupations where metal and glass are heated to the molten state. In these processes, there may be a concomitant exposure to ultraviolet rays and to excessive light radiation. Infrared rays are utilized in industry in the heating and drying of many materials, e.g., painted and lacquered objects and automobiles.

Infrared radiation causes a vasodilation of the skin and stimulation of cellular activity. In excessive doses, it produces an erythema followed by pigmentation and freckling. The most serious effect of prolonged exposure to infrared radiation is the development of a cortical cataract at the posterior pole. This cataract form is found in workers over 35 years of age who have been exposed for some years to the glare from molten glass or metal or from furnaces.

Video Display Terminals (VDTs). In a policy statement, the Canadian Medical Association declared: "Many reputable scientific surveys have shown that VDTs do not emit ionizing radiation (x-radiation). The health problems experienced by many VDT operators are, according to the best knowledge available, essentially ergonomic, being related to the physical characteristics of the workplace. VDT users more often have visual, musculoskeletal, and stress-related complaints than other workers. Proper ergonomic standards (e.g., appropriately designed work spaces, approved office furniture and machines, adequate lighting and glare reduction, regular rest breaks, and suitable environmental conditions) should be encouraged in the workplace to maximize comfort of VDT operators" (17).

3.2.5. Electricity
The effects of electrical currents upon the body depend on external and individual conditions. The severity of the damage is proportional to the strength and duration of the current. In general, the higher the voltage, the greater will be the current passing through the body. The strength of the current will be increased if the skin is wet or damp. The current chiefly affects the organs through which it passes. When the current passes through the brain, the patient may be rendered unconscious. Death is caused by ventricular fibrillation, failure of the respiratory centre, or prolonged tetanus of the respiratory muscles resulting in suffocation. Voltage as low as 35 volts have been known to cause death. If the current does not pass through any of the vital organs, other parts of the body may be affected. This may result in functional or structural damage, which may be either temporary or permanent.

Permanent disability is usually the result of electrical burns in tissues directly affected by the current. A discussion of electromagnetic fields that are generated by electric current and are indirect effects of electricity to which workers may be exposed is given in Chapter Nine.

3.3. BIOLOGICAL AGENTS

These include bacteria, rickettsia, viruses, fungi, and protozoa. Diseases caused by such agents may be regarded as occupational in origin when the nature of the work involves exposure to the organism. Thus tuberculosis may be accepted as an occupational disease when it occurs in health care professionals whose daily work has caused them to be exposed to *Mycobacterium tuberculosis*. The majority of occupational diseases of infectious origin occur in groups of employees exposed to animals or birds, such as abattoir workers, veterinarian, and pet shop workers. An example of this type of biological disease (undulant fever) is given below. Of more recent concern, however, are blood-borne infections such as AIDS and hepatitis B in the workplace, particularly (but not exclusively) in the health care setting. Blood is increasingly being recognized as a potentially toxic substance.

Blood-Borne Occupational Diseases
The occurrence of occupationally acquired blood-borne infection depends on the frequency and types of hazardous exposures, the risk associated with each type of discrete exposure and the prevalence of infection in the patient population. The prevalence of blood-borne infective agents in persons admitted to one Canadian hospital were as follows: hepatitis B surface antigen, 2.1%; HIV antibodies 0.6%; antibodies to the hepatitis C virus 0.5% (18). The generalizability of these results cannot be assumed. The other factors are discussed below.

The risk of a health care worker contracting hepatitis B from an occupational exposure is significant. Risks among U.S. health care workers (from the Occupational Health and Safety Administration, or OSHA, and the Federal Register) are quoted, as insufficient data are available from Canada (19). OSHA's risk assessment yields an estimated 20 to 31 cases of clinical hepatitis per 1,000 and risk of death of 2 to 3 per 1,000 on the basis of a 45-year working life.

In regard to HIV infection, although the proportion of health care workers infected is similar to the general population, there is a statistically greater proportion of infected health care workers with no known risk factors or an undetermined transmission category. The risk of seroconversion among cohorts of health care workers with parenteral exposures has been shown to be small, less than 0.5%. In relation to occupational exposure to HIV in Canada, no seroconversions have been documented in the national surveillance program on occupational exposure to HIV among 317 health care workers with percutaneous, mucous membrane, and skin exposures as of April 5, 1992 (20).

Universal precautions, intended to prevent parenteral, mucous membrane, and non-intact skin exposures of health care workers to blood-borne pathogens, have been recommended and widely introduced (21). There is some concern, however, about the effectiveness of universal precautions in preventing occupational spread of HIV. A surveillance study by the Federal Centre for AIDS indicated that health care workers were exposed to blood despite protection, but seroconversions did not result (22). The basic tenet of universal precautions is that every specimen should be regarded as hazardous and treated with equal care. The reader is advised to review the recommendations made by the National Committee for Clinical Laboratory Standards. No attempt is made here to reproduce these, but the following salient points from the recommendations are made. Universal precautions include prevention of sharp instrument injuries, use of protective barriers, and immediate washing of hands and surfaces contaminated by blood and other fluids to which universal precautions apply. These measures are intended to supplement existing practices of hand washing and use of gloves to prevent infection. Universal precautions apply to blood and other body fluids containing visible blood and tissues, but do not apply to faeces, nasal secretions, sputum, sweat, tears, urine, and vomit unless they contain visible blood.

A further current issue in relation to occupational spread of HIV is the reciprocity of the rights of patients and health care workers with regard to HIV testing (23). Attention was drawn to the potential risk for patients contracting HIV from infected practitioners by reasonable evidence that three patients were infected with HIV by a dentist (24). This type of transmission is, however, regarded as a rare occurrence. Guidelines for the continuing practice of HIV-positive physicians have been produced in a number of jurisdictions. The Laboratory Centre for Disease Control has advised that mandatory testing of health care workers and patients for HIV is not currently warranted due to the extremely small risk of HIV transmission in this setting and the impracticality of this measure.

As an adjunctive measure to prevent blood-borne infection, recommendation has been made for pre-exposure hepatitis B vaccination for health care workers potentially exposed to blood. Compliance among health care workers for hepatitis B vaccination has been high. Protocol for appropriate post-exposure hepatitis B, testing, passive immunization, and active vaccination have been developed (25). Protocols have been designed to reduce the incidence of blood-borne infections in hospitals and other health care settings (26).

Undulant Fever (Brucellosis, Malta Fever)

Undulant fever is an acute infectious disease characterized by a prolonged febrile course with irregular remissions and exacerbations. It is caused by a member of the *Brucella* group of microorganisms. The causative agent is ingested from contaminated food and drink, particularly milk, butter, and cheese from infected goats and cows. It is also contracted by those who handle infected meat and meat products. The majority of cases occur in farmers, milkers, and abattoir workers. The average incubation period is two weeks, with the onset being gradual. Fever, anorexia, constipation, loss of weight, and generalized muscle and joint pains are common characteristics.

3.4. MECHANICAL AND ERGONOMIC AGENTS

Soft-tissue injuries from repetitive use or static loading are of increasing importance because of the increase use of computer keyboarding.

Tenosynovitis and Bursitis
The inflammation of tissues near joints occurs as a result of chronic repetitive movements, exertions, impacts, pressure, or the resumption of aggressive work after an extended break (e.g., winter layoff for bricklayers). The resulting inflammation often manifests clinically as tenosynovitis, bursitis, and myositis, causing pain and swelling in the tendons, joints, or muscles subjected to the strains. In the treatment of occupational tenosynovitis and bursitis, transfer to other work or removal from the job is important so that the affected part can be put at rest.

Hand-Arm Vibration Syndrome (Raynaud's Phenomenon)
The clinical effects resulting from prolonged use of piston-operated vibrating tools have been recognized for some years. Portable vibrating tools are of two main types: the piston-operated pneumatic tools, such as road and rock drills, chipping hammers, or riveting hammers, and the newer rotating tools that consist of a handle through the centre, which is a rotating spindle, and are driven by an electric motor or compressed air. Both types of tools may be carried in the hands. In either case, the vibrations of the tool are transmitted to the hands and arms of the operator.

The most common effect is a disturbance of the blood vessels of the fingers, which is quite similar clinically to Raynaud's disease. The condition may develop as early as months of exposure to the vibrations but usually requires longer exposure. Sometimes the condition first becomes apparent after exposure to vibration has ceased. Exposure to cold is the precipitating factor inducing the vasospastic attacks. Another associated feature of traumatic vasospastic disease is the effect on the neurological system, which includes pain and tingling in the extremities, and loss of grip strength. Both the vascular and neurological symptoms may be lessened by the use of calcium channel-blocking medication. It is imperative that the worker be removed from the offending environment to prevent further progression of the disease.

Carpal Tunnel Syndrome
Carpal tunnel syndrome is characterized by pain in the hand and lower arm associated with disturbances in sensation and grip strength. It is caused by compression of the median nerve as it passed through the wrist (carpal) tunnel formed by bones of the wrist and transcarpal ligament. The worker often complains that the pain is worse at night or when driving, and is relieved by shaking the hands vigorously. In the

workplace it is associated with jobs involving repetitive wrist flexon and extension with forceful gripping and vibration. Typical jobs are meat packers, seamstresses, automobile and aircraft assembly line workers, and clerical workers. Simple therapy includes wrist splints and anti-inflammatory drugs but if these provide no relief a surgical procedure may be required to release wrist pressure. A change in the way that a worker performs the work is essential to avoid recurrence. Many other common conditions may be responsible for carpal tunnel syndrome including pregnancy, diabetes, rheumatoid arthritis, and hypothyroidism.

3.5. PSYCHOSOCIAL AGENTS

Stress-induced illness in the workplace is becoming increasingly recognized as a serious problem with at least one workers' compensation board compensating for workplace stress-inducing illness. Regardless of whether or not stress is considered to cause a compensable illness, workplace-induced stress is increasingly being seen to have high indirect costs in terms of decreased productivity due to job dissatisfaction, mental illness, and increased absenteeism. Stress may be attributable to increase in work load, responsibility, and fear of loss of job security, all of which are characteristic of the downsizing that has occurred in North American industry in the 1980s and 1990s. Additionally, there are the stressors specific to particular jobs such as working in geographical isolation (such as at a remote outpost) or working shift work.

Post-traumatic stress disorder is a recognized condition in those workers who have experienced a near-death accident or witnessed an accident resulting in a death. It is characterized by irritability, depression, "video-replay", and nightmares.

3.6. SKIN DISEASES

Skin diseases are notable in that they may be the result of chemical, physical, or biological classes of environmental exposures. Consequently, they are discussed separately here. The skin forms a major component of the interface between the work environment and the worker unless the worker is completely protected by barrier clothing. Skin diseases constitute a major portion of compensated occupational disease. Occupational skin disease may be categorized into contact dermatitis, occupational acne, pigmentation disorders, neoplastic disorders, and miscellaneous disorders.

Contact dermatitis may be irritant or allergic. Irritant contact dermatitis is a result of direct injury to the skin as with many industrial materials including but not limited to acids, alkalis, metal compounds, detergents, petroleum products, oxidizing agents, solvents, and frequent hand washing with water with or without soap. Immunology does not play a role in the development of irritant contact dermatitis. On the other hand, an allergic contact dermatitis is the result of an immunologic reaction to a chemical agent. The presence of allergic contact dermatitis is usually confirmed by patch testing.

Occupational acne is the result of exposure to various agents that causes a chronic inflammatory process in the pilosebaceous follicles. Agents implicated in the development of occupational acne include oil, fats, and tars. Chloracne is the pathognomonic marker of exposure to halogenated aromatic hydrocarbons, including PCBs, dioxins, and organochlorine pesticides. Pigmentation disorders may be staining, hyperpigmentation, or hypopigmentation. Examples of exposures that result in staining include aniline dyes, picric acid, nitric acid, coal tar, and silver. Exposure to phytotoxins, ionizing radiation, or ultraviolet light may result in hyperpigmentation. Phenols and hydroquinones, on the other hand, may result in hypopigmentation. Radiation, ultraviolet light, arsenic, and polyaromatic hydrocarbons are some of the agents associated with the development of skin cancer.

Exposure to different extremes of temperature may result in miscellaneous skin disorders, for example, chilblains, immersion foot, and frostbite as a result of exposure to cold, and sunburn and toasted skin syndrome as a result of exposure to heat.

4.   SUMMARY

Occupational health may be defined as the maintenance and promotion of health in the working environment. The annual incidence of occupational injuries and illnesses in the Canadian workforce is about 12%. Injuries account for 97% of all compensated cases by workers' compensation boards; the remainder comprises occupational diseases. In 1994 alone, $2.33 billion was paid out by Ontario's WCB. The most common kind of occupational injury or illness is back injuries, according to WCB data.

Primary prevention in occupational health first involves substitution, and, if this is not possible, then segregation is attempted, including ventilation. Personal hygiene and protective equipment are used if the measures outlined above are not feasible. *Secondary prevention* in occupational health involves the use of preplacement and periodic examinations. Another aspect of secondary prevention in the workplace is the issue of employee screening for substance abuse. *Tertiary prevention* involves treatment, rehabilitation, and retraining under the auspices of workers' compensation. *Health promotion* in the workplace has emerged as an effective approach enabling access to the substantial numbers of persons in the workplace not only for the prevention of work-associated health problems, but for the introduction of wellness programs incorporating attention to lifestyle and other health determinants.

The agents causing occupational disease may be divided into five broad groups: chemical, physical, biological, mechanical or ergonomic, and psychosocial. In order to establish causality between the workplace and the health problem there must be adequate concentration and duration of exposure, absorption into the body, appropriate temporal sequence, and consistency of ill health effects with the putative exposure.

Chemical agents consist of organic dusts, mineral dusts and metallic dusts and fumes. Mineral dusts include silica, asbestos, and coal. Prolonged inhalation of "free" silica leads to silicosis. The most serious feature of silicosis is that it predisposes one to tuberculosis infection. In asbestosis, the essential lesion is a diffuse fibrosis, which probably begins around the terminal bronchioles. Metallic dusts and fumes incorporate lead, mercury, cadmium, and nickel. Lead is perhaps the most important metallic dust because it is the most used and because of the serious disability that may result from poisoning. There are two types of poisoning: acute and chronic. Acute lead poisoning results from a single exposure to a large dose, usually occurring as a result of accidental ingestion of lead salts. Chronic lead poisoning occurs from the inhalation or ingestion of small amounts of lead dust, fumes, or vapours over a relatively long period of time.

Volatile solvents and organic materials also affect the health of the worker. The three important classes of solvents are aromatic hydrocarbons, chlorinated hydrocarbons, and alcohol, esters, and ketones. Among the aromatic hydrocarbons, benzene is the most dangerous solvent used commercially. Poisoning can be both acute and chronic. The toxicity of chlorinated hydrocarbons varies from very high to very low, attacking the liver and kidney. Carbon tetrachloride is the most toxic of the group. Methyl alcohol may cause dizziness, unconsciousness, cardiac depression, and eventually death. Gases used in industry are either irritating to the upper respiratory tract (e.g., ammonia, chlorine) or are not irritating (e.g., carbon monoxide, hydrocyanic acid).

Physical agents have the potential of creating ill health for the worker. The effects produced by excessive noise may include fatigue, impaired hearing, increased blood pressure, decreased efficiency, and emotional disturbances. Industrial noise is a combination of sounds of different frequencies. Very high temperatures may bring about heat cramps, heat exhaustion, or heat stroke. Exposure of hands, feet, ears, and nose to the cold can cause chilblains or precipitate attacks of Raynaud's disease. Frostbite is a more severe and largely irreversible form of local cell injury. The most common effect resulting from repeated vibration is a disturbance of the blood vessels of the fingers. Muscular stiffness, soreness, blisters, and "occupational cramps" are clinical signs of the adverse effects of repeated motion on certain body parts. Decompression sickness and barotrauma are examples of the body's reaction to abnormalities of air pressure.

Another physical agent is ionizing or non-ionizing radiation. The ultimate effect of ionization is damage to, or death of, the cells. The type and severity of the injury depends on the extent of the tissue exposed and on the particular tissue that absorbs the radiation. Non-ionizing radiation comprises UV, infrared, microwave, and radio and television waves. Electrical currents travelling through the body damage tissues through which they pass. Hence, excessive noise, temperature and humidity, repeated motion and vibration, abnormalities of air pressure, radiation, and electricity all pose threats to human health.

Biological agents include bacteria, viruses, fungi, protozoa, and rickettsia. Disease caused by these organisms maybe regarded as occupational in origin when the nature of the work involves exposure to the organism. Since quite a few diseases are spread via blood (e.g., AIDS, hepatitis B, hepatitis C), it is beginning to be recognized as a toxic substance. The occurrence of occupationally acquired blood-borne infection depends on the frequency and types of hazardous exposures, the risk associated with each type of discrete exposure and the prevalence of infection in the patient population.

Mechanical and ergonomic agents cause soft-tissue injuries such as tenosynovitis and bursitis. They can also cause hand-arm vibration syndrome (Raynaud's phenomenon) and carpal tunnel syndrome. Many of these conditions are the result of repetitive movements or poorly designed physical working environments, and can be prevented or alleviated by change of job or change in the way tasks are performed, or by medication.

Psychosocial agents, like mechanical and ergonomic agents, are becoming increasingly recognized as contributing to health-related problems in the workplace. Stress may be attributed to workload, responsibility, or fear of job loss, or to geographical isolation or shiftwork. However, regardless of whether stress causes compensable illness, it clearly incurs high indirect costs in the form of absenteeism, poor productivity, and mental illness. Post-traumatic stress disorder is also a recognized condition that can be related to occupation.

Skin diseases comprise a major portion of compensated occupational disease. Occupational skin disease may be categorized into contact dermatitis, occupational acne, pigmentation disorders, and neoplastic disorders.

5. REFERENCES

1.   Statistics Canada, Household Division. The Labour Force, Catalogue no. 71-001-XPB. Ottawa: Ministry of Industry, 1996.
2.   Statistics Canada, Labour Division. Work Injuries, 1992-1994, Catalogue no. 72-208. Ottawa: Ministry of Industry, 1995.
3.   Ministry of Labour. Occupational Injuries and Their Cost in Canada 1990-1994. Ottawa: Statistics and Analysis Unit, Legislation Development and Liaison, Occupational Health and Safety Branch, 1995.
4.   Statistics Canada, Household Surveys Division. Historical Labour Force Statistics, Catalogue no. 71-201. Ottawa: Ministry of Industry, 1996.
5.   Markham JW, Kirkbride J, Pelmear P. Health Surveillance Data. Occupational Health in Ontario 1986;7(4):192-204.
6.   Ross JB. Prevention of Occupational Disease: Problems of Data Collection for Adequate Surveillance. Canadian Medical Association Journal 1992;147(10):1443-1445.
7.   Spiegel S, Yassi A. Occupational Disease Surveillance in Canada: A Framework for Considering Options and Opportunities. Canadian Journal of Public Health 1991;82:294-299.
8.   American Conference of Governmental Industrial Hygienists. Threshold Limit Values and Biological Exposure Indices for 1996-1997 Cincinnati: American Conference of Governmental Industrial Hygienists, 1997.
9.   Derouche F. Promoting Health in the Workplace. Ontario Prevention Clearinghouse News 1992;3(4):1-2.
10.   Erfurt J, Foote A, Mex A, Heirich M, Gregg W. Improving Participation in Worksite Wellness Programs: Comparing Health Education Classes, a Menu Approach, and

Follow-Up Counselling. American Journal of Health Promotion 1990;4(4):270-278.

11. Health Promotion and Programs Branch. Corporate Model of Workplace Health System. Ottawa: Health Canada, Ministry of Supply and Services, 1996.

12. Canadian Medical Association Policy Summary. Drug Testing in the Workplace. Canadian Medical Association Journal 1992; 146(12):223A-B.

13. Canadian Medical Association Policy Summary. The Physician's Role in Helping Patients Return to Work After an Illness or Injury. Canadian Medical Association Journal 1997; 156(5):680A-C.

14. LaDou J. Occupational Medicine (2nd ed.). Norwalk; Appleton & Lange, 1996.

15. Brooks S. Environmental Medicine. St. Louis: Mosby, 1995.

16. Rosenstock L, Cullen M. Textbook of Clinical Occupational and Environmental Medicine. Philadelphia: W.B. Saunders Company, 1994.

17. Video Display Terminals (Policy Statement). Canadian Medical Association Journal 1986; 135(6):688A.

18. Louie M, Low DE, Feinman SV, McLaughin B, Simor AE. Prevalence of Bloodborne Infective Agents among People Admitted to a Canadian Hospital. Canadian Medical Association Journal 1992;146(8):1331-1334.

19. Liss G. Estimated of the Burden of Illness Due to Occupational Exposure to Bloodborne Infections. Ottawa: Health Studies Service, Ministry of Labour, 1990.

20. Wallace E. Update: National Surveillance of Occupational Exposure to the Human Immunodeficiency Virus (HIV) April 15, 1992. Public Health and Epidemiology Reports Ontario 1992;3(13):210.

21. Update: Universal Precautions for the Prevention of Human Immunodeficiency Virus, Hepatitis B Virus, and Other Blood-Borne Pathogens in Health Care Settings. Canadian Disease Weekly Report 1988;14(27):117-123.

22. Federal Centre for AIDS. National Surveillance of Occupational Exposure to the Human Immunodeficiency Virus. Ottawa: Federal Centre for AIDS, 1992.

23. McQueen M. Conflicting Rights of Patients and Health Care Workers Exposed to Blood-borne Infection. Canadian Medical Association Journal 1992;147(3):299-302.

24. Update: Transmission of HIV Infection During Invasive Dental Procedures. Canadian Medical Association Journal 1992;146(4):519-521.

25. Ministry of Supply and Services. Canadian Immunization Guide (3rd ed.). Ottawa: Health and Welfare Canada, 1989.

26. Ministry of Health Ontario. Ontario Hospital Association and Ontario Medical Association Communicable Disease Protocols. Public Health and Epidemiology Reports Ontario 1992;3(12):187.

Chapter

11

Periodic Health Examinations

Since the release of Lalonde's *A New Perspective on Health of Canadians* (1), there has been increased emphasis on disease prevention and health promotion through various strategies such as health education, taxation, regulations, and modification of lifestyles. Physicians have focused their activities on early detection of diseases and early interventions. In this chapter, major clinical activities, specifically the periodic health examination, are discussed.

The annual check-up is an attempt to integrate preventive activities into clinical practice. The presumed reasons for annual examinations include prevention of specific diseases by risk-factor identification and intervention, early identification and treatment of disease, establishment of a baseline examination, and development of the patient-doctor relationship. However, effectiveness was never fully established. The practice of the annual examination has never been fully examined, yet it could be criticized on many grounds, such as its ritualistic nature, content and frequency, low yield, irrelevance to the needs of different age groups, and the inclusion of tests and procedures with scanty evidence of effectiveness or efficacy. It was in this context that the Canadian Task Force on the Periodic Health Examination was established by the Conference of Deputy Ministers of Health in 1976.

1. CANADIAN TASK FORCE ON PERIODIC HEALTH EXAMINATION

The terms of reference for which the Task Force (2) worked were relatively straight-forward:

- To identify the main killing or disabling conditions, unhealthy states, and unhealthy behaviours that affect Canadians and to determine which could possibly be prevented according to current knowledge.

- To consider evidence for the benefit of early detection or prevention of killing or disabling conditions, unhealthy states, and unhealthy behaviours in the non-complaining individual. (If early detection or prevention was judged to be beneficial, the particular condition was termed preventable.)
- To define groups at high risk for specific preventable conditions, states, and behaviours.
- To design health protection "packages" shown to be effective — or, in special circumstances, desirable on other grounds — that should become part of periodic health examinations at defined ages and for defined population groups.
- To make recommendations on the procedures, content, frequency, and appropriate providers of periodic health examinations and preventive interventions at defined ages and for defined population groups.
- To propose specific measures for evaluating the effectiveness and efficiency of the recommended plan for periodic health examinations that would permit recurring reassessment and improvement.

The Task Force concluded that it would be better to identify preventable conditions of importance to each age group, and to assess the detection manoeuvres and preventive interventions related to each condition. Its main recommendation is therefore that the routine annual check-up be abandoned in favour of a selective approach that is determined by a person's age and sex. The Task Force recommends a specific strategy comprising a lifetime health care plan based on a set of age- and sex-related health protection packages. This is an innovative approach, and other countries have since adopted similar approaches. For example, the recent publication by the U.S. Preventive Services Task Force called *The Guide to Clinical Preventive Services* assesses the effectiveness of 169 interventions in clinical practice (3). Another impressive aspect of the Task Force was its recognition that new scientific information is constantly emerging and could result in the Task Force altering its recommendations or including new conditions in health protection packages.

The Task Force received many submissions and held several discussions with different groups. Based on these, the Task Force has made recommendations over the past 20 years and published a compendium of all the topics and recommendations in *The Canadian Guide to Clinical Preventive Health Care* (4). As new information becomes available, the updates made by the Task Force are added to its recommendations, which are published in the *Canadian Medical Association Journal* and on the Internet (see the Appendix B).

2.   DEFINITIONS

The Task Force used the following key words and terms.

Beneficial Manoeuvre. An intervention or manoeuvre is considered beneficial when more good than harm accrues to the individual or to the groups of individuals to whom it is applied.

Early Detection. Early detection of a condition or a disorder refers to its identification in an individual before symptoms and signs make the condition apparent to the affected individual, the immediate family, or a non-professional observer. Early detection is also referred to as pre-symptomatic detection.

Effectiveness. Effectiveness is the attribute of an intervention or manoeuvre that results in more good than harm to those to whom it is offered. Effectiveness is determined by both the efficacy of the intervention and actual compliance.

Efficacy. Efficacy is the attribute of an intervention or clinical procedure that results in more good than harm to those who accept and comply with the intervention and subsequent treatment.

Efficiency. Efficiency is the attribute of an effective intervention or manoeuvre when it is made available to those who can benefit from it with optimal use of the resources required.

Groups at High Risk for Preventable Conditions, States, and Behaviour. These are groups in which the frequency of preventable conditions, states, or behaviour is demonstrably higher than in the general Canadian population. It may be justified to institute detection manoeuvres for these groups that are not judged necessary or feasible for the general population.

Health Protection Packages. These are sets of procedures that particularly apply to the periodic health examination at certain ages and in certain at-risk groups.

Periodic Health Examination. This is a group of tasks designed either to determine the risk of subsequent disease or to identify disease in its early, symptomless stage. Simple interventions are covered by this definition, such as injections for immunization, application of laboratory tests for early detection, administration of screening instruments, and counselling. The periodic health examination is applied to the patient who is asymptomatic for the preventable condition.

Preventable Condition, State, or Behaviour. This is a condition that has been demonstrated by well-designed clinical investigations to be either completely preventable or detectable at a stage when its progress or the impact of its consequences can be favourably affected by treatment.

Preventive Intervention. This is any intervention that reduces the likelihood of a disease or disorder affecting a person (primary prevention), that interrupts or slows the progress of a disease or the irreversible damage from a disease through early detection and treatment (secondary prevention), or that slows the progress of the disease and reduces resultant disability through treatment of established disease (tertiary prevention).

The criteria used to assess potentially preventable conditions and classify recommendations for their inclusion or exclusion were the current burden of suffering (impact on the individual and on society), the manoeuvre (risks and benefits; sensitivity, specificity, and predictive values; and safety, simplicity, cost, and acceptability), and the effectiveness of the intervention.

2.1. EFFECTIVENESS OF INTERVENTION

The effectiveness of intervention was graded according to the quality of evidence obtained, as follows:

I-1:   Evidence obtained from at least one properly randomized controlled trial.

II-1: Evidence obtained from well-designed controlled trials without randomization.

II-2: Evidence obtained from well-designed cohort or case-control analytic studies, preferably from more than one centre or research group.

II-3: Evidence obtained from comparisons between times or places with or without the interventions. Dramatic results from uncontrolled experiments (such as the results of the introduction of penicillin in the 1940s) could also be regarded as this type of evidence.

III: Opinions of respected authorities, based on clinical experience, descriptive studies or reports of expert committees.

2.2. CLASSIFICATION OF RECOMMENDATIONS

On the basis of these considerations, the Task Force made a clear recommendation for each condition as to whether it should be specifically included in a periodic health examination. Recommendations were classified as follows:

A: There is good evidence to support the recommendation that the condition be specifically considered in a periodic health examination.

B: There is fair evidence to support the recommendation that the condition be specifically considered in a periodic health examination.

C: There is poor evidence regarding the inclusion of the condition in a periodic health examination, but recommendations may be made on other grounds.

D: There is fair evidence to support the recommendation that the condition be excluded from consideration in a periodic health examination.

E: There is good evidence to support the recommendation that the condition be excluded from consideration in a periodic health examination.

Because the effectiveness of treatment or of the preventive measure for a condition was of such importance to the Task Force, the final recommendation for each condition relied heavily on an assessment of the evidence. Thus a class A recommendation was rarely made in the absence of grade I evidence regarding effectiveness of treatment or prevention. However, there is one exception to this rule: when a clinical intervention was shown, in grade II terms, to save the lives of victims of a previously universally fatal condition. For example, if malignant hypertension is left untreated, all affected patients will die; if treated, most will survive. Thus grade II evidence is sufficient for a class A recommendation. Such examples are rare, however, and grade I evidence was required for the highest recommendation for most conditions.

3.   HEALTH PROTECTION PACKAGES

Appendix A at the end of the book contains health protection packages that are up to date as of April 1998, for various age groups, and for both sexes. In some instances, the recommendation is intended only for a designated high-risk group.

4.   COMPLIANCE

A number of studies of compliance with the Canadian Task Force on the Periodic Health Examination have been undertaken (5-7). For example, one recent study concluded that most (90%) primary care physicians complied with the recommendations of the Task Force for breast examination, mammography, cervical smears, and initial counselling against smoking (8). Most of the physicians who participated in the study stated that they perform preventive manoeuvres in the context of an annual general physical examination rather than integrating them into routine patient care.

5.   SUMMARY

Since 1974, increased emphasis has been placed on disease prevention and health promotion through various strategies. These strategies include health education, modification of lifestyle, and early detection and intervention by physicians.

This chapter discussed the periodic health examination and the Canadian Task Force on the Periodic Health Examination. The Task Force was established in 1976 to assess the effectiveness of the annual check-up, which has been criticized on several grounds. Some of the terms of reference for the Task Force included the design of effective health protection packages, the definition of groups in the population at high risk for specific preventable conditions, and the consideration of the benefits of early detection. The Task Force concluded that it would be more efficient to identify preventable conditions of importance to each age group and the appropriate intervention for these conditions. Hence, it recommended that routine annual check-ups be abandoned in favour of a selective approach determined by a person's age and sex. The Task Force also recognized that since there is constantly new scientific information that may alter its recommendations, new conditions to the health protection packages may have to be added.

Some of the terms used by the Task Force were defined, in particular early detection, efficacy, efficiency, periodic health examination, and preventive intervention.

Methods for grading the effectiveness of an intervention and for classifying the Task Force's recommendations were also established.

The Task Force created health promotion packages for various age groups and for both sexes are outlined in Appendix A. Recent studies have demonstrated that most primary care physicians are complying with some of the recommendations most of the time.

6. REFERENCES

1. Lalonde M. A New Perspective on the Health of Canadians. Ottawa: Ministry of Supply and Services, 1975.

2. The Canadian Task Force on Periodic Health Examination: The Periodic Health Examination. Canadian Medical Association Journal 1979;121(99):1193-1254.

3. Report of the U.S. Preventive Services Task Force. Guide to Clinical Preventive Services (2nd ed.). Baltimore: Williams & Wilkins, 1995.

4. Canadian Task Force on the Periodic Health Examination. The Canadian Guide to Clinical Preventive Health Care. Ottawa: Health Canada, Canada Communication Group Publishing, 1994.

5. Battista RN. Adult Cancer Prevention in Primary Care. Canadian Medical Association Journal 1983;73(1036-1039).

6. Battista RN, Palmer CS, Marchand BM, et al. Patterns of Preventive Practices in New Brunswick. Canadian Medical Association Journal 1985;132:1013-1015.

7. Battista RN. Practice Guidelines for Preventive Care: The Canadian Experience. Canadian Task Force on the Periodic Health Examination. Canadian Medical Association Journal 1993;149(12):1795-1800.

8. Smith HE, Herbert CP. Preventive Practice among Primary Care Physicians in British Columbia: Relation to Recommendations of the Canadian Task Force on the Periodic Health Examination [see comments]. Canadian Medical Association Journal 1994;150(6):871-879.

Part Three

Canada's Health Care System

Chapter

12

Evolution of National Health Insurance

The choices each country makes with respect to health policy reflect the extent to which it is a just and caring society (1). Accordingly, political leaders and health ministries of every country are faced with a series of decisions about how best to meet the health care needs of their population. Conceptually, the organization of health care systems can be divided into how health services are *delivered* to those in need, and how payment for the provision of these services are *financed*. Decisions about the delivery and financing of care focus on whether the public sector or the private sector is predominantly responsible for each function and in what combination.

At a secondary level, the decision about the public-private distinction is repeated for each specific health sub-sector (e.g., acute care, chronic/long-term care, pharmaceuticals, mental health). "Public" can refer to the national (federal), provincial (state), regional or local level (2). "Private" may refer to corporate for-profit entities, small businesses, individual and their families, or charitable not-for-profit entities, which in turn may rely on a mixture of volunteers and paid labour and act as mediating structures to carry out public objectives. In this context, there are three other items that must be understood: financing, i.e., how services are paid; delivery, i.e., how services are provided to recipients of care; and allocation, i.e., how resources flow from those who finance care to those who deliver it.

It is this exact combination of varying delivery and financing models that makes each individuals health system unique. This chapter provides an overview of the organization of delivery and financing of the Canadian medicare system, reviews its historical evolution, and, finally, compares it with the configurations and current reforms in several other industrialized nations.

The contemporary Canadian health care system is unique among all industrialized nations because it combines a system of private service delivery (where health providers are self-employed rather than employees of the state) with publicly financed care through a single-source provincial government payer. Additionally, due to the way federal-provincial responsibilities were divided at the time of Confederation, Canada does not have a single health system, but rather ten provincial and two territorial health systems with uniform federal guidelines. To understand these uniquely Canadian features, and how they evolved from a free enterprise system of medicine, we must examine the historical development of health care in Canada (3, 4). While reading this chapter, readers are advised to keep in mind that the current legal foundation of Canada's health system is based on three statutes: the *Constitution Act, 1982*, which deals primarily with the jurisdictional power between federal and provincial governments, the *Canada Health Act* (CHA), and *Canada Health and Social Transfer Act (CHST)* (see Table 12.1). The CHA outlines the national terms and conditions, whereas the *CHST Act* sets conditions for fiscal transfers from the federal government to provinces.

1.   HEALTH CARE PRIOR TO 1950

1.1. HEALTH AND THE BRITISH NORTH AMERICA ACT

In 1867, Canada's Confederation was proclaimed in the *British North America Act* (*BNA Act,* now known as the *Constitution Act, 1982*), our most fundamental constitutional document. At that time, the government's role in the health care system was minimal. Most of the Canadian population had to rely on its own resources for medical care, and hospital services were provided only by charitable trusts and religious organizations. Naturally, those who drafted the *BNA Act* and the Fathers of Confederation could not predict the volume of industrial and technological growth, or the health care needs for the coming years. The only references to health matters in the *BNA Act* are found in section 91, which enumerates the power of the federal government, and section 92, which enumerates provincial powers:

> *Section 91* It shall be lawful for the Queen, by and with the Advice and Consent of the Senate and House of Commons, to make Laws for the Peace, Order, and good Government of Canada, in relation to all Matters not coming within the Classes of Subjects by this Act assigned exclusively to the Legislatures of the Provinces; and for greater Certainty, but not so as to restrict the Generality of the foregoing Terms of this Section, it is hereby declared that (notwithstanding anything in this Act) the exclusive Legislative Authority of the Parliament of Canada extends to all Matters coming within the Classes of Subjects next hereinafter enumerated; that is to say...
> *Sub-section 6* The Census and Statistics.
> *Sub-section 11* Quarantine and the Establishment and Maintenance of Marine Hospitals.

Table 12.1:   Historical Evolution of Federal Government Involvement in Personal Health Care

Year	Events
1867 Confederation	*British North American Act* (now *Constitution Act*, 1982); no involvement.
1935-1945	Proposed national health care and security legislation; legislation rejected by provinces.
1948	National Health Grants; beginnings of infrastructure for national health insurance.
1957	*Hospital Insurance and Diagnostic Services Act*; universal hospitalization for acute care.
1966	*Medical Care Act*; universal coverage for physicians' services.
1977	*Established Programs Financing Act* and Extended Health Care Services; revised financial arrangements and coverage for additional services.
1984	*Canada Health Act*; consolidation of previous three acts with some revisions.
1989	Devolution of financial contributions.
1996	*Canada Health and Social Transfer Act;* consolidation of finances under previous arrangement of *Established Programs Financing Act*, Canada Assistance Plan, and postsecondary education.

Section 92 In each Province the Legislature may exclusively make Laws in relation to Matters coming within the Classes of Subjects next hereinafter enumerated; that is to say...

Sub-section 7 The Establishment, Maintenance, and Management of Hospitals, Asylums, Charities, and Eleemosynary Institutions in and for the Province, other than Marine Hospitals.

The sections on the preceding page are quoted in detail because of the frequency of current discussions on the relative responsibilities of the federal and provincial governments in health care. Health is primarily a provincial responsibility, but the federal government also has specific responsibilities, which are described in the next chapter. With regard to health care for Aboriginal peoples, one of the early treaties mentioned a "medicine chest" to be provided by the federal government, a provision that has been supported by the courts over the years (5).

1.2. 1867 TO 1948

The origin of public medical care and hospital insurance can be traced to Saskatchewan, which became a province in 1905 when it was still emerging from the frontier stages of development. In 1914, the rural municipality of Sarnia, Saskatchewan, experimented with a form of medical care insurance by offering physicians a retainer to practise in the area. This plan guaranteed the physician certain remuneration and allowed for a practice on a fee-for-service basis. The experiment was so successful that, two years later, the provincial government passed the *Rural Municipality Act*. It permitted any rural municipality in Saskatchewan to levy property taxes to retain doctors who provided primary medical care and public health services in the area. This legislation encouraged doctors to settle in Saskatchewan. These sorts of publicly supported plans continued to operate for some years, numbering about 100 by 1946. Similar but less extensive plans were adopted by Manitoba in 1921 and by Alberta in 1926.

In 1916, Saskatchewan took one of the first steps to break down the tradition of municipal responsibility for hospital care by passing the *Union Hospital Act*, which permitted municipalities to merge into hospital districts for building and maintaining hospitals. In the following year, legislation gave municipalities the right to collect taxes to finance hospital care for their residents. By 1946, many local plans were operating in the province.

The first attempt to develop a national health insurance program was in 1935, when the federal government passed the *Employment and Social Insurance Act* to collect taxes in order to provide certain social security benefits, including health benefits. However, the provinces challenged this act, because it encroached on their jurisdiction. Their position was later upheld by the Supreme Court of Canada. After World War II, the world sought "reconstruction". This goal brought about certain promising changes that bettered the lives of people in some countries, particularly in the western world. The provision of social services — especially in the areas of health, education, and welfare — was influenced by this concept.

At the same time, it was extremely difficult for provincial governments and major Canadian hospitals to find adequate financial resources to provide health services.

Health costs were rising. There were technological advances and the union movement was influencing the hospital work force. Attempts by the federal government to deal with the problem failed because the issue became entangled with a jurisdictional dispute between the federal and provincial governments. Between 1942 and 1944, the Select Committee on Social Security of the House of Commons received reports on social security, the Report of the Advisory Committee on Health Insurance and a draft bill for comprehensive national health insurance. After considering these reports, the Select Committee produced a specific proposal for a broad program of social security, including health insurance on a cost-share and phased-introduction basis. It was presented to the provincial governments in 1945 at the Dominion-Provincial Conference on Post-War Reconstruction. This proposal was rejected because the provinces and federal government could not agree on the financial arrangements.

Saskatchewan decided to proceed on its own, and, in 1947, it introduced a hospitalization plan for all residents, financed by a combination of premiums and general taxes. Other provinces followed. British Columbia introduced its universal hospital insurance program in 1949, and Alberta initiated a limited plan in 1950. Newfoundland and Labrador joined Confederation in 1949 with their own health insurance plan.

2.   THE HEALTH CARE SYSTEM BETWEEN 1948 AND 1977

2.1. NATIONAL HEALTH GRANTS

A step towards the development of a national insurance program was the enactment of the *National Health Grants Act of 1948*. This act marked the entry of the federal government into the health field. Under it, grants-in-aid were provided to the provinces for a variety of public health services: hospital construction, laboratory services, and professional training for public health. These grants were viewed as "fundamental prerequisites of a nationwide system of health insurance". Later, other grants were added, but, except for Professional Training Grants and Public Health Research Grants, they were all gradually abolished after the introduction of Canadian medicare and the contemporary provincial health insurance programs.

Since provinces had jurisdiction over health, the role of the federal government was restricted to assistance in paying the bills. However, the federal government could steer the health care system by imposing conditions whenever it shared the cost of programs.

2.2. HOSPITAL INSURANCE AND DIAGNOSTIC SERVICES ACT OF 1957

There have been a number of federal acts passed since 1950; one of the first was the *Hospital Insurance and Diagnostic Services Act* (HIDS), passed by Parliament in 1957 and enacted in 1958. The *HIDS Act* provided for federal cost sharing of all services delivered in hospital (except for those provided by physicians) for those provinces with a universal hospital insurance plan. Five provinces immediately agreed to the terms of the act. By 1961, it was operating in all provinces and territories and covered 99% of the population of Canada. Its main purposes were to establish and maintain services and facilities that would lead to better health and health care for the population as a whole by providing, as its name implies, hospital care and diagnostic services. Although all residents of Canada were eligible for hospital insurance coverage, the federal law excluded services for those already eligible for similar benefits under other federal or provincial legislation such as workers covered by workers' compensation legislation or veterans covered by the *Pensions Act.*

A basic principle that influenced the development of hospital insurance legislation was the belief that existing traditions should be maintained as far as possible. Therefore, the pattern of hospital care and ownership that existed before 1957 was retained, and provincial autonomy in health care was not infringed. The policy of provincial autonomy allowed each province to decide on its own administrative methods, while ensuring a basic uniformity of coverage throughout the country.

2.2.1. Terms and Conditions

HIDS stipulated that the following must be insured services provided to inpatients:

- Accommodation and meals at the standard or public ward level;
- Necessary nursing service;
- Laboratory, radiology, and other diagnostic procedures;
- Drugs, biologicals, and related preparations;
- Use of operating room, case room, and anaesthetic facilities, including necessary equipment and supplies;
- Routine surgical supplies;
- Use of radiotherapy facilities, where available;
- Use of physiotherapy facilities, where available;
- Such other services as specified in the agreement.

At the option of each province, any of the above could also be provided as insured outpatient services. A fairly comprehensive range is now provided by hospitals in all provinces. Provinces may include additional benefits in their plans without affecting the federal-provincial agreements. The act also made hospital insurance portable for residents who temporarily left their home province, although coverage was subject to provincially regulated limits. In many cases, elective hospitalization outside the province required prior approval, which could be withheld in some provinces if equivalent services were available.

2.2.2. Methods of Financing

The federal contribution paid to the provinces for insured services amounted to approximately 50% of the costs of those services. Shared costs under the agreements with the provinces excluded most hospital construction costs and could also include the cost of movable equipment and most fixed equipment specifically required by hospitals. Each province determined how its share of the costs would be financed; most financed their share out of general revenue, but some provinces also imposed premiums or certain authorized charges.

HIDS was replaced by the *Canada Health Act* in 1984, which has similar provisions.

2.3. MEDICAL CARE ACT OF 1966

2.3.1. Events Leading to the Medical Care Act of 1966

Hospital insurance paved the way for medical care insurance. Saskatchewan once again was the first province to experiment with a compulsory, government-sponsored medical care insurance program. The program's principles were prepayment, universal coverage, and acceptability both to providers and receivers of services. The legislation received royal assent in November 1961, and, despite a strike by physicians, the program was implemented on July 1, 1962. British Columbia, Alberta, and Ontario adopted their own medical insurance programs between 1963 and 1966.

In 1965, the federal government's Royal Commission on Health Services (appointed in 1960, with the Honourable Emmett M. Hall, Justice of the Supreme Court of Canada, as chair) completed the most comprehensive assessment of health services undertaken to that date. It found that nearly 60% of Canadians had some form of insurance against the costs of medical care, but for approximately 30% of those insured, this coverage was inadequate. The Commission recommended strong federal government leadership and financial support for medical care. However, it also recommended that the operating controls of the program be decentralized under the provincial governments. General standards and guidelines were suggested as part of the federal government's conditions, but the Commission recommended that each province should be permitted wide latitude in its program. Closely related were recommendations for greatly expanded support for teaching, research, and other facilities for training health care personnel. In the summer of 1965, a new federal proposal based on the recommendations of the Hall Commission was introduced at a federal-provincial conference.

2.3.2. Enactment of the Medical Care Act of 1966

After a series of discussions between the federal and provincial governments, the *Medical Care Act* of 1966 was enacted and implemented in 1968. By 1971, all provinces had set up programs that complied with the act. Under the *Medical Care Act*, each province received a federal government contribution equal to half of the average per capita medical care costs incurred by all provinces, multiplied by the number of insured people in that province. As the average cost in poorer provinces was lower than in richer provinces, these cost-sharing arrangements gave larger proportion of payments to the poorer provinces. Hence, the federal contribution as a proportion of the total cost for medical care varied among provinces. In 1975/76, the proportion ranged from 40.8% in British Columbia and 49.2% in Ontario, to 67.7% in Prince Edward Island and 75.6% in Newfoundland. Under the act, all physicians' services and some additional services provided by dentists and chiropractors were covered. To be eligible for federal contributions, the provincial medical services plan was required to meet criteria that is very similar to HIDS, and were called the "Four Points": medical insurance must be comprehensive, universal, portable, and publicly administered.

2.3.3. Terms and Conditions
Comprehensive Coverage
At a minimum, the plan was to provide coverage for all services rendered by medical practitioners, without dollar limit or exclusions, provided there was medical need, unless coverage was available under other legislation. The plan was to be administered so that no financial limitation prevented an insured person from receiving necessary medical care. Certain surgical-dental procedures by dental surgeons (when rendered in hospital) were included from the beginning, and other professional services were added as the federal government considered fit. Each province could provide additional insured benefits but without federal cost sharing.

Universality
The plan was to be uniformly available to all eligible residents (no fewer than 95% of the population must be covered). Each province determined whether its residents should be insured on a voluntary or compulsory basis. Provinces were allowed to charge premiums to the enrollees in the program. No discrimination according to previous health, race, age, or non-membership in a group was permitted, but partial or complete premium subsidization for low-income groups or the elderly was allowed, if all qualifying residents were treated equally. Similarly, utilization charges at the time of service were not precluded by the federal legislation if they did not impede, either by their amount or by the way they were applied, reasonable access to necessary medical care, particularly for low-income groups.

Portability
Under the *Medical Care Act,* benefits were portable when the insured person was temporarily absent from the province, whether travelling anywhere in the world or changing jobs, retiring or moving from one province to another, provided the individual remained enrolled in the program and paid premiums in those provinces where premiums were charged. When an insured resident moved to another province, the province of origin would provide medical care benefits during any waiting period imposed by the medical insurance plan of the destinations. No province could impose a waiting period

longer than three months before a new resident was entitled to obtain coverage. Some provinces required that people obtain approval before having elective (i.e., non-emergency) care outside their province. In general, provinces limited the amount payable for medical services received out of province to the amount payable for similar services in the person's province.

Public Administration

The plan was non-profit and administered by a public agency accountable to the provincial government for its financial transactions.

The above criteria gave each province substantial flexibility in determining the administrative arrangements for the operation of its medical care insurance plan and in choosing its financing plan (through premiums, sales tax, or other provincial revenues, or a combination thereof). Federal contributions to the provinces under this program totalled $1.7 billion by the fiscal year 1975/76.

Like HIDS, this act was replaced by the *Canada Health Act* in 1984, which has similar provisions.

3.   1977-1984: NEW FINANCING OF HEALTH CARE PROGRAMS AND THE CANADA HEALTH ACT

By the 1970s, the shared-cost health programs had become a critical problem for both the federal and provincial governments. The chief bone of contention between the two levels of government was increasing health care costs as the cost was transferred from the private sector to public sector. In 1976, total health expenditures in Canada exceeded $13 billion. Because these programs were "open-ended" (i.e., the federal government paid the provinces about half of the cost for insured hospital and medical care costs), they impeded federal governmental program planning in other fields. The provincial governments were also dissatisfied because, while the most expensive costs of health care were shared, other important and innovative aspects (e.g., development of community-based services instead of general hospital care) were not shared. To alleviate this, a new agreement on financing arrangements was reached at the Conference of First Ministers in December 1976. The legislation was enacted on March 31, 1977, as the *Federal-Provincial Fiscal Arrangements and Established Programs Financing Act* (*EPF Act*), 1977, and included extended health care services.

3.1.   ESTABLISHED PROGRAMS FINANCING ACT, 1977

3.1.1. Description of Financing Arrangements

Commencing April 1, 1977, federal contributions to the provinces for the established programs of hospital insurance, medical care and postsecondary education were no longer directly related to provincial costs. Rather, the new arrangements made room within the tax-point system for the provinces to increase their tax revenue without necessarily increasing the burden on the taxpayer, and allowed for associated equalization and cash payments.

In general terms, the total federal contributions for the above three programs were now based on the current value of the 1975/76 federal contributions for these programs. The tax room vacated by the federal government consisted of a reduction in the federal tax schedule of 13.5 personal and 1.0 corporate income tax points. An equalization payment was available to all provinces to raise the value of the tax points to the national average. At that time, it was believed that the yield from the new provincial taxes would increase faster than the rate of growth of the gross national product (GNP). The yearly cash payments to the provinces had approximately the same value as the tax room transferred. The formula for the cash payments is complex, and interested readers may consult the original act.

These financing arrangements initially provided each province with more money than it might have received with the previous cost-sharing formula, but the increase was tied to the GNP and population growth. There was greater equality among the provinces in what they received from the federal government per capita, and they had greater flexibility in the use of their own funds and federal contributions. The arrangements were more stable for both levels of government. Program administration was simplified because federal auditing of provincial records was no longer required. The terms of the program's financing arrangements were to be indefinite, but a provision in the legislation permitted the federal government to terminate the arrangements with three years' notice.

The federal government had attached broad conditions to its cash payments in order to guarantee adequate standards of health care across the country. The conditions were the same as those used for hospital and medical care insurance since the beginning: comprehensiveness, universal coverage, portability of benefits and nonprofit administration by a public agency.

This act was replaced by the *Canada Health and Social Transfer Act* in 1996, which has similar provisions.

3.1.2. Extended Health Care Services

Under the *EPF Act,* a financial contribution was made by the federal government for extended health care services. Payments began on April 1, 1977. The Extended Health Care Services Program allowed the federal government to make block-funded contributions (one payment to cover all services) to the provinces to assist them in providing the following:

- Nursing homes (intermediate care);
- Adult residential care;
- Converted mental hospitals;
- Health-related aspects of home care;
- Ambulatory health care.

This program had three purposes:

- To provide the provinces with financial assistance for providing less costly forms of health care in conjunction with the insured services of the *Hospital Insurance and Diagnostic Services Act* and the *Medical Care Act*;
- To encompass most of health and institutional health services within a similar block-funding financial arrangement;
- To provide the provinces with greater flexibility.

Funding for 1988/89 was approximately $48 per capita ($1.27 billion), with the same terms as those of the EPF (i.e., based on the growth of GNP and the population). Since this program was viewed as complementary to basic hospital and medical care insurance, the only condition of payment was that the province furnish the federal minister of health with information required by the federal government for its international obligations, national planning and standards, and information exchanges with the provinces.

This arrangement was replaced by the *Canada Health and Social Transfer Act* in 1996, which has similar provisions.

3.2. EVENTS LEADING TO THE CANADA HEALTH ACT

The EPF no longer tied federal payments to particular forms of health services, which reduced the federal steering effect. During the late 1970s, health care costs increased faster than the GNP, leading the provinces to bear greater costs. As a result, the provinces introduced measures of cost containment such as restraints on raising physicians' fees. An increasing number of physicians responded to this by "extra-billing" their patients (6) that is, billing patients above the fee schedules which were negotiated with their provincial health insurance plans. These factors led to charges from the public and interest groups that medicare was being "eroded". The federal government established another commission to review the Canadian health care system led again by the Honourable Emmett M. Hall, who had reviewed the health care system in 1964.

In 1980, Mr. Justice Hall published the results of this review (7). This health services review emphasized the issue of accessibility of services. Hall concluded that extra-billing was threatening to violate the principle of uniform terms and conditions and would prevent access to services for some people. He therefore recommended that this practice be banned and that fair compensation for physicians' services be determined through negotiation between physicians and governments, with binding arbitration if negotiations failed. Those physicians unwilling to accept the plan as payment in full would be required to practise entirely outside the plan, as was already the case in Quebec. They would bill their patients directly, and patients would be responsible for the full cost of the service.

In 1981, the Parliamentary Task Force on Federal-Provincial Fiscal Arrangements, an all-party task force of Members of Parliament, published a review of the EPF, entitled *Fiscal Federalism in Canada* (8), This report included a review of the problems in delivering health care and fulfilling various program conditions outlined in the original hospital and medical care insurance acts. As well, it addressed the question of whether health care in Canada was underfunded and recommended, as had Mr. Justice Hall, that a national health council be formed that would be independent of government and of health care providers; this council would act as a coordinating body for defining, planning, and implementing health policy for Canada. Such a council could monitor whether the conditions of the various health care programs were being met.

3.2.1. Enactment of the Canada Health Act, 1984

Following these two major reports, the federal government introduced proposals for a new *Canada Health Act* in May 1982, which was enacted in April 1984 with support from all political parties.

3.2.2. Terms and Conditions of the Canada Health Act

The following are the major features of the *Canada Health Act* (CHA):

1. The CHA replaced two existing acts, the *Hospital Insurance and Diagnostic Services Act* and the *Medical Care Act*.
2. The CHA maintained the program criteria and conditions of payment to the provinces of the cash portions of the federal contributions for insured health services for extended health care services.
3. The CHA covers the following insured health services: necessary hospital services, medically necessary services by physician, and surgical-dental services performed in a hospital. These are almost identical to those in the previous acts.
4. The CHA covers the following extended health care services: nursing home intermediate care, adult residential care, home care, and ambulatory health care as defined in the previous act.
5. To be eligible for the full cash portion of the contribution, a provincial health care program must meet the following criteria:
   a) *Public Administration.* The program must be administered by a public authority accountable to the provincial government.
   b) *Comprehensiveness.* The program must cover all necessary hospital and medical services, and surgical-dental services rendered in hospitals.
   c) *Universality.* One hundred per cent of the eligible residents must be entitled to insured health services.
   d) *Portability* The waiting period for new residents must not exceed three months. Emergency insured health services must be made available to Canadians temporarily out of their own province at no extra charge to them. The home province must pay for out-of-province services at the host province rates and must pay for out-of-country services at the home province rates.
   e) *Accessibility.* Reasonable access to insured health services must not be obstructed, either directly or indirectly, by charges or other mechanisms. Extra-billing and user charges are not permitted except as outlined in the regulations attached to the CHA.
6. The CHA stipulates that physicians and dentists must receive reasonable compensation. Adequate payments must be made to hospitals in respect of insured health

services. Provinces may designate non-physicians' as "health care practitioners".

7. The CHA also stipulates that to be eligible for full cash portion of the federal contribution and payment, provinces must meet conditions of payment including the *Provision of Information* (reasonable information on the operation of the program supplied by the provinces to the federal Minister of Health), and *visibility* (federal contributions to the programs are to be given appropriate visibility).

If a provincial plan fails to satisfy any of the program criteria except for those related to extra-billing or user charges, or the province fails to comply with the conditions of payment, the cash portion of the federal contribution or payment may be reduced. This reduction is discretionary and requires consultation with the province. If a province fails to comply with the condition of payment relating to extra-billing and user charges, the act provides for a non-discretionary reduction of the cash portion by the amount charged through extra-billing or user charges. Because few provinces were allowing extra-billing or user charges, the act made certain provisions so that provinces can pass necessary legislation to ban these practices. Hence, for the first three years after proclamation, any funds withheld because of extra-billing or user charges were to be held in Public Accounts of Canada, and were to be paid to the province if the practices of extra-billing or user charges were eliminated during those three years. The act came into force on April 1, 1984.

4.   BEYOND THE CANADA HEALTH ACT

As indicated above, one of the conditions of the *Canada Health Act* was a partial withholding of funds from provinces that allowed extra-billing and hospital user charges. Ontario, Alberta, Manitoba, Saskatchewan, and New Brunswick allowed extra-billing. With the introduction of the *Canada Health Act*, these provincial governments had to enact legislation to ban extra-billing, or else they would lose revenue from the federal government. This, in turn, strained relations between the two levels of governments and also between provincial governments and their respective medical associations. For example, in 1986, when Ontario introduced legislation banning extra-billing, some physicians in that province went on strike. But by 1987, all provinces had banned extra-billing. The Canadian health care system was moving toward an increased federal role, especially in the areas of formulation, monitoring, and enforcing of program conditions.

4.1.   BILLS C-96, C-69, AND C-20

The federal government, however, has since been forced into a position of progressive withdrawal of transfer payments for health care and postsecondary education to the provinces as a result of budgetary deficit pressure and political squabbles related to jurisdictional disputes (9). These transfer payments, which were established under the EPF arrangements in 1977, are given to the provinces partly as tax credits and partly as cash. The total grant was to be revised annually according to changes in population and GNP. Subsequent to the *Canada Health Act*, the federal government stabilized its financial commitment by amending the funding formula in its favour. Bill C-96, introduced in 1986, reduced the annual per capita escalator to 2% below GNP growth. In 1991, Bill C-69, also known as the *Government Expenditures Restraint Act*, was proclaimed, further reducing the escalator. It also froze transfer payments for two years (1990/1991 and 1991/1992) and reduced further increases to 3% below GNP growth. Bill C-20, passed in 1991, extended the freeze to 1994/1995 and allowed the federal government to withhold any federal transfer payment for breach of the *Canada Health Act*. It was anticipated that the cash component of the transfer payments would be nonexistent by the year 2000.

The only way the federal government can control how the provinces implement the CHA criteria is by withholding cash. As federal cash payments are likely to diminish and disappear (as predicted) and provinces face increasing financial constraints, provincially implemented universal health insurance as presented by the *Canada Health Act* 1984 may be eroded.

5.   OTHER HEALTH PROGRAMS FINANCED BY THE GOVERNMENT

5.1. CANADA ASSISTANCE PLAN (1966)

Under the Canada Assistance Plan (CAP), the federal government paid 50% of the cost of cash assistance and health and welfare services to people in need. The program was administered by provincial governments, which were free to offer a wide range of health care benefits. The range of benefits varied from province to province, but could include such services as eyeglasses, prosthetic appliances, dental services, prescribed drugs, home care services, and nursing home care. The only eligibility requirement specified was that of need, determined through an assessment of budgetary requirements, client income, and resources. A province could not demand previous residence as a condition for initial or continued assistance. The eligibility requirements and rates of assistance were set by the provinces and adjusted to the local conditions and needs of special groups. The provinces had to establish appeal procedures for decisions relating to the provision of assistance.

The reduction of federal transfer payments in relation to health care also affected the CAP. Bill C-69 capped the growth of the payments at 5%. A reduction of the financing of social assistance in this manner would likely have adverse effects on the health of marginalized groups that depend on CAP payments for their daily needs.

CAP was replaced by the *Canada Health and Social Transfer Act* in 1996.

5.2. VOCATIONAL REHABILITATION OF DISABLED PERSONS (1952)

The Vocational Rehabilitation of Disabled Persons program has been administered by Health Canada since April 1, 1973. Under it, the federal government contributes 50% of the costs to all provinces (except Quebec) of providing a comprehensive range of services for the vocational rehabilitation of physically and mentally disabled people. Services include social and vocational assessment; counselling; training; maintenance allowances; the provision of tools, books, and other equipment; remedial and restorative treatments; and the provision of prosthetic and orthotic appliances, wheelchairs, and other mobility aids.

5.3. CANADA HEALTH AND SOCIAL TRANSFER ACT (1996)

In 1996, the *Canada Health and Social Transfer Act* (CHST) replaced federal transfers for social assistance under the CAP, and for health and postsecondary education under the EPF (described in section 5.1) (10). The CHST is a block fund designed to give provinces enhanced flexibility in designing and administering efficient health care and social programs while upholding basic principles of medicare and safeguarding social programs. The block grant supports health care, social programs and higher education. Unlike the EPF, the CHST does not delineate a "health" portion and a "postsecondary education" portion; the appropriate division of the federal transfer is entirely at provincial discretion.

The CHST consists of both a direct cash transfer from the federal government and federal tax concessions that allow provincial governments to raise additional revenues from taxes without increasing the overall tax burden on taxpayers. CHST entitlements were set at $26.9 billion for 1996/97 and $25.1 billion for 1997/98. The 1997/98 entitlement level continues for 1998/99 and 1999/2000. Thereafter, the entitlement level will grow at 2% less than the growth of the GDP (for 2000/2001) and 1% less than GDP (2002/03). There is a legislated cash limit to ensure that the cash component of CHST will total at least $12.5 billion in each of the five years covered by the arrangement. The CHST transfer is initially allocated to the provinces based on provincial shares under the former EPF and CAP programs.

6.   DESCRIPTION OF NATIONAL HEALTH INSURANCE PROGRAMS OF SELECTED COUNTRIES

The first sections of this chapter traced the evolution of Canada's medicare system from Confederation in 1867 to the present. What started with a minimal state role in a privately financed and mostly privately delivered system has evolved into a largely publicly funded system that has been referred to by many as Canada's public policy success story (1). The evolution of the Canadian health care system as it faces its many current challenges, however, is not yet over. Some of the main issues facing the system at present are described in Chapters 13 to 16 and are summarized in the final chapter of the book. In this section, the health care systems of several advanced industrialized nations are described to allow the reader to compare and contrast the Canadian health care system within an international context.

The 1990s have been a decade of the universal restructuring of health care systems, both in North America and abroad. Triggered largely by fiscal considerations and concerns about increases in health care costs, virtually every government in the industrialized world has sought to reform its health care system (11). In its review of recent health system reforms, the Organization for Economic Cooperation and Development (OECD) lists the following key goals of health care reform (12):

- Adequacy and equity in access to health services;
- Income protection;
- Macro-economic efficiency;
- Micro-economic efficiency;
- Appropriate provider autonomy;
- Freedom of choice for consumers.

Striking a balance among the needs of consumers, providers, payers, and governments has created the need for compromises. Each country (and province) has chosen to structure its compromises in its own unique way, reflecting the political, social, historical, and economic realities of its own culture. The following brief overview describes how several very different countries have sought a balance between equity and efficiency, between individual provider and consumer needs and societal needs, between public sector priorities and private sector priorities, and between national standards and local flexibility and responsiveness. Table 12.2 provides a comparison of health infrastructure and health outcome statistics for selected countries (11).

6.1. UNITED KINGDOM (A PUBLIC/PUBLIC MODEL)

The British National Health Service (NHS) has existed since 1948, when it was created as part of the United Kingdom's post-war restructuring. It was the first publicly funded and publicly owned health system to appear in western Europe. With 6.9% of GDP spent on health in 1995, the U.K. spends consistently less on health care than most of its European or North American neighbours.

6.1.1. Finance
The NHS is a universal system of national health insurance financed from general tax revenues. It provides comprehensive coverage not only of professional services, but also of hospitalization and other benefits such as drugs, dental care, eyeglasses, and hearing aids. Eligibility for medical benefits is universal based only on citizenship,

and care is provided free of charge at time of delivery. Because of concerns raised in the 1970s about waiting lists for elective surgery and other non-emergency care, the government allowed the development of a small private health insurance sector to cover these services. Approximately 10% of the population has private insurance. Prior to the 1989 reforms, hospitals were run by District Health Authorities (DHAs) and received global lump-sum budgets, set ultimately by the central government.

With NHS, people register with general practitioners (GPs), who provide primary care and referrals to specialists. Just over one third of all physicians are GPs who work as independent contractors to the NHS. Until recently, GPs were paid largely through capitation (a payment mechanism for paying physicians an agreed amount per person per year no matter how often people use the services) with some mixed reimbursement to encourage certain procedures (e.g., preventive exams and screenings). Hospital staff physicians (specialists) are salaried, but are allowed part-time private practice. They bill the private health insurance plans for the services of their private practice.

6.1.2. Delivery

Until recently, the system in the U.K. was almost entirely public delivery, with the National Health Service owning and operating most health facilities. Since the introduction of White Paper reforms in 1989, ownership of many hospitals has shifted from the public sector (i.e., state ownership) to independent, self-governing trusts. GPs remain independent contractors.

6.1.3. Health System Reforms

Although largely successful in keeping down macro-level costs, the U.K. health care system had been criticized for being overtly bureaucratic and unresponsive to patient needs — complaints frequently heard about public delivery systems. These shortcomings were addressed in the 1989 White Paper "Putting People First", which sought to introduce an element of managed competition into the delivery side of the U.K. health care system while maintaining the public financing role (13).

The reforms of the 1990s have separated the purchaser and provider functions of the NHS. The NHS allocates money for health services to 14 Regional Health Boards, which, in turn, disburse funds among the District Health Authorities in their region. There are roughly 15 DHAs per region, each served by four or five hospitals. The DHA becomes the purchasing agent for health services for its population, entering into service contracts with local self-governing hospital trusts. These contracts are awarded on a competitive basis based on service cost and quality. Large groups of GPs (serving 7,000 or more people) can also form fund-holding groups and purchase services from public and private hospitals. DHAs and GP fund-holders contract with the hospital trusts for the quantity and type of services to be provided and for the fees that the hospitals will be paid.

An announcement in January 1998 appears to sweep away the internal market and family practitioner fund-holding. One key point for new reform is the formation of some 500 primary care group teams of family practitioners (FPs) and community nurses who will take over the bulk of the NHS budget. Each team will provide care for approximately

Table 12.2: International Comparisons of Health System Inputs and Outputs: Part I

==COUNTRY	% GDP spent on health (1995)	Per capita health spending[a]	% Public sector spending[a]	Hospital beds per 1,000 population[b]	Hospital admission rate[b] (% of population)	Average length of stay[b] (days)	Physicians per 1,000 population[b]	Physician contacts per capita[b]
Australia	8.4	$1,571	68.5	8.9	23.0	10.0	2.2	10.6
New Zealand	7.5	$1,096	76.9	7.3	13.9	7.7	2.0	3.8
Canada	9.5	$1,819	71.8	6.0	14.1	12.6	2.2	6.9
U.S.	14.5	$3,516	44.3	4.4	13.7	8.8	2.5	5.9
Denmark	6.5	$1,867	83.0	5.0	21.1	7.6	2.8	4.8
Finland	8.2	$1,601	75.2	10.0	22.8	14.8	2.6	3.9
Norway	7.3	$2,074	94.5	14.5	16.7	9.1	3.3	3.8
Sweden	7.7	$1,732	83.4	7.0	19.9	9.4	3.0	2.9
France	9.9	$2,229	78.4	9.3	23.3	11.7	2.8	6.3
Germany	9.6	$2,388	73.5	9.7	21.1	16.1	3.2	12.8
The Netherlands	8.8	$1,921	77.6	11.3	10.9	33.3	2.5	5.7
United Kingdom	6.9	$1,211	84.1	5.1	19.3	10.2	1.5	5.8
Japan	7.2	$2,607	79.1	15.6	8.3	46.4	1.7	15.9
OECD average	8.6	$1,374	72.7	8.4	16.2	14.4	2.5	6.1

[a] 1992 OECD data

[b] 1991 OECD data

[c] 1989-90 OECD data

Source: Schieber GJ, Poullier JP, Greenwald LM (1994). Health System Performance in OECD Countries, 1980-1992. Health Affairs. 13(4):100-12, and OECD (1992) U.S. Health Care at the Crossroads, OECD, Paris.

Table 12.2: International Comparisons of Health System Inputs and Outputs: Part II

COUNTRY	1993 population (millions)	Infant mortality rate	Percent low birth weight	Life expectancy at birth		Life expectancy at age 60	
				males	females	males	females
Australia	17.7	6.1	6.3	75.0	80.9	19.5	23.7
New Zealand	3.5	6.8	5.9	73.1	78.9	18.6	22.6
Canada	28.7	7.3	5.5	74.9	81.2	19.6	24.3
U.S.	268.0	8.4	7.1	72.2	78.8	18.8	22.7
Denmark	5.2	5.4	5.3	72.3	77.6	17.6	21.4
Finland	5.1	4.4	4.0	72.1	79.5	17.6	22.2
Norway	4.3	5.1	4.4	74.2	80.2	18.4	22.9
Sweden	8.7	4.8	4.3	75.5	80.8	19.4	23.4
France	57.5	6.4	5.8	73.3	81.4	19.4	24.6
Germany	81.0	5.8	5.8	73.8	79.3	18.0	22.4
The Netherlands	15.3	6.3	4.9	74.0	80.0	17.7	22.5
United Kingdom	58.2	6.3	6.9	73.6	78.9	17.8	21.9
Japan	124.6	4.3	6.8	76.3	82.5	20.2	24.9
OECD average		7.2	5.4	72.9	79.2	18.0	22.3

• 1992 OECD data
• 1991 OECD data
• 1989-90 OECD data

Source: Schieber GJ, Poullier JP, Greenwald LM (1994). Health System Performance in OECD Countries, 1980-1992. *Health Affairs*. 13(4):100-12, and OECD (1992) U.S. *Health Care at the Crossroads*, OECD, Paris.

100,000 people. The team system will be implemented in April 1999, and all FPs will be required to join a team. Another key point is a 24-hour NHS nation-wide telephone service staffed by experienced nurses offering callers practical advice, to begin in 2000. It is aimed in particular at people who cannot contact or reach their FP or who cannot go to a hospital emergency room. Other significant aspects of the reform include a guaranteed reduction in waiting periods for cancer care, starting immediately; the establishment of the National Institute of Clinical Excellence to develop best practice guidelines based on evidence for all physicians and other health care professionals; and the appointment of the Commission for Health Improvement, to monitor how well the guidelines are being followed and act as a troubleshooter. These developments indicate the rapidity with which changes are occurring in the U.K. and the lack of evaluation of the changes being made.

6.2. UNITED STATES (A PRIVATE/PRIVATE MODEL)

At the other end of the public/private continuum from the United Kingdom's largely public sector health care system lies the United States. The U.S. health care system is a very fragmented, pluralistic system with health services provided by a loosely structured system organized at the local level. More recently, private insurance companies have set up vertically integrated networks of care for their subscribers. Although several publicly funded and delivered health care programs exist in the U.S., 55% of American health care is financed and delivered privately.

The U.S. spends more on health care than any other industrialized country in the world. In 1995, the U.S. spent 14.5% of its GDP, or $3,094 per capita on health (more than twice the per capita average of the countries surveyed by the OECD).

6.2.1. Finance
There are multiple methods of financing health services in the U.S. Key elements include the following:
- The private health insurance industry, which covers three quarters of the population (e.g., Blue Cross/Blue Shield, private insurance companies, corporate self-insurance, managed care plans);
- Two publicly funded government plans — Medicare and Medicaid. **Medicare** is a federally subsidized program for those over age 65, for some people with disabilities under age 65, and for people with chronic renal diseases. Benefits that are not generally transferable outside the U.S. medicare fall into two parts: part A, a hospital insurance program for the population mentioned above, and generally requiring contributions by participants for a minimal period of their working lives; and part B, an optional, social security arrangement for medical care insurance and covering part of the costs of services provided by medical practitioners and certain other benefits. **Medicaid** is a series of state programs with federal cost-sharing. Eligibility for medicaid benefits is based on income and means criteria,

and is determined by county welfare boards. Benefits cover inpatient and outpatient hospital services, laboratory and radiology, basic physician medical services, and skilled nursing facility coverage for people over age 21;

- Individual out-of-pocket payments; and
- A growing proportion of the population that is uninsured. It is currently estimated that 39 million people in the U.S. are uninsured or under-insured. Insurance coverage is largely employment-based and is entirely voluntary. Small employers generally cannot afford to offer their employees insurance coverage, and most part-time and contractual workers are not covered even by large companies.

Ambulatory care physicians in private practice are paid fee-for-service, usually by their patients who are subsequently reimbursed by their insurance plans. Physicians working in private practice can, and usually do, extra-bill above levels reimbursed by insurance companies. Those physicians working in managed care organizations, such as Health Maintenance Organizations (HMOs) or Preferred Provider Networks, are generally paid on a capitation or salary basis, but a wide assortment of plans and payment arrangements are possible. Most recently, there has been a rapid movement toward integrated delivery structures, and the managed care portion of the market has grown.

6.2.2. Delivery

In the U.S., the dominant system of health services delivery is private and usually for-profit. Public services are usually limited to providing care to special groups such as veterans, the mentally ill, or the poor. Some jurisdictions (cities or counties) operate public hospitals and community health centres as a social safety net, although many such institutions are now under fiscal pressure and are being downsized or closed.

6.2.3. Health System Reforms

There are two main concerns driving recent health reform efforts in the U.S. (12). The first, as in the majority of OECD countries, is a concern with rapidly growing health care expenditures. The difference between the U.S. and other OECD countries is not one of substance, but of degree. The second major trend, unique to the U.S., is the growing proportion of the American population that is entirely uninsured. For this reason, the *Health Security Act* of 1993 was proposed in the U.S. by President Bill Clinton (14). The Clinton Reform Plan would have included mandatory, universal health care coverage for all U.S. citizens and legal residents with public- private mix, but the plan was defeated by Congress. On August 21, 1996, President Clinton signed a law prohibiting insurance companies from denying coverage to any applicant based on pre-existing medical conditions. Although still a far cry from the original, more ambitious plan, the Clinton administration felt that this was the first step in an ongoing reform process.

In addition to the national reforms proposed by President Clinton and others, individual states have also undertaken significant reform efforts. Most notable among these efforts are the Oregon Plan and health reforms in California.

Briefly, the State of Oregon's reform efforts centred on extending medicaid coverage to a wider net of the state's poor, while at the same time limiting the number and type of services that would be covered. Service rationing was decided through a process of broad public consultation, and was based on the social value and perceived effectiveness assigned to each service. For a more detailed discussion of the Oregon Plan see Chapter 15.

6.3. FRANCE (A MIXED MODEL)

France is a comparatively big spender on health care (11, 15). With 9.9% of its GDP spent on health care in 1995, France spends more on health care than any other western European country. Its system is complex and pluralistic and charges more in the form of individual user fees than other European countries.

6.3.1. Finance
Health system finance in France is the responsibility of several entities and organizations, both public and private. In general, health services in France are paid for through open-ended, compulsory health insurance funds called the *Caisses nationales,* which operate within the national social security scheme. These insurance funds are financed by compulsory, income-related payroll taxes and provide almost universal (99% of the population) coverage. The payroll tax is split between employers, who contribute 12.6% of the employees' income to the *Caisse*, and employees, who contribute 6.8% of their income. The *Caisses* are semi-autonomous, non-governmental bodies responsible for administering the insurance scheme. Membership is based on occupation. There is one large fund called the Sickness Fund for Salaried Workers, covering the majority (80%) of all workers and their dependants, and pensioners. The remaining 20% of workers are covered by 15 smaller *Caisses* for self-employed workers, farmers, and special groups such as miners and transport workers.

In addition to the compulsory coverage provided by the *Caisses nationales*, 80% of the population purchases supplementary private insurance on a voluntary basis to "top up" the coverage provided through the universal system. Supplementary health insurance is provided by private insurance companies or by non-profit, charitable societies called *Mutuelles*. *Mutuelles* provide reimbursement for user charges (called *ticket moderateur)*, extra billing, and a few benefits not covered by the *Caisses*. They are financed through a voluntary payroll deduction of 2.5% of income. Supplementary private insurance is paid for through actuarial based, voluntary premiums.

Mutuelles also finance a system of safety-net care for the very poor in France or those with unstable employment. This comprises roughly 5% of the population.

The Ministry of Health provides funds from general taxes for community health services (e.g., immunizations) and for capital development of public hospitals.

Insurance companies offer payment in the form of reimbursement to patients for most ambulatory care, while paying most physicians directly for hospital care. The health insurance is comprehensive, including services rendered at home, at a doctor's office, or in a hospital. Included are home care, dental and nursing care, drugs and prostheses, and replacement income during illness. No disease is excluded. Cost sharing applies to most services provided by public programs, comprising approximately 17% of all health care expenditures in France. Of all the western European countries, only France requires such a high level of cost sharing by individuals for the health services they receive. As part of this cost-sharing scheme, there is a *ticket moderateur* levied for every service provided; this user fee is set at 25% of the negotiated fee for physician visits, at 30% for "necessary drugs", and at 60% for "comfort drugs". About 10% of insured people who are chronically ill or receiving long-term care do not have to pay the user fees for prescription drugs and those individuals with supplementary private insurance can be reimbursed.

6.3.2. Delivery

Health care services in France are provided through a mixed public and private delivery system. Seventy per cent of hospitals are public and 30% are private — some private, non-profit; others private, for-profit. Public hospitals in France are large, well equipped, and designed to offer comprehensive care including emergency and trauma care. Private hospitals, conversely, are usually much smaller and designed to provide specialist care such as obstetric services, elective surgery, or long-term care. Public hospitals are supported by global budgets set according to the workload of the hospital using a formula based on diagnostic-related groups (DRGs). Private hospitals, however, are paid on a per diem rate.

Physicians in private hospitals are considered private entrepreneurs, getting paid on a fee-for-service basis by their patients, and comprise about two-thirds of all hospital physicians. The remaining one third of physicians work in public hospitals or in private non-profit hospitals, are public employees who receive a salary, and are also allowed a private practice on a part-time basis outside their hospital practice. The majority (80%) of ambulatory physicians work in private practice. The remainder are employed by the health insurance scheme, by charitable societies, or by official authorities responsible for providing services to the poor. People can choose their primary care physician and public or private hospitals freely. There is no gatekeeper role for GPs.

6.3.3. Health System Reforms

The French have been tinkering with their system since the early 1980s in an effort to bring down health care costs while maintaining accessibility and equity. The 1980s had witnessed the introduction of physicians into the private sector, who had the right to extra-bill. This privatization of health is currently being reformed in order to:

- Freeze entry into the private sector except for specified sub-groups of junior hospital doctors;
- Increase the amount of time devoted to public sector delivery by doctors already in the private sector to 25%;
- Increase by 5 francs the fees for physicians in the public system; and
- Finance continuing medical education for doctors via a small levy on physician fees.

The Hospital Reform Law of 1991 was also passed with the intention of curbing some of the advantages enjoyed by private hospitals and creating a more level playing field between the two sectors. It covered the following issues:
* Regional hospital planning (including both public and private hospitals);
* Greater autonomy for public hospitals in setting their own investment budgets and in determining the number of positions allocated for practising physicians;
* Increased regulatory control over acquisition of expensive equipment, and the use of expensive medical techniques;
* Utilization review and accreditation of private hospitals;
* Agreements and contracts between private hospitals and the *Caisses*, to specify the expected volume of service.

Other more minor reforms in the 1990s have focused on containing health care system costs through fee limits and a variety of pharmaceuticals and services, as well as by controlling the number and fees of health care professionals. Most recently, there has been some discussion of major structural reforms to the French health care system such as changing from the current system of sickness funds supplemented with private insurance to a system of managed competition that would allow care to be purchased and provided by *Reseaux de soins coordinées* (Centres of Coordinated Care) similar to HMOs.

6.4. GERMANY (A MIXED MODEL WITH INCREASING GOVERNMENT REGULATIONS) (16, 17)

Germany spends 9.6% of its GDP, or $1,775 per capita, on health care expenditures. Public sector expenditures comprise 71.5% of all health care spending. This is slightly lower than the OECD average. Germany has the largest economy in Europe.

6.4.1. Finance
Health care in Germany is financed primarily through a system of compulsory, open-ended non-governmental social insurance funds called sickness funds. There are approximately 1,100 such funds covering the health care costs of roughly 90% of the population. Money for the sickness funds is collected through income-related payroll taxes at a rate of 12.8% of individual income; half of the contribution is paid by the employer and half by the employee. Contributions for individuals who are unemployed, retired, disabled, or below the poverty line are made by local sickness funds and local governments.

Membership in these sickness funds is compulsory for the vast majority of the population. Although the most affluent Germans (10% of the population) can choose not to participate in the sickness funds and can buy private health insurance instead from roughly 45 non-profit, private insurance companies, individuals usually cannot freely choose which sickness fund to join. This decision is made according to the individual's place of residence and occupation. These funds are called *Reichversicherungsordnung* (RVO) funds (State Insurance Regulation) and include, for example, local/regional sickness funds, industrial funds, crafts funds, rural funds, sailors' funds, miners' funds, and blue-collar or white-collar workers' funds.

Individuals who have stable employment and earn over a certain income per month can actually choose which sickness fund to join. Their membership is usually in voluntary sickness funds called *Ersatzkassen*. The compulsory funds (RVO) cover approximately 60% of the population; the voluntary *Ersatzkassen* cover roughly 28% of the population and private insurance covers roughly 10%. The remaining 2% of the population includes employees such as police and armed forces and some individuals on social welfare who receive free health care. Less than half a per cent of the most wealthy Germans remain uninsured and all residents of the former East Germany are covered through the mandatory RVOs.

Contribution to a sickness fund includes coverage for unemployed spouses and all dependants, whether children or adults. This is called the "solidarity principle". According to this principle, a member's contribution to a sickness fund remains the same whether that person is single or has dependants or non-working family members who are co-insured.

German sickness funds cover a comprehensive array of health services mandated by federal legislation to prevent different levels of coverage. Benefits include preventive services, family planning, maternity care, prescription drugs, ambulatory medical care, dental care, transport, inpatient care, home nursing service, rehabilitation services (including treatment at spas), and income support during sick leave. There are small co-payments for dentures and other dental prosthetics, eyeglasses, non-emergency transport, prescription drugs, and a small daily fee for the first 14 days of inpatient care and for inpatient rehabilitation. Nursing home care and care in homes for the elderly are not covered. Individual out-of-pocket expenses comprise 11% of total health expenditures. Physicians are allowed to extra-bill only their private patients; the practice of extra-billing remains very limited.

6.4.2. Delivery

The German delivery system is a mixed public and private one that is fairly heavily regulated. There are three types of hospitals: publicly owned hospitals (51%); private, voluntary, non-profit hospitals usually owned by charities or religious groups (35%); and private, proprietary, for-profit hospitals usually owned by doctors individually or in groups (14%). Ambulatory care and inpatient care are completely separate.

Ambulatory physicians — both GPs and specialists — do not generally have admitting privileges to hospitals, while hospital physicians generally cannot provide outpatient care. An exception to this strict division exists in the private sector, where ambulatory care physicians (mostly specialists) can rent hospital beds from private hospitals to allow for inpatient treatment of their patients. Individuals are allowed free choice of GPs and specialists, and are admitted to hospitals by referral from an ambulatory care doctor; the hospital is usually the closest one to the person's residence. Physicians are paid on a fee-for-service basis by the sickness funds rather than by their patients. Thus, as in Canada, individuals are usually not aware of the costs of health care services. The sickness fund negotiates with regional professional associations to set the so-called "relative point value index" for each service. For example, a telephone consultation is assigned 80 points, a home visit 360 points, and lab/diagnostic work between 360 and 900 points. The physician is paid quarterly by the sickness fund based on caseload — that is on the volume and mix of services provided. The fees are calculated not in absolute terms, but according to the number of value-point services provided in comparison with other physicians. Thus, at the time of service provision, the physician *also* does not know the actual cost. Usually, value points are set higher for the voluntary *Ersatzkassen* than for the RVOs funds.

6.4.3. Health System Reforms

The 1993 reform of the German health care system was considerably more comprehensive than earlier reforms, at least in part because the central government now had to contend with equalizing services and health outcomes in the former East German regions (which had used a total public approach) with those in West Germany. It was designed to limit overall expenditures by controlling the volume as well as the price of physician services and pharmaceuticals. Additionally, reforms sought to increase the power of the sickness funds and state (*Länder*) governments with regard to the power of professional organizations. Key elements of the reform included the following:

- Increased co-payments for pharmaceuticals;
- Controlled/decreased prices for pharmaceuticals — both manufacturing prices and prices reimbursed by sickness funds;
- An income penalty for physicians who prescribe drugs at higher rates than set by pharmaceutical budgets;
- Growth in physician expenditures capped at the growth rate of incomes of members of the sickness funds (outpatient surgery, preventive care, and services provided by physicians in the former East Germany are given more room to grow);
- Reduced fees for dental services,
- Limited rights of physicians to boycott or strike;
- Increased government control over the number of medical school admissions and the number of new practising specialists, and a mandatory retirement age of 68;
- Hospital payments changed from per diem rates to prospective budgets based on specific rates for individual procedures and conditions;
- Unlimited choice of sickness funds for certain groups and creation of a risk-equalization scheme.

6.5. NEW ZEALAND (PRIVATIZATION OF A PUBLIC/PUBLIC MODEL)

New Zealand spends roughly 7.5% of its GDP or $1,079 per capita on health care, of which 77.2% comes from the public sector. It is important to note that the public sector role in health care system financing has decreased from 88% just ten years ago.

A particular challenge for the New Zealand health system lies with the health of the country's Aboriginal population (Maori Polynesians, 12% of the population, and Pacific Island Polynesians, 6% of the population). Studies have repeatedly concluded that the level of the health of the Aboriginal population is significantly lower than that of the remainder of the New Zealand population.

New Zealand's health care system is still very much in transition (18). Its original health care system, established in 1938, is quite similar to the British NHS-providing universal health care coverage for care in the public hospital system. Health care services were financed through general tax revenues. Some administrative reforms occurred in the late 1980s (discussed below), but the original system remained largely unchanged. Major structural reforms were planned and developed by the National (conservative) Party in 1991 as part of a broader general restructuring of government and its role in society. The planned reforms led to widespread opposition among health care providers and the public. As a result, the health care reform had to be more gradual and less all-encompassing than originally envisioned. New Zealand's health care system, as it looks today, is still evolving to include various aspects of the reform planned in the early 1990s.

6.5.1. Finance

Like most other industrialized nations, New Zealand's health care system is financed through a combination of public and private sources of funds. Originally, the system provided universal health coverage for public hospital care to all New Zealanders, financed through general taxes. The system remained largely unchanged until the 1970s, when worsening economic conditions led to constraint on public spending for health care and other social services and, paradoxically eroded cost control.

Currently, 80% of New Zealand's health care budget is financed through general taxes allocated from the central government to Regional Health Authorities (RHAs). These funds finance the public hospital system, subsidize care in private hospitals, and pay for ambulatory physician services. Private hospital care is partially subsidized through RHA budgets (at approximately 20% of costs), with the remainder financed by the patient.

Increasing proportions of New Zealanders carry some type of supplementary private health insurance, mostly to speed up access to elective medical and surgical procedures and for reimbursement of fees not covered by the public system. Private health insurance is financed through voluntary premiums and is usually purchased through the workplace. Premiums are tax deductible. Increasing budgetary pressures have led to increased cost shifting for ambulatory care. Currently, the public health insurance scheme covers only 10% of the costs of adult ambulatory care visits. The remainder must be paid for by the individual or by private insurance. Children's ambulatory care visits are reimbursed at higher rates, with public subsidies covering 76% of the costs of routine visits. For visits requiring more than routine care, physicians can charge extra fees.

6.5.2. Delivery

New Zealand's health services delivery system combines public, private and voluntary services. The majority of hospital beds are public (77%). As in France, the public and private hospital systems are not parallel: private hospitals are much smaller and less comprehensive than public hospitals, and usually limit their services to highly specialized procedures. For example, some hip replacement surgery and almost all hernia operations are conducted at private hospitals, while neurological and cardiac surgery are almost exclusively provided by public hospitals. Public hospitals provide complex laboratory services and blood supplies to private hospitals. Private hospitals are also frequently used for geriatric care. With increasing budgetary pressures in the public system, the New Zealand government has encouraged the private sector to increase its provision of less serious and less urgent care. Ambulatory physicians in New Zealand can currently choose to serve under contract to RHAs or remain in private practice and be paid on a fee-for-service basis. The majority have remained in independent private practices. Individuals have free choice of primary care physicians and specialists, and free choice between public and private hospitals. GPs in New Zealand do not have a gatekeeper role.

6.5.3. Health System Reforms (19)

Prior to 1989, hospital and related services were almost entirely provided by elected hospital boards, which received budgets from the central government based on their population size and population characteristics (age and gender composition, mortality, fertility). In 1989, these boards were converted to 14 Area Health Boards (AHBs), partly elected, partly appointed, in order to integrate the provision of hospital and related services with public health services that had previously been provided by the Department of Health. The overall goal of the boards was to improve the health of their communities, to provide a balanced range of health services, and to coordinate the public sector with the private sector. At this time, the funding envelope also changed. Instead of being paid a fixed sum each year based on population characteristics, the AHBs began to submit long-term strategic plans and requested commensurate budgets, but without adding budget increases. In other words, they were free to set their own health services priorities specific to their population needs, but funding for new programs had to be found at the expense of existing ones.

With the 1991 Reform Plan prepared by the conservative government (and implemented in 1993), the AHBs were replaced by four Regional Health Authorities (RHAs), which were given the responsibility for purchasing a broad spectrum of care for their population (averaging 750,000 each), including acute and long-term hospital services, general practice/primary care services, services for the mentally ill, and services for the disabled. Parallelling the internal market reform approach in England, New Zealand separated purchasing responsibilities from providing responsibilities. RHAs receive funding from the central government based on a capped and capitated budget for the region. The publicly owned acute care hospitals of the 14 AHBs were transformed into 23 commercial entities called Crown Health Enterprises (CHEs). The RHAs contract with the CHEs to provide health services. Needs assessment of the health care needs of the regional population is the responsibility of the RHAs, while providing a comprehensive array of health services for an agreed-upon budget is the responsibility of the CHE. RHA payment to the CHEs is based on volume and type of services provided.

The direction of this recent reform has been toward decreased government involvement in both financing health care (to lighten the fiscal burden on overtaxed public budgets) and in health services delivery (to promote greater efficiency and cost containment). The solution was to increase co-payments for all outpatient hospital care (the Conservative Party had wanted to introduce co-payments for inpatient care as well, but this was abandoned due to extreme public protest), and to implement a system of internal markets following the U.K. model. The internal market system implemented in 1993 included a comprehensive set of new health care structures, integrated all purchasing through the four RHAs, established contracts as the means of resource allocation, and favoured competition and incentives over regulation. It also brought elements of private sector, corporate-type functioning into the health care system by subjecting CHEs to the *Company Act*, *Commerce Act*, and taxation provisions, and by appointing CHE chief executive officers largely from the business sector.

Health care systems of different industrialized nations are described above and comparisons are made between each other and with that of Canada. As can be seen all of these nations have a different mix of public and private financing and delivery of care. Many of them are reforming their system to achieve ideal balance according to the political ideology of the time.

7. SUMMARY

The *Constitution Act* of 1982 gave the federal government a minimal role in the health care system. Section 91 of the act states that the federal government has power with respect to census, statistics, and quarantine, whereas section 92 gives provinces the primary responsibility in health matters. However the federal government has become involved in health care by sharing the cost of programs and thus steering the health care system. Since 1950, a number of federal acts have been passed most significantly, the *Hospital Insurance and Diagnostic Services Act* of 1957 (which provided universal hospitalization) and the *Medical Care Act* of 1966 (which provided universal coverage of necessary medical services). The federal government shared 50% of the cost of these programs with the participating provinces, provided the provinces met four criteria: universality, portability, comprehensiveness, and public administration. All provinces participated in these programs. In the 1970s, the shared cost of health programs became a critical problem for the federal and provincial governments alike and this led to the legislation of the *Federal-Provincial Fiscal Arrangements and Established Program Financing Act* (EPF) of 1977. In this act, the federal government agreed to pay the provinces through transfer of income tax points and by cash contribution linked to an increase in the GNP instead of the previous 50% cost sharing. The EPF no longer tied federal payments to a particular form of health services, thus reducing the federal steering effect.

During the early 1980s, critical reviews of national health insurance programs and financing arrangements led to the 1984 enactment of the *Canada Health Act*. This act amalgamated the *Hospital Insurance and Diagnostic Services Act* and the *Medical Care Act*. It also established five criteria that provincial health programs must meet in order to be eligible for the full cash portion of the federal government contribution, namely public administration, comprehensiveness, universality, portability, and accessibility. The act also banned extra-billing, and by 1987 all the provinces had complied. It appeared that the Canadian health care system was moving toward an increased federal role, especially in the areas of formulation, monitoring, and enforcing of program conditions. However, as a result of budgetary deficits, the federal government was forced to reduce transfer payments for health care and postsecondary education to the provinces. Bills C-96, C-69, and C-20 were enacted to freeze the cash flow to the provinces, resulting in a diminished federal role in enforcing health care policy. In an attempt to stabilize the amount of federal health and social transfers to the provinces and maintain a role in health, the federal government passed the *Canada Health and Social Transfer Act* in 1996 — a block grant to the provinces covering health care, higher education, and social programs.

Although it appears that Canada has a national medicare program, this is incorrect, because health care is actually a provincial responsibility. The involvement of the federal government is through financial contributions, which enables the federal government to establish national standards. As a result, Canada has ten provincial and two territorial health care systems that are structured on federal guidelines and provide mainly sickness care and, to a lesser extent, preventive practices carried out by physicians. However, the jurisdictional dispute between the provinces and the federal government in the health sector has become a source of increasing tension.

The health care systems of the United Kingdom, the United States, France, Germany, and New Zealand are described and similarities and differences with Canada's health care system are highlighted.

8. REFERENCES

1.   Mhatre S, Deber R. From Equal Access to Health Care to Equitable Access to Health: A Review of Canadian Provincial Health Commissions and Reports. International Journal of Health Services 1992;22(4):645-666.
2.   Deber R, Narine L, Baranek P, et al. The Public-Private Mix in Health Care. 1998;4:419-542.
3.   Vayda E, Deber R. The Canadian Health Care System: An Overview. Social Science and Medicine 1984;18(3):191-197.

4. Department of National Health and Welfare. Review of Health Services in Canada 1976. Ottawa: Government of Canada, 1976.
5. Young T. Health Care and Cultural Change: The Indian Experience in the Central Subarctic. Toronto: University of Toronto Press, 1988.
6. Heiber S, Deber R. Banning Extra-Billing in Canada: Just What the Doctor Didn't Order. Canadian Public Policy 1987;13:62-74.
7. Hall EM. Canada's National-Provincial Health Program for the 1980's. A Commitment for Renewal. Ottawa: Health and Welfare Canada, Special Commissioner, 1980.
8. Parliamentary Task Force on Federal-Provincial Fiscal Arrangements. Fiscal Federalism in Canada. Ottawa: Ministry of Supply and Services, 1981.
9. Poulin C. The History of Health Care Funding in Canada and the Implications of Bill C-20. Public Health and Epidemiology Reports Ontario 1992;3(10):160-164.
10. Health System and Policy Division. Canada Health and Social Transfer: Backgrounder. Ottawa: Health Canada, Policy and Consultation Branch, 1996.
11. Abel-Smith B, Mossialos E. Cost-Containment and Health Care Reform: A Study of the European Union. Health Policy 1994;28:89-132.
12. Organization for Economic Cooperation and Development (Paris). Health Policy Studies No. 1: U.S. Health Care at the Crossroads. Washington: OECD Publications, 1992.
13. Health Policy: Special Issue on Health Reform in the NHS. Health Policy 1993;25:1-183.
14. Angell M. The Beginning of Health Care Reform: The Clinton Plan. New England Journal of Medicine 1993;329(21):1569-1570.
15. Weill C. Health Care Technology in France. Health Policy 1994;30:123-162.
16. Henke KD, Murray M, Ade C. Global Budgeting in Germany: Lessons for the United States. Health Affairs 1994;13(4):7-21.
17. Kirkman-Liff BL. Physician Payment and Cost-Containment Strategies in West Germany: Suggestion for Medicare Reform. Journal of Health Politics, Policy and Law 1990;15(1):69-99.
18. Raffel MW, Raffel NK. The Effect of Economic Constraints on the Health Care System in New Zealand. Health Policy 1987;8:171-81.
19. MacLeod GK. Health Care Financing Reform in New Zealand. Health Affairs 1994;13(4):210-215.

Chapter
13

Federal and Provincial Health Organizations

Under the *Constitution Act 1867*, the federal government had almost no power in personal health care. However, through a number of financial arrangements, the federal government influenced two major areas of health care: medical care and hospital care. This chapter deals with the major functions of federal and provincial governments in this context. It describes how both levels of government cooperated to work at arm's length so as to avoid intruding on each other's jurisdiction. These joint ventures have particularly benefited the smaller provinces, which do not always have the resources to mount in-depth studies or planning processes.

1. FEDERAL HEALTH ORGANIZATION

As seen in Chapter 12, under the terms of Confederation the federal government had relatively little jurisdiction over health care. In 1872, the Department of Agriculture had primary responsibility for federal health activities which were gradually dispersed among several departments: Agriculture, Inland Revenue, and Marine and Fisheries. In 1919, the Department of Health was established by an act stating that its duties, powers, and functions "extend to and include all matters relating to the promotion or preservation of the health, social security and social welfare of the people of Canada over which the Parliament of Canada has jurisdiction". In 1929, the Department of Soldiers' Civil Reestablishment was discontinued and the Department of National Health became the Department of Pensions and National Health. In 1945, it was split into Health and Welfare Canada and the Department of Veterans' Affairs. At that time, the task of Health and Welfare Canada was two-fold: to promote, preserve, and restore the health of Canadians, and to provide social security and social welfare to Canadians. In June 1993, the department was reorganized and welfare responsibilities were moved to what is now called Human Resources Development. The remaining department is now known as Health Canada. Its mission (as stated in 1995) is "to help the people of Canada maintain and improve their health" through "a renewed national health system, national leadership and partnerships on health; and the provision of timely, responsive and evidence-based advice and action on health issues" (1). Health Canada lists the following as its chief goals:

- To foster active partnerships with provinces, territories, and others;
- To develop a more effective health intelligence network;
- To improve knowledge management and dissemination, as well as evidence-based decision making;
- To give increased priority to initiatives that redress the most significant health inequalities in Canada;
- To renew its relationship with First Nations peoples;
- To provide leadership on health promotion, disease prevention, and health strategies; and
- To create innovative, targeted, and effective programs.

2. HEALTH PROGRAMS

As of 1997, Health Canada is composed of five branches and a departmental secretariat. It is also represented in five regional offices throughout Canada — the Atlantic region, Quebec, Ontario, Manitoba/Saskatchewan, and the Pacific West. The five branches are the Health Promotion and Programs Branch (HPPB), the Health Protection Branch (HPB), the Medical Services Branch (MSB), the Policy and Consultation Branch (PCB), and the Corporate Services Branch (CSB). The federal Minister of Health is responsible for these branches. Under the Minister, there are Deputy Ministers and Associate Deputy Ministers, a number of Assistant Deputy Ministers, as well as Regional Director Generals who report to the Minister through the Deputy Ministers. The Minister of Health is also accountable to Parliament for:

- The Medical Research Council;
- The National Advisory Committee on AIDS;
- The National Advisory Council on Aging;
- The Canadian Centre on Substance Abuse; and
- The Patented Medicine Prices Review Board.

Although Health Canada branches, divisions, and units are frequently reorganized in an effort to streamline operations and reduce waste, the basic priorities have remained fairly stable over the past several years. The following section outlines some of the functions and activities carried out by each branch and its subdivisions (unless otherwise indicated, subdivision and unit names are accurate up to 1995) (1, 2). For the most up-to-date and accurate information on Health Canada's organizational structure, the reader is urged to refer to the Health Canada web site listed at the end of the book.

2.1. HEALTH PROMOTION AND PROGRAMS BRANCH (HPPB)

The Health Promotion and Programs Branch provides financial and technical support to the provinces and territories for insured health care services and certain extended health care services, as well as promotes the adoption and maintenance of healthy lifestyles and supports public health research. This branch is made up of three main directorates:
- The Population Health Directorate;
- The Strategies and Systems for Health Directorate; and
- The Regional Operations and Branch Management Planning Directorate.

2.1.1. Population Health Directorate

The objective of the Population Health Directorate (previously called the Health Promotion Directorate) is to help Canadians achieve healthy lifestyles. It uses four strategies for health promotion: equipping the public to deal with lifestyle issues; promoting a social climate that supports healthy lifestyles; supporting self-help and citizen participation in health promotion; and lobbying for social welfare and other established programs. As of July 1997, the Directorate has four divisions: the Population Health Development Division, the Childhood and Youth Division, the Division on Aging and Seniors, the Adult Health Division, and the Partnerships and Marketing Division. Responsibilities of each of three life-stage divisions (e.g., childhood and youth, adult, and aging and seniors) include:
- Serving as the specialist within Health Canada for issues relating to their particular age group, including providing expertise on issues related to appropriate environments, e.g., where we learn and play (children), where we work (adults), and where we live (seniors);
- Providing expertise, leadership, and coordination regarding overall program and policy development for their age group;
- Managing and supporting cross-sectorial work regarding their age group;
- Advising on the needs, priorities, strategies, and program gaps for their age group; and
- Running federal/provincial/territorial groups and cross-departmental/cross-federal committees for their age group.

These divisions are supported by the Population Health Development Division, which is responsible for overall program support, coordination, and program grants, and by the Partnerships and Marketing Division, which is responsible for disseminating information through the Population Health Clearinghouse and for expertise in social marketing.

2.1.2. Strategies and Systems for Health Directorate

The primary focus of the Strategies and Systems for Health Directorate is to promote the continuing development and maintenance of reasonable standards of health care and parity among provincial health programs. This program includes five sub-programs: Research and Knowledge Development, Policy Development and Coordination, HIV/AIDS Policy Coordination and Programs, Health Issues, and Health Systems. In all of these programs, the Directorate assists the provinces by assuming leadership and coordinating functions through the Federal/Provincial Advisory Committee structure, which was established to assist the Conference of Deputy Ministers in fulfilling its mandate. Directorate activities include developing information resources, facilitating national consensus and action plans, and providing grants to national voluntary agencies and non-governmental organizations. Two recent key initiatives of the Health Systems Division are the National Action Plan for Physician Resource Management and the National Strategy on Quality and Effectiveness in Health Care. The Health Issues Division focuses on national programs regarding tobacco, drugs/alcohol, violence, fitness, nutrition, mental health, and sexual and reproductive health.

2.1.3. Extramural Research Program

The main component of the Research and Knowledge Development Division is the Extramural Research Program, which is delivered by the National Health Research and Development Program (NHRDP). Through this program, Health Canada obtains information and develops and evaluates innovations related to its broad departmental objectives. Applications for grants are accepted from any appropriately qualified individual or institution or, in special cases, from provincial and municipal governments.

The NHRDP underwent an extensive review and consultation process in 1995. As a result, some of the programs have been limited or discontinued. Currently, the greatest emphasis is on the relevance and applicability of research to current health policy debates in Canada. The following areas are targeted for research grants until the year 2000:

- Population health (including the determinants of health and the effects of equity on health);
- Impact of public policies on health (including health, economic, environmental, employment, and immigration policies);
- Renewal and restructuring of health systems;
- Research on new methodologies; and
- Research on the transfer and acquisition of knowledge.

Clinical outcomes research, demonstration projects, community needs assessments, basic research, and research into the effects of biology or the effects of the physical environment on health will no longer be funded by the NHRDP. The NHRDP supports health research through career scientist awards, master's and doctoral level fellowships, post-doctoral fellowships, and its Personnel Support Program. The total amount of funds allocated to research projects through all of NHRDP's funding programs equalled $22.5 million in 1997, but this amount will be halved in the future as money for special initiatives such as projects on seniors' health finish. Because such initiatives are of a specialized, one-time nature, most will not be refunded.

2.2. HEALTH PROTECTION BRANCH (HPB)

The Health Protection Branch is responsible for protecting the public against unsafe foods, pharmaceuticals, cosmetics, medical and radiation-emitting devices, harmful microbes, technological and social environments as they relate to health, environmental pollutants and contaminants of all kinds, and fraudulent drugs and devices. This branch also monitors the occurrence and causes of communicable and non-communicable diseases, and establishes laboratory medicine standards.

The HPB has five operational directorates: Food, Pharmaceutical Drug, Environmental Health, National Health Surveillance, and Field Operations. It is responsible for enforcing the *Food and Drugs Act and Regulations*, the *Narcotic Control Act and Regulations*, the *Proprietary or Patent Medicine Act*, and the *Radiation Emitting Devices Act and Regulations*. In addition, under the *Hazardous Products Act and Regulations*, the HPB has joint responsibility with Consumer and Corporate Affairs Canada for product safety.

2.2.1. Food Directorate

Standards of safety and purity of food products are developed through laboratory research and maintained by a regular and widespread inspection program. The inspection of food-manufacturing operations plays a major role in assuring that clean, wholesome foods and ingredients meet recognized standards. Changing food technology requires the development of laboratory methods to ensure the purity of new ingredients and the quality of packaging material. The Food and Drugs Regulations list chemical additives that may be used in foods, the amounts that may be added to each food, and the underlying reasons for the additives, such as preservation. Information on a new additive must be submitted to the directorate and reviewed carefully before it can be included in the permitted list. Considerable emphasis is placed on studies to ensure that the levels of pesticide residue in foods are not a health hazard. The effect of new packaging and processing techniques on food spoilage is also of special concern.

2.2.2. Pharmaceutical Drug Directorate

The Pharmaceutical Drug Directorate regulates both the manufacture and distribution of pharmaceutical drugs in Canada. The conditions described in the Manufacturing Facilities and Control Regulations, which relate to facilities, employment qualifications, quality control procedures, maintenance of records, and a recall system for withdrawing any batch of drugs from the market. Inspectors regularly visit pharmaceutical facilities to ensure that the drugs produced meet the standards required for sale in Canada. Facilities that manufacture biological products to be sold in Canada, such as serums and vaccines, must be licensed according to the specifications of the *Food and Drugs Act and Regulations*, whether they are located in Canada or abroad.

When a new drug is to be placed on the market, the manufacturer is required by law to provide the Directorate with specific information, including a quantitative list of its ingredients, evidence of its safety and effectiveness, the formulation of dosages, and reports of any adverse effects. This information is studied to ensure that the drug is safe and effective for the purposes claimed. Even after a new drug is on the market, its sale can be banned by the HPB if the Drug Adverse Reaction Reporting Program indicates that it is unsafe or injurious.

Another major activity of HPB is the Quality Assessment of Drugs Program, which enables the public to purchase high-quality drugs at reasonable prices. This program includes inspection of manufacturing facilities, assessment of claims and clinical equivalency of competing brands, and provision of information to professionals and to the general public.

2.2.3. Environmental Health Directorate

The Environmental Health Directorate is responsible for studying the adverse effects of the chemical and physical environment on human health, and for ensuring the safety, effectiveness, and non-fraudulent nature of medical devices. The Directorate has the responsibility of developing assessments of health hazards for the work and home environments and for household products, and for developing criteria for assessing air and water quality. Research is conducted on radiation hazards, and environmental and occupational exposures are monitored. Health Canada has taken new initiatives and extended programs under the Action Plan for Health and the Environment as part of the Federal Environmental Agenda (Green Plan). The Great Lakes Health Effects Program involves health surveillance, human-exposure monitoring, and toxicological testing.

2.2.4. National Health Surveillance Directorate

One of the directorates of Health Canada's Health Protection Branch is the Laboratory Centre for Disease Control (LCDC), which works closely with provinces and their public health laboratories. The LCDC is Canada's national centre for the identification, investigation, prevention, and control of human diseases. The Centre's core activities include disease surveillance, disease prevention, and disease control. It monitors and investigates outbreaks of both infectious and non-infectious diseases and injuries, studies their associated risk factors, and evaluates related prevention and control programs.

Disease Surveillance. Activities include developing surveillance programs and analysing the occurrence of particular diseases; studying and evaluating data on communicable and non-communicable diseases in hospitals, laboratories, communities, and internationally; and developing policies to control communicable and non-communicable diseases. Analysing provincial and national data, the LCDC produces publications such as *The Canada Communicable Disease Report, Chronic Diseases in Canada,* and others targeted to a variety of audiences. It also responds to requests from provinces to investigate outbreaks.

Disease Prevention. Activities include the study of risk factors associated with infectious and non-infectious diseases, and the development and evaluation of prevention and control programs.

Disease Control. The Disease Control Services of LCDC carry out a range of laboratory work including identifying infectious diseases in clinical specimens submitted by provincial public health or university and teaching hospital laboratories for the diagnosis of individuals; developing methods and reagents for the early, rapid, and reliable detection of infectious diseases; promoting high levels of quality assurance in laboratory diagnoses through national programs in evaluation, proficiency testing; characterizing human pathogens and evaluating their role in human infectious diseases from a national perspective for the prevention and control of epidemics; and developing biotechnology for transfer to industry for commercialization of diagnostic commodities.

The LCDC currently operates nine bureaus: Cancer, Cardiovascular/ Respiratory Disease and Diabetes, HIV/AIDS and Sexually Transmitted Diseases, Infectious Diseases, Microbiology, Special Health Initiatives, Reproductive and Child Health, Surveillance and Field Epidemiology, and Strategic Planning and Risk Management. The Bureau of Surveillance and Field Epidemiology, and the Bureau of Strategic Planning and Risk Management support the other seven programs. The LCDC was recently reorganized to assume responsibilities previously held by the Bureau of Chronic Disease Epidemiology and the Bureau of Infectious Disease Epidemiology. Current priorities for study and development include antibiotic-resistant pathogens, especially those implicated in hospital outbreaks; diabetes and cardiorespiratory diseases such as heart attack and asthma; tuberculosis; cancer risk assessment, prevention, early detection and treatment, and environmental risk assessment and surveillance; sexually transmitted disease prevention and control; perinatal diseases; and vaccine-preventable diseases in children (3).

2.3. MEDICAL SERVICES BRANCH (MSB)

The Medical Services Branch is responsible for providing mainly those health services assigned to the federal government in the *Constitution Act, 1867,* which were quarantine services, health services to civil servants, health services to travelling Canadians, a national prosthetics service, civil aviation medicine, and emergency health services to all Canadians in the event of civil or natural disasters. It also provides health services to the Aboriginal peoples that were considered part of the treaty obligations; these services include health care and public health. The MSB provides services through its six divisions described below.

2.3.1. First Nations and Inuit Health Programs Directorate
The basic objective of this directorate is to assist Aboriginal peoples to attain a standard of health comparable to that of other Canadians. In Yukon, insured hospital and medical care programs for Aboriginal peoples are administered by the Yukon government, whereas the MSB manages other health services, including a comprehensive public health program, special arrangements to facilitate communication between health

stations, and the transportation of people referred from isolated communities to medical centres. In certain zones, several universities provide medical personnel and students on rotation. As residents of a province or territory, First Nations people are entitled to the benefits of the cost-shared provincially operated medical and hospital insurance plans on the same terms and conditions as other Canadians. As many of the First Nations communities are small and often located in remote and isolated areas, these insured benefits are supplemented by the MSB, which assists First Nations bands to arrange transportation, and obtain drugs and prostheses. A comprehensive public health program provides dental care for children, immunization, school health services, health education, and prenatal, postnatal, and healthy baby clinics. Direct financial assistance to Aboriginal organizations supports First Nations programs directed toward improving their quality of life.

Since Aboriginal peoples live all over Canada, there is a network of 510 specially designed health facilities that operate in all provinces: 72 nursing stations, 189 health stations, 94 health offices, 104 health centres, five hospitals, and 46 other facilities. The MSB is in the process of transferring control of health services to the First Nations. At the time of writing, 26% of the Aboriginal bands across the country now control their health services, while an additional 26% are at a "pre-transfer" stage. The remaining bands are in the process of acquiring control. Also, under the Community Health Representative Program, increasing numbers of Aboriginal people are being trained and employed in public health and medical care programs.

2.3.2. Quarantine and Regulatory Service

The MSB is responsible for the inspection of all vessels, aircraft, and other conveyances, as well as their crews and passengers arriving in Canada from foreign countries, in order to prevent the entry of diseases such as cholera, plague, and yellow fever. Fully equipped quarantine stations are located at all major seaports and airports. The MSB is also responsible for enforcing standards of hygiene on federal property including ports and terminals, vehicles travelling interprovincially, and Canadian ships and aircraft.

2.3.3. Occupational and Environmental Health Services Directorate

The MSB oversees a comprehensive occupational health program for federal employees (public servants) throughout Canada and abroad. This service includes health counselling; surveillance of the occupational environment; pre-employment, periodic, and special examinations; first aid and emergency treatment; and a wide range of advisory services and special health programs. The Directorate also provides environmental and contaminant health services on Aboriginal reserves, and provides emergency health services for visiting dignitaries.

2.3.4. Civil Aviation Medicine

The MSB advises Transport Canada on the health and safety of all involved in Canadian civil aviation. Aviation medical officers at regional and central headquarters review all medical examinations, participate in aviation safety programs, and assist in air accident investigations. Close liaison with authorities responsible for foreign aviation medicine is maintained, because standards are usually based upon international agreements.

2.3.5. Prosthetic Services

The objectives of the Prosthetic Services are to make available high-quality prosthetic and orthotic rehabilitation, under the terms of agreements with most provinces and with Veterans' Affairs Canada, and to provide expertise in this field.

2.3.6. Health Advisory Services Directorate

The Health Advisory Services Directorate provides emergency health services in the event of civil or natural disasters. It prepares plans to ensure that the health component of the MSB would be able to operate in the event or threat of nuclear attack, and to advise, assist, and stimulate provincial and municipal health departments in emergency health planning for both peacetime and wartime emergencies.

Certain divisions, such as Immigration Medical Services and Disability Assessment, that were previously administered by Health and Welfare Canada, have recently been moved to other ministries (see Section 3).

2.4. POLICY AND CONSULTATION BRANCH (PCB)

The objective of the Policy and Consultation Branch is to provide advice to the Minister of Health, Deputy Minister, and other branches on trends and issues, policy requirements, and communications and information needs relative to departmental objectives, priorities, and programs. It has three main roles designed to meet that objective. First, it undertakes research analysis and advises on health policy issues. Second, it acts as a resource for policy development and communications activities of other branches. Finally, it provides information on health-related matters to the Ministry, its provincial counterparts, and national and international organizations. Programs are the PCB Communications, Health Insurance, Health Information, International Affairs Directorate, and the Women's Health Bureau.

2.4.1. Communications Directorate

The Communications Directorate provides senior managers and staff of Health Canada with strategic communications advice, carries out media and public environmental research and analysis to ascertain public attitudes and reactions to policy, develops communications plans and action plans for program issues, including organizing conferences and mass media campaigns, and implements and evaluates communications activities. Regional staff also provide information concerning Health Canada's programs and activities to the general public and distribute departmental publications.

2.4.2. Health Insurance

This program ensures that all residents of Canada have reasonable access to insured health care services on a prepaid basis and supports extended health care services. The program monitors and enforces the adherence of the provinces to the established criteria and conditions for federal contribution as outlined in the *Canada Health Act* (see Chapter 12).

2.4.3. Health Information Division

The Health Information Division of the PCB develops initiatives for new health information systems that mirror major trends or developments in health. It also maintains a number of health-related databases. It provides analytic and reporting services to the PCB, program branches, other departments, the provinces, and non-governmental clients. Most recently, it has been instrumental in the creation of the Canadian Institute for Health Information (CIHI), and now works closely with CIHI on health information initiatives.

CIHI is a federally chartered, independent, not-for-profit organization. It consolidates the programs, functions, and activities of the Hospital Medical Research Institute, the MIS Group, the Health Information Division of Health Canada and the Health Statistics Division of Statistics Canada into one body. Its primary functions are to collect, process, and maintain a comprehensive number of databases and registries that cover health-related human resources, services, and expenditures, and to set national standards for financial, statistical, and clinical data as well as for health information technology.

2.4.4. International Affairs Directorate

The International Affairs Directorate coordinates Canada's participation in international health and social affairs, and promotes networking between international, intergovernmental, and non-governmental organizations. One of its principal responsibilities is coordinating, monitoring, and, where required, initiating policies and strategies on issues that affect more than one branch or require interdepartmental consultation. It also maintains a centre for gathering and disseminating information on international trends in health and welfare matters.

2.4.5. Women's Health Bureau

The Women's Health Bureau is the key advisory and coordinating program responsible for the development, assessment, implementation, and integration of a range of policies and programs that ensure the promotion and preservation of the health, social security, and social welfare of Canadian women and their families. The Bureau's Director chairs the standing Departmental Advisory Committee on the Status of Women's Concerns to that all branches cooperate to achieve departmental and federal goals. The Bureau has been designated the Canadian focal point for the Pan-American Health Organization's Program on Women, Health, and Development.

2.5. CORPORATE SERVICES BRANCH (CSB)

The Corporate Services Branch supports the development and delivery of Health Canada programs through financial planning and administration, human resources support, information systems, office accommodation, internal audit, facilities management, and general administrative direction in line with departmental and government-wide policies.

3.   RELEVANT SOCIAL PROGRAMS (4-6)

Under the general government reorganization in June 1993, a series of social and income security programs that directly and indirectly affect health were transferred from Health and Welfare Canada to the newly formed Ministry of Human Resources Development. Additionally, the Child Tax Benefit Program (formerly the Family Allowance and Child Tax Credit) was transferred to the Department of Revenue, while medical assessment of immigrants was transferred to the Department of Citizenship and Immigration. The social programs described briefly below have the goals of promoting and strengthening the income security of Canadians, sharing in the cost of provincial and territorial social assistance, welfare services and rehabilitation programs, and assisting in the development of social services to meet changing social needs.

3.1.   INCOME SECURITY PROGRAMS

The income security programs promote and preserve the social security and social welfare of Canadians through the administration of the *Old Age Security Act*, the Canada Assistance Plan, and Parts II and III of the *Canada Pension Plan Act*. Through a network of regional offices and client service centres, these programs provide financial assistance to people with disabilities, the elderly, single-parent families, orphans, the unemployed, and low-income individuals. These programs complement existing social welfare, provincial, and local programs.

3.2.   SOCIAL SERVICE PROGRAMS

These programs consist of major federal-provincial cost-sharing programs that provide basic assistance for those whose budgetary needs exceed available resources (for whatever reason). They also provide consultation on social and welfare-related issues, including employability and vocational rehabilitation; alcohol and drug treatment and rehabilitation; services to people with physical and mental impairment; child welfare, child abuse, and family violence; family and community services; and voluntary action. Contributions are provided to help seniors maintain and improve their quality of life and independence, as well as to encourage seniors to utilize their skills, talents, and experience within the community. The National Adoption Desk has also been incorporated into this division to coordinate the adoption of children from other countries into Canada.

4.   OTHER RELEVANT PROGRAMS (1)

Health Canada is also involved in a number of other interdepartmental activities related to health. The tasks of these relevant advisory councils are given below.

Initiated in 1985, the National Strategy to Decrease Tobacco Use in Canada (7) coordinates federal, provincial, and local government efforts as well as programs and activities of health and non-governmental organizations that work to decrease smoking among Canadians. Health Canada administers federal tobacco legislation that restricts the sale of tobacco products to minors, and prohibits the advertising and promotion of these products. Other legislation requires that warning messages be printed clearly on tobacco product labels. Apart from legislative activities, the Strategy coordinates and facilitates health promotion programs, disseminates information through the National Tobacco Clearinghouse, operates prevention/protection/cessation programs, engages in research, and funds local initiatives.

4.1.   NATIONAL AIDS SECRETARIAT

The National AIDS Secretariat coordinates and monitors federal HIV/AIDS activities in Health Canada and other federal departments, and in the provinces and territories. It supports the National Advisory Committee on AIDS and the Federal/Provincial/ Territorial Committee on HIV/AIDS. The Secretariat focuses on financial accountability, monitors and provides strategic advice, facilitates the assessment of the Strategy and its initiatives, encourages private sector involvement in HIV/AIDS programs and activities, supports national HIV/AIDS research planning, and ensures effective and coordinated federal communication on HIV/AIDS through the National AIDS Clearinghouse.

4.2.   NATIONAL ADVISORY COUNCIL ON AGING

The National Advisory Council on Aging was created by Order-in-Council on May 1, 1980, to advise the Minister of Health Canada on issues related to the aging of the Canadian population and the quality of life of seniors. The Council has members from all parts of the country as well as a mix of language, ethnic groups, and occupational backgrounds. The Council reviews the needs of seniors, recommends remedial action, acts as liaison with other groups, encourages public discussion, and disseminates information. In carrying out its responsibilities, the Council works closely with the Minister of State for Seniors.

4.3. PATENTED MEDICINE PRICES REVIEW BOARD

The Patented Medicine Prices Review Board (PMPRB) was established by Parliament in 1987 as part of the *Patented Medicines Act*. The PMPRB monitors and regulates the prices of all patented medicines in Canada: first, by limiting the introduction of new patented medicines onto the market, and second, by limiting the introductory prices of new patented drugs. Since its establishment, patented medicine price increases have been limited to the rate of increase in the consumer price index. Additionally, with respect to its monitoring function, the PMPRB maintains a comprehensive database on all manufacturers' prices for patented medicines and has created a Patented Medicines Price Index.

4.4. NATIONAL FORUM ON HEALTH

The National Forum on Health was officially launched on October 20, 1994. It was created to address the issues relating to the reform of the Canadian health care system so as to maintain a strong commitment to the five pillars of medicare while increasing efficiency, cost effectiveness, access and high-quality care. The Forum was chaired by the Prime Minister of Canada and vice-chaired by the Minister of Health. The 24 members were chosen from across Canada based on their expertise and perspective on health policy, and included academics, health care professionals, and consumers. The issues addressed by the Forum included the determinants of health, evidence-based decision making, Canadian values governing health and health care, and striking a balance between the public and private sectors with regard to health. Public participation and consultation were central to the Forum's mandate and activities (8-13). In the final report of the National Health Forum, which was published in February 1997, the members of the Forum concluded that "the health care system [of Canada] is fundamentally sound", that it receives an adequate amount of funding, and that there is room for improving certain aspects of its functioning (14). The relevant chief recommendations of the report are discussed in Chapter 17.

5.   PROVINCIAL HEALTH SYSTEMS (15)

Constitutionally, the provincial governments have primary responsibility for all personal health matters, such as disease prevention, treatment, and maintenance of health — a right that provinces increasingly cite in order to exercise greater freedom in health system restructuring and reform without perceived federal interference. For example, in August 1996 at the Premiers Conference in Jasper, Alberta, premiers Ralph Klein (Alberta) and Mike Harris (Ontario) called for decentralization of all health matters. Citing the *Constitution Act*, both premiers claimed that health, education, and social services are provincial responsibilities rather than federal, and called for a decreased federal government role in enforcing the terms and condition of the *Canada Health Act*. This has become an increasingly contentious issue, as federal guidelines and requirements continue while the cash portion of funding transfers decrease.

However, the financing of services such as preventive health services, hospital services, treatment services for tuberculosis and other chronic diseases, and rehabilitation and care for people who are chronically ill and disabled depends chiefly on provincial and municipal governments. Provincial administrations work closely with hospitals and voluntary community health associations, the health care professions, and teaching and research institutions. Methods of organizing, financing, and administering health ministries vary from province to province. For instance, in some provinces, programs such as hospital insurance, medical care insurance, tuberculosis control, cancer control, and alcoholism are administered directly by the provincial ministry of health. In other provinces, the same programs may be the responsibility of separate public agencies directly accountable to a provincial minister of health. In some provinces, such as Quebec and Prince Edward Island, the ministry of health is amalgamated with the ministry of community and social services, an emerging trend across the country.

Other ministries can also finance some of the health-related services. For example, in some provinces, the ministry of labour is responsible for occupational health, the ministry of community and social services is responsible for people with cognitive impairment, and the ministry of education is responsible for the management and treatment of children with physical disabilities. Voluntary associations such as the Victorian Order of Nurses and the Arthritis Society may provide specialized health services, which are often largely supported by government financing. This diversity stems from traditional and financial considerations. In many provinces, one third to one half of the total budget is allocated to health services.

There are several explanations for these divisions. It may be that, to reduce the power of a minister with such a large budget, the functions of the health ministries are distributed across different ministries. Or many of the special services provided by other ministries are viewed as health services. However, the end result is the fragmentation and duplication of services. More recently, fiscal constraints and political/ideological shifts have also increased the amount of privatization of both financing and delivery of services within the health sector.

5.1. LOCAL AND REGIONAL HEALTH BOARDS AND COUNCILS

Beginning for the most part in the early 1990s, many provincial ministries of health have undergone extensive public consultations and reviews in an effort to improve the functioning of their health systems. A key component of these recent reforms is the devolution and decentralization of decision making for health to the regional and local levels. Based on the premise of increased community and consumer empowerment through increased participation in health, and on the belief that the health sector needed greater flexibility and responsiveness to local needs, regionalization has proceeded swiftly in every province except Ontario. However, within the health community, there is a growing suspicion that regionalization has been created to cut health care costs and to shift "blame" from the provincial government to the local level.

Each province is divided into regions, ranging from four in Nova Scotia and Newfoundland to 30 in Saskatchewan, based partly on population size and natural geographic and administrative boundaries. Each region's health needs are managed by a regional or district health board comprised of roughly 10 to 15 members. The composition and process of choosing board members varies from province to province, but generally includes both elected and appointed officials who represent a wide variety of constituencies and interests. They are usually drawn from consumer or special-needs groups, hospitals and health services centres, professional groups, voluntary agencies, and elected officials. This mix of membership increases the board's accountability before its community while it simultaneously ensures the inclusion of particular areas of expertise or the representation of particular cultural backgrounds that may not already be represented. Several provinces, such as Alberta and Saskatchewan, have provided for direct links between regional boards and organizations of physicians to ensure that physicians have a voice in regional planning and resource allocation decisions.

The exact functions of regional health boards across provinces vary, but in general include the following:

- Assessment of health needs of the population in its region;
- Development of policy and program priorities within the region and related allocation of resources;
- Administration of funding, including allocation of funds to community and nongovernmental organizations for primary care;
- Planning and coordinating service delivery, including planning of capital projects;
- Guaranteeing reasonable access to high-quality health services in a coordinated and integrated system of care;
- Liaison with community agencies and with the provincial ministry of health;
- Management and operation of service delivery and financing of institutions, including hospitals, long-term care, and other health services centres;
- Evaluation of health system outputs and outcomes; and
- Promotion of public participation in the decision-making process.

In all the provinces that have regionalized structures, except New Brunswick and Newfoundland, regional health boards have replaced individual hospital boards. New Brunswick and Newfoundland have set up separate regional hospital boards (eight such institutional/hospital boards in each province) in addition to their regional health boards, which are responsible for the administration of health services provided by hospitals.

5.1.1. Funding Formulas

In order to increase the effectiveness of regional health boards, which were usually only advisory in nature, most provinces have passed legislation to restructure their ministries of health and devolve financial decision making and planning and prioritizing activities. With recent cuts at all levesl of government, one potential reason for restructuring was to transfer difficult funding decisions to the regional level during a time of downsizing so the provincial government does not have to bear the blame for unpopular decisions.

In general, recent provincial legislation has changed funding formulas to allow for the devolution of decision-making. While the provincial ministries collect taxes to finance the health care system and develop regional funding envelopes, regional health boards allocate funds to service organizations based on their own needs assessments and policy priorities. Health insurance claims covering physician remuneration remain, for the most part, under the administrative auspices of the province. For example, government funding in Saskatchewan to district boards is based on needs assessments and population counts. Each district can borrow the money but is not allowed to tax local communities. Other provinces are also moving toward funding formulas based on population needs. Currently, only Saskatchewan, Quebec, and New Brunswick have functioning budget formulas in place. British Columbia, Alberta, Manitoba, and Nova Scotia are in the preparatory/planning phases of implementing population-based funding. Funding for physician remuneration through provincial health insurance plans is, as a rule, maintained as a separate budget category within ministry (not regional board) budgets.

Table 13.1 summarizes the structure and functions of regional health boards throughout Canada.

In many cases, regionalization plans and implementation are still in various stages of implementation. For example, in British Columbia, the New Democratic Party (NDP) government recently reviewed the successes and failures of the regionalization process, which led to changes in the number of boards, in the selection of board members, and in the geographical jurisdiction of each board. Nova Scotia recently confirmed the boundaries of its four local community boards and chose chief executive officers to head each region, but has not yet transferred all health services to these boards. And Ontario has had a system of local planning and advisory boards called District Health Councils in place for two decades, but these councils have no fiscal authority; plans for further devolution of ministry tasks are currently being considered.

In general, concerns over regionalization include the notions that regional boards will create more government bureaucracy instead of increasing responsiveness to local needs and that appointed rather than elected board members cause the positive aspects of accountability to be lost. There are also concerns about regional boundaries and the maintenance of freedom for consumers to choose their health care provider regardless of region, and about funding envelopes and resource allocation mechanisms, especially with regard to specialized tertiary and quaternary care centres (e.g., does a region with highly specialized hospitals pay for the services of those hospitals that serve multiple regions?). In addition, in an era of fiscal restraint, many public health activists fear that public health and community services will lose in the funding allocation struggle as each board identifies which services it can and will fund.

5.2. FUNCTIONAL ORGANIZATION OF PROVINCIAL MINISTRIES OF HEALTH

The role of the provincial ministries of health, in most cases, has been revised to meet the increased role of regional and local boards. In most cases, provincial ministries have devolved service delivery responsibilities to regional boards while maintaining responsibility for:

- Policy formation and standard setting;
- Overall health sector planning;
- Corporate services;
- Financing and the administration of funding envelopes;
- The administration of provincial insurance plans covering physician remuneration;
- Evaluation and monitoring; and
- The management of computerized information systems.

The main exception to this trend is the Ontario Ministry of Health, where the organizational structure remains more or less unchanged and oriented toward financing individual hospitals and agencies rather than regional boards.

Since the administrative structures of provincial health ministries are constantly changing, no organizational chart of the ministries is included here; for up-to-date information, readers are advised to visit the web site of each provincial ministry of health listed in the Appendix B. However, the functional organization remains stable. Provincial health responsibilities fall into three areas: direct delivery of health services, financing of health services, and administrative services (see Table 13.2 for a summary).

5.2.1. Service Delivery

Service delivery involves those services that, in most provinces, fall under the jurisdiction of the ministry of health with regard to budget, policies, and control. For the most part, the actual delivery of health services is now the responsibility of regional health boards, with the function of the ministry of health at the provincial level limited to financing health services, administration, and planning (covered below). Thus, regionalization represents the centralization of most services to regional levels from local bodies.

Aboriginal and Northern Health Services

In the provinces with sparsely settled northern areas, the provincial health departments provide both treatment and preventive health services. Saskatchewan, Manitoba, and the Yukon have set up northern health services, and other provinces have similar services.

In British Columbia, the health needs of Aboriginal groups are now a responsibility of each regional health board. A special Aboriginal Policy Framework, which addresses issues particular to Aboriginal health, has been developed by the province's

Table 13.1:   Regional Structures by Province

Province (Population) Year of legislation	Number of districts	Size of district (average)	Board membership	Comments
Newfoundland (547,160) 1994	4 Community Health Boards; 8 Regional Institutional Boards	2,600 - 17,200	Community Boards: 10-15 members, appointed by the Minister of Health to serve a three-year term, with a limit of three consecutive terms. Board members serve on a voluntary basis. Institutional Boards: 12-18 members, appointed by the Minister of Health based on community agency nominations.	Community Boards are responsible for the delivery of community health services in five areas, including health promotion, health protection, continuing care (including home support services, recently transferred from the Department of Social Services), mental health, and alcohol and drug dependency. Responsibilities do not include integration of Regional Institutional Boards with Community Boards except in Northern Newfoundland and Labrador. Eight Regional Institutional Boards replace individual hospital boards.
Prince Edward Island (132,855) 1993	5 Regional Health Boards	7,800 - 67,600	Regional Boards are composed of 7-10 members. They are currently appointed by the Minister of Health from nominations in the community, but will transfer to elected positions.	Regional Boards are responsible for community health and social services including mental health, hospitals, home care, long-term care, seniors' residences, addiction services, public health nursing, dental care, housing, child and family services, social assistance, employment development services, physician services, correctional services and probation, and youth centres.
Nova Scotia (899,970) 1994	4 Regional Health Boards; undetermined number of local Community Health Boards	15,000 - 35,000	Interim Board members appointed by the Minister of Health to serve on a volunteer basis for a two-year term. Permanent governance structures were determined in 1996.	Regional Boards have replaced individual hospital boards. Additional responsibilities include the planning and provision of long-term care, public health, and home care services.

Province	Boards	Population	Composition	Description
New Brunswick (729,630) 1992	8 Regional Hospital Boards	35,800 - 180,000	Each Regional Hospital Board has 12-16 members. Three or four Board members are appointed by the Minister of Health, two or three are appointed by the Board itself, and the remaining members are selected or appointed in accordance with the region's hospital bylaws.	Regional Hospital Boards have replaced individual hospital boards, but there are no regional or community health boards planned.
Quebec (7,045,080) originally in 1971, reconfigured in 1991	Originally 12 Health and Social Service Boards; replaced by 17 Regional Health Boards plus one HSSB for the Cree population of James Bay	36,000 - 1,111,000	20 Board members are elected by regional assemblies from among their members.	Regional Health Boards are responsible for planning, coordination, and resource allocation of health and social services. Additionally, Boards specify Specific Medical Activities (SMAs) to be completed by young/new GPs. Some hospital administrations have merged with Regional Boards.
Ontario (10,642,790)	discussions regarding regionalization, but no restructuring as yet	N/A	N/A	N/A
Manitoba (1,100,300) work in progress; as of 1994-95	10 Regional Health Advisory Boards for rural/northern regions and 2 urban regions (Winnipeg and Brandon)	25,000 - 96,000	Recommendations are for boards to be composed of 15 members serving three-year terms, with a limit of 2 consecutive terms. The majority of Board members will be elected from district health councils, but will also allow for appointments by the Minister of Health based on nominations from the community. Board members are paid a yearly stipend.	At this time, there are no provisions for linking health and social services.

Table 13.1:   Regional Structures by Province *(cont'd)*

Province (Population) Year of legislation	Number of districts	Size of district (average)	Board membership	Comments
Saskatchewan (976,615) 1993	30 District Health Authorities	9,000 – 224,000	District health boards include no more than 12 members, of which eight are elected. Up to 4 more members (including physicians) can be nominated by the community and appointed to the board by the Minister of Health. Members serve a two-year term and are not paid a salary.	Acute and long-term care, home care, mental health, addiction services, ambulance services, and public health services are the responsibility of district boards. Hospital-, health centre-, ambulance- and some home care boards have amalgamated functions with District Health Authorities. Each district board works closely with an affiliated branch of the Saskatchewan Medical Association.
Alberta (2,669,195) 1994	17 Regional Health Authorities	15,000– 754,000	Regional Health Authority members are appointed by the Minister of Health. Beginning 1998, 1/3 of board members will be appointed, while 2/3 will be elected. Twelve to 15 members serve on each board for a two-year term. No health professionals can be voting members of regional boards due to conflict of interest laws, but each board must have a physician liaison council responsible for representing physicians' interests and concerns.	Regional Health Authorities have replaced hospital boards with the exception of Catholic Hospitals. Acute care, community care and support, residential and long-term care (including mental health services) and health promotion are administered at the regional level while specialized care, provincial labs, communicable disease monitoring, and services provided by the Alberta Cancer Board have remained at the provincial level.

Province (Population) Year	System	Population	Board Composition	Notes
British Columbia (3,689,755) 1993	2-level regional system: 20 Regional Health Boards; 80 Community Health Boards (70 established, 10 more planned)	62,000 - 517,000 (183,000)	*Regional level:* appointed by the government. Planned for 1/3 appointed, 2/3 elected, but plans temporarily delayed. 2/3 of membership is from Community Boards. Board members chosen on two key principles: 1) they should take reasonable account of representation by population; 2) they should protect the interest of small communities. *Community level:* mixed - 1/3 elected officials (e.g. from school boards, city councils); 1/3 elected from public; 1/3 ministerial appointees.	Regional Health Boards have replaced individual hospital boards in British Columbia. The system was recently reviewed by the NDP government to assess what changes would be necessary. The government decided to change the number of Regional Boards to 11 from the original number of 20, and only 34 Community Health Councils instead of the originally planned 82. Additionally, each geographic region to be served by only one board – either an RHB or an CHC – and not both as previously envisioned. Finally, the Ministry has proposed to temporarily suspend the election of board members. Board members, representing a broad range of skills and experience, will be appointed by the Ministry of Health until the transitional period is over. The Ministry of Health still plans to implement Board elections at a later date.
Northwest Territories (64,125)	5 Regional Health Boards; 3 Hospital Boards	10,000	Board members are appointed by the Minister of Health.	Boards to cross geographic lines and be based on Aboriginal status.
Yukon Territory (30,650)	Discussions underway; no regionalization as yet	N/A	N/A	N/A

Table 13.2:   Functions of the Provincial Health System

Service Delivery	Service Financing (direct or via Regional Health Boards)	Administrative services
Services for tuberculosis and cancer patients	Public health services*	Health services planning
Health services in remote areas	Home care programs	Health manpower planning, training, and regulation
Ambulance services	Mental health services	Standard setting for health institutions and public places
Public health laboratories	Hospital and medical care	Health research
	Dental care	Health surveillance (communicable disease control)
	Prescription drugs	
	Services for allied health professionals	Emergency health services
	Other services, e.g., health appliances and equipment	Vital statistics
	Services for welfare recipients	

* Most provinces except Ontario

New Directions Development Division and has been delivered to regional boards for implementation. Regional boards are encouraged to include Aboriginal members.

Alberta has no Native health branch. Its Population Health and Program Development Division is responsible for developing policy with regard to Aboriginal health issues. During the process of planning and implementing regional health boards, Aboriginal participation was encouraged on regional boards and in policy consultations. Many of the northern regions of Alberta have substantial Aboriginal representation. Additionally, the Division recently released the Aboriginal Health Strategy to regional boards to assist the Regional Health Authorities (RHAs) and the Provincial Mental Health Board to consult with Aboriginal leaders and communities to provide health services in an appropriate, culturally sensitive way.

The Community and Mental Health Services Division in Manitoba has a Rural and Northern Operations branch. Primary care and public health nursing are provided by Manitoba Health to 23 northern and remote areas with limited access to other medical services and facilities. A 1964 Memorandum of Agreement divides responsibility between Manitoba Health and the Medical Services Division of Health Canada for providing health care services to northern communities that are distant from major medical centres. Clinical and community health services are provided under federal jurisdiction to communities with a majority Status Indian population, and under provincial jurisdiction to communities with a majority non-Status Indian and Métis population. Most recently, Manitoba Health has become involved in the development of the Aboriginal Health and Wellness Centre in Winnipeg. Aboriginal leaders play a key role in planning service delivery through this centre in a wellness-oriented and culturally appropriate manner.

Saskatchewan's Strategic Services Division has a Northern Health Services Branch, which provides primary care, public health nursing, mental health services, physician services, children's dental services, home care, public health inspection, nutrition counselling, speech and language pathology, and health education to residents of Northern Saskatchewan. Community mental health nurses and mental health social workers maintain regular contact with all northern communities including First Nations band offices to ensure that northern residents with mental health problems receive assistance and counselling. As well, community health educators provide interpretive services to people who speak Cree and Dene.

Ontario has established the Aboriginal Health Office responsible for implementing the Aboriginal Health Policy Framework and, with the Ministry of Community and Social Services, the Aboriginal Healing and Wellness Strategy. There are three basic directions for the development of a sound health policy for Aboriginal communities in Ontario. The first direction deals with the health status of Aboriginal groups, and relates to health promotion and illness prevention, wellness, addictions, mental health, long-term care, and disability. The second direction deals with access to health services, including issues of language and communication, patient advocacy, transportation to health facilities, the existence of appropriate and effective health facilities, training of health personnel, and the coordination of health services with traditional healing. The third direction deals with planning and representation, which includes participation of Aboriginal communities, representation on planning boards and boards of services delivery agencies, and public appointments to liaise with government. Ontario's Aboriginal Healing and Wellness Strategy is built on a framework of holistic health and well-being based on the presupposition that health must be addressed throughout the four life stages of an individual's life (infancy, youth, adulthood, and old age) in a holistic way (including physical, mental, emotional, spiritual, and cultural health) and within a continuum of care (including health promotion, prevention, treatment, and rehabilitation).

Occupational Health

Services designed to prevent accidents and occupational diseases and to maintain the health of employees are the common concern of provincial health departments, labour departments, workers' compensation boards, industrial management, and unions.

Provincial agencies regulate working conditions and offer consultant and educational services to industries. All provinces have legislation (covering factories, shops, mines, and workers' compensation) that set standards for work-related health, safety, and accident prevention. Most provinces maintain environmental health laboratories that study industrial health problems such as the effects of noise on workers.

The nature and extent of occupational health services vary from province to province depending on the type of industry. In provinces with large-scale mining operations, for example, there are usually strong programs to provide experts in dust control, toxicology, and industrial diseases. In other provinces, there may be a different mix of expertise as in provinces where insecticides or industrial chemicals are problems.

Public Health Laboratories

Public health laboratories assist with the identification and control of epidemic and endemic diseases. All provinces maintain a central public health laboratory, and most have branch laboratories to assist local health agencies and the medical profession in the protection of community health and the control of infectious diseases.

Women's Health

Women's health services range from involvement in breast screening programs, genetic services, and family violence to the health care needs of immigrant, refugee, and racial minority women. Currently, British Columbia, Ontario, Quebec, New Brunswick, Prince Edward Island, and Nova Scotia provide provincially funded breast cancer screening or mammography programs to some or all of their female residents.

5.2.2. Service Financing

As indicated above, all of the services listed here are financed totally or partially by the provincial government. As a result, provinces exert pressure on professionals and institutions for setting standards for the services and controlling costs. Recently, provinces are trying to manage the system through their financial clout.

Health Insurance Programs

The basic principles of hospital and medical insurance stated by the federal government were described in Chapter 11, so only the relevant features of the provincial insurance programs are described here. In some provinces, administration of the hospital insurance plan and the medical insurance plan is combined, whereas in others, the two plans have separate administrative structures.

Health insurance coverage is automatic and compulsory in all provinces, requiring only some form of registration. All provinces, except Alberta and British Columbia, fund their health care only through general revenues and/or a levy on payrolls. Alberta and British Columbia also have a component of premiums based on income. The *Canada Health Act Annual Report* published by Health Canada is an excellent source of details on the functioning of the health insurance plans in each province (the reader can also refer to the web sites listed in Appendix B) (16). Coverage for insured services is available to all Canadian residents on equal terms and conditions, and cannot be denied on grounds of age, income, or pre-existing conditions.

The federal government has established a Health Insurance Supplementary Fund (administered by the Health Insurance Division of Health Canada's Policy and Consultation Branch) with provincial contributions to provide for payment of claims for hospital or medical services for residents of Canada who have lost coverage through no fault of their own. This might occur, for example, if someone changing residence was not recognized as eligible under the rules of any province. It would not apply if coverage was lost through the individual's own fault, as in non-payment of premiums.

Those provinces that charge premiums make some provision to cover those unable to pay (such as welfare recipients and those whose incomes are slightly above the poverty level) through full and partial subsidies. All provinces also provide additional services for recipients of public assistance and for those over age 65. These commonly include prescription drugs and may also include dental services, eyeglasses, prostheses, home care services, and nursing home care, depending on the province. Additionally, provinces such as Ontario, Manitoba, Saskatchewan, Alberta, and British Columbia provide some money for the services of chiropractors, podiatrists, and optometrists. Usually there is a dollar limit on these services covered.

The Alberta Health Care Insurance Plan offers additional health insurance to residents who cannot obtain Alberta Blue Cross coverage through an employer on an individual basis at special rates. Non-group Blue Cross provides additional benefits for approved prescription drugs, accidental dental care, ambulance services, registered clinical psychological services, home nursing care, and so on. Blue Cross coverage is also provided at no charge to registrants aged 65 and older and their dependents, as well as to eligible widows and widowers aged 55 to 64 and their dependents. The Alberta Health Care Insurance Plan is partially funded by premiums. Medical and non-medical practitioners registered with the Plan are monitored by the Professional Review Board.

Drug Plans

The majority of Canadians have some form of coverage for prescription medicines. In 1995, it is estimated that 88% of Canadians had coverage: 62% were covered under private plans, 19% under provincial plans, and 7% were covered under both. Of the 12% of the population with no drug coverage, more than half were employees and their dependants whose employers do not provide a supplementary drug benefit plan. Fewer than 4% of Canadians without access to a drug benefit plan were self-employed and their dependants, and 2% were without employment and did not qualify for government or private plans (17). All provinces and territories provide drug coverage for residents receiving social assistance. Most provinces require that residents share at least some of the cost. In most provinces and territories, residents are enrolled in the government-sponsored seniors drug plan. When they reach age 65, residents are also usually expected to pay some of the costs, depending on income. In New Brunswick and Newfoundland, seniors' eligibility in the government-sponsored drug plan is based on income. In Saskatchewan, the eligibility requirements for seniors are the same as for other residents using the Saskatchewan Prescription Drug Plan. In Quebec, seniors who have access to group coverage can choose to maintain the group coverage rather than enrolling in the government plan.

Most provinces provide drug insurance for residents under age 65. Manitoba, Saskatchewan, and British Columbia have universal pharmacare programs. In Quebec, residents must have prescription drug coverage either by a group plan or the government plan administered by the Régie de l'assurance-maladie du Québec. In Alberta, residents under age 65 have access to a government-subsidized drug plan by paying premiums and enrolling. In Ontario, the Trillium Drug Plan provides relief for drug costs that are high relative to a recipient's income. Prince Edward Island, the Yukon, and Northwest Territories have programs for chronic disease and disabilities that provide prescription drugs for most chronic conditions. In addition, most provinces provide drugs for the treatment of venereal disease, tuberculosis, and other infections for which a public health hazard exists, and for which treatment costs are very high (for example, cystic fibrosis or AIDS).

The *Canada Health Act* includes drugs and biological and related preparations that are administered in the hospital within the definition of hospital services. However, prescription drug coverage in nursing homes or long-term care facilities across Canada differs. In British Columbia, Alberta, and Manitoba, costs are not shared with the resident. In Saskatchewan, Nova Scotia, Newfoundland, Yukon, and the Northwest Territories, residents of nursing homes are eligible for government-sponsored drug plans in the same manner as other residents in the community. In New Brunswick and Ontario, low-income residents of nursing homes do not share the costs or pay reduced amounts. In Quebec and Prince Edward Island, residents of publicly owned or sponsored nursing homes and long-term care facilities receive drugs without charge, while those in private facilities are responsible for their drug costs.

Dental Plans

Most provinces provide emergency basic dental health services to children, adults, and seniors on social assistance (18). Few provinces, such as British Columbia, Quebec, and Newfoundland, have special provision for children's dental programs, mainly in the area of preventive dentistry. The federal government provides basic dental services to Status Indians and Inuit with three delivery options: fee for service, contract session, or salaried staff.

Appliances and Equipment

Appliances and equipment comprise devices and equipment necessary or complementary to medical treatment. Provinces differ in the benefits provided, and the following examples illustrate inter-provincial variations.

The Alberta Aids to Daily Living (AADL) program is coordinated by the Public Health Division. AADL assists with the provision of program-approved medical equipment and supplies to Albertans living at home with a chronic or terminal illness or disability. Those over age 65 do not pay, while those under age 65 do — a discrepancy noted in the "Action Plan" of the Premier's Council on the Status of Persons with Disabilities.

The Medical Supply Services program in the British Columbia's Community and Family Health Division provides support to patients receiving specialized home maintenance care. The kidney dialysis service, for all home and community dialysis procedures, is the core operation of the program. Medical and nutritional supplies are also coordinated to address haemophilia, parenteral nutrition, and enteral nutrition. All of the program's services are provided with quality assurance and provincial advisory committees that cooperate closely with each patient's hospital. The Services to the Handicapped Branch has an At Home Program that provides respite support, medical equipment, and supplies to families caring for a child with severe disabilities. The Hearing Services Branch operates the British Columbia Hearing Aid Program to provide selection, fitting, repair, and sale of hearing devices at competitive prices.

Saskatchewan's Community Health Treatment Services Branch has the Saskatchewan Aids to Independent Living program, which provides equipment and other support to people with disabilities. People referred by designated health care professionals are eligible for benefits such as mobility and environmental aids and other special equipment, as well as for support for the costs of drugs and supplies required by certain conditions.

Within its Continuing Care Branch, Manitoba has a Home Care Equipment and Supplies Branch that provides a support service by acquiring, warehousing, distributing, maintaining, and repairing a range of medical supplies and equipment required in order to support the care and independent living of people with physical disabilities within their own communities. The equipment is purchased in bulk and provided on loan to eligible Manitoba residents under the authorization of a health care professional. People who are eligible include those who are physically disabled because of disease, traumatic injury, or the natural aging process, and need medical equipment to support their care and independence in the community. In 1994/95, there were 23,699 clients registered with the program. This number has been fairly steady for the past five years.

Ontario's Assistive Devices Program pays up to 75% of the price of goods such as electric wheelchairs, myoelectric limbs, hearing aids, and respiratory equipment. In 1993/94, just under 117,000 people were served by the program with a total expenditure of $82.25 million.

The Seniors Rehabilitation Equipment Program is run by the Community and Environmental Health Branch of the New Brunswick Public Health and Medical Services Division. Seniors may borrow, at no charge, standard and specialized equipment to assist in the activities of daily living. The equipment is loaned by the Canadian Red Cross Society and funded by the Department of Health and Community Services.

5.2.3. Administrative Services

Administrative Services are those operational functions that government undertakes to plan, forecast, and evaluate necessary services.

Planning of Health Services

All provincial ministries of health have a group of civil servants who, with the help of outside consultants, do short- and long-range planning of health services. These groups may be loosely structured or have a defined status within the ministry, such as the division of strategic planning and research within the Ministry of Health in Ontario.

Often the minister, recognizing the deficit in services, appoints a special committee composed of selected citizens and professionals who receive support from civil servants. The task of these committees is to recommend mechanisms for delivering health services to the population or sub-groups of the population. Some examples of these committees' reports are the *Rochon Commission Report* in Quebec, outlining the blueprint of health and social welfare services, the *Rainbow Report: Our Vision of Health* by the Premier's Commission on Future Health Care for Albertans, and *Nurturing Health: A Framework on the Determinants of Health* by the Ontario Premier's Council on Health Strategy.

Planning and Training of Health Human Resources.

The ministry of health in many provinces actively assesses the future needs for health human resources. In cases where there is an oversupply of health care professionals (for example, doctors and nurses), some of the provinces have taken active steps to reduce the number of students admitted into these professional schools, or to discourage immigration of these professionals. In situations where there is a lack of human resources, subsidies have been provided to students entering that profession. Several provincial governments have proposed a ban on any new billing numbers for new medical school graduates wishing to practice in the urban areas of their provinces or any areas where there is an oversupply of physicians. Frequently, such proposals are met with extremely negative reactions on the part of provincial medical associations. Nevertheless, the trend remains that new graduates choosing not to practise in underserved areas receive substantial cuts to their remuneration levels.

Regulation of Health Professions

The established health professions, including medicine, dentistry, and pharmacy, are regulated by their respective licensing bodies, which are mandated by provincial legislation. Other health care professionals and technicians are also usually regulated or certified (for details see Chapter 17).

Standard Setting for Health Institutions and Public Places

All of the acute, chronic, rehabilitation, extended care, and mental health hospitals are governed by specific legislation. Standards are set for nursing homes in many provinces as well. There are definite standards and guidelines for public places such as restaurants, food-handling places, industries, and factories. Legislation usually emanates from within the civil service or from concerned members of the legislature.

Health Research

Most provinces have intramural health research to help long-range planning of health services. Wealthier provinces, such as Alberta, British Columbia, Quebec, and Ontario, earmark funds for extramural research. These research grants are usually peer-reviewed and span from basic research to demonstration grants for updating health care systems. In some provinces, there has been a recent trend for the Ministry of Health to invite tenders for the areas to be researched.

Emergency Health Services

The Health Advisory Services Directorate, established in 1959 as part of Health Canada, encourages the provinces to develop their own emergency health services divisions, with the support of an advisory committee. These are organized under a provincial director who is generally assisted by a medical, paramedical, and a nursing consultant. Federal emergency health services are represented in the provinces by the Regional Director of the Medical Services Branch.

The four-fold tasks of provincial emergency health services are to ensure that vital health functions are maintained during or reorganized after emergency or disaster, to encourage and assist local planners in the establishment of emergency medical units, to train health care professionals and the general public in emergency health procedures, and to place emergency medical units from the national stockpile in strategic locations.

Vital Statistics

Each province has a registrar-general who is responsible for keeping records of vital events such as births, marriages, and deaths. This department usually provides statistical information pertaining to these vital events. The reporting of births, deaths, and marriages is mandatory in all provinces and specific forms are designed to record these events (see Chapter Two for information about birth and death certificates). These data are also provided to the federal government, which publishes national statistics. However, due to financial constraints, Statistics Canada recently announced that it will no longer publish nor require the collection of information on marriages. Statistics Canada asserts that, due to changing family structures in contemporary society, information on marriages is no longer relevant for health programs. Marriage statistics will continue to be collected through the Bureau of the Census.

6. PROVINCIAL HEALTH REFORMS

Faced with the similar pressures of growing government deficits, weakening economies, aging population, and increasing consumer demand, all ten provinces and the two territories are undergoing restructuring and reform in an effort to make the most of limited resources and still meet their population's health needs (19). The timing of the reform varies from province to province — some provinces, such as Alberta or Saskatchewan, began reform in the early 1990s, while others, such as Nova Scotia, started in the mid 1990s. Nevertheless, they are discovering common solutions to common problems. (The reports even use the same metaphors for health reform — a house undergoing construction or renovation, blueprints for reform, architects, and on!)

There is a general consensus among all the provinces for the following key aspects of reform.

6.1. REGIONALIZATION

As discussed in greater length in an earlier section, in an effort to increase flexibility and be more responsive to community needs, every province except Ontario has devolved decision making for health services delivery and financing allocation to the local level.

6.2. INCREASED FOCUS ON PREVENTION AND HEALTH PROMOTION

Every provincial reform report recognizes health as being more than the absence of disease and calls for greater emphasis on wellness through health promotion and disease prevention. Programs dealing with alcohol and drug abuse, AIDS and sexually transmitted diseases, healthy lifestyles and cancer, and high blood pressure screening will receive increased attention and funding in the future. This is particularly important in the Yukon, where preventable morbidity and mortality from accidents, injuries, and poisonings is the second leading cause of death. However, on a larger scale, it appears that emphasis for prevention and health promotion is rhetoric rather than reality as a very small proportion of health care expenditures are devoted to disease prevention and health promotion.

6.3. HEALTHY PUBLIC POLICY

Related to the increased focus on health promotion is the realization that the health sector does not exist in a vacuum. Most provincial reports called for increased cooperation and coordination among all government departments for their optimal effect on health; as the *Provincial Health System Reform Report* states: "Public policy designed to achieve province-wide health objectives must be written in cooperation with other government departments" (15). An example of this type of work is British Columbia's Ministry for Children and Families, which coordinates policy among the Ministries of Health, Social Services, Education, Skills and Training, and Women's Equality, and the Attorney General's Office.

6.4. FOCUS ON SPECIAL NEEDS GROUPS

With increasing fiscal pressures and the need to cut back, all provinces mention certain special needs groups as high priorities. In the Yukon, Alberta, and Manitoba, reports focus on the special needs of Aboriginal groups. Other examples include people with disabilities, single-parent families, and the poor. It is the expressed desire of provincial ministries that by shifting decision making to the local level, regional and district boards can identify the special needs groups particular to each community and develop programs to meet their needs.

6.5. MENTAL HEALTH REFORM

One special needs group consistently identified by every province in need of urgent reforms is people who are mentally ill. Paralleling the provincial reforms that focus on moving care closer to communities, most mental health reform proposes an integrated, community-based system of care. In addition, many provinces recognize that the needs of people who are mentally ill do not end with the provision of health services, and demand greater attention to and coordination of such issues as housing, income, and employment for this group.

6.6. LONG-TERM CARE AND HOME CARE REFORM

Recently, there has been a shift toward prevention and promotion activities and non-institutional alternatives to care; this is different from the past institutional focus of long-term care. Motivated largely by financial need and consumer preference for accessible health services closer to home or in a community setting, rather than in the more traditional and more expensive institutional setting, all provinces are planning to reform long-term care and home care. In an era of fiscal constraints, these two programs consistently receive increased funding.

6.7. INFORMATION SYSTEMS

In order to facilitate greater ease of informed decision making, there is increased interest in the development of integrated, system-wide information systems to be managed by provincial health ministries. Manitoba, building on its Drug Information System, is the farthest along in creating such a comprehensive system. Saskatchewan, Ontario, and Nova Scotia are currently conducting provincial consultations to assess system feasibility. Such an information system would give health care providers immediate access to patient information and medical history, thereby decreasing costly duplication of services, increasing the quality of care by providing complete medical histories, avoiding dangerous drug interactions, and making it easier for providers to assess possibilities for patient treatment and support services in the community. In addition, planners at the provincial, regional, and district levels would have access to complete, accurate information about service utilization patterns and outcomes. Concerns focus on confidentiality and security issues of such a large and comprehensive database.

Recently, a number of provinces have introduced unique identifier systems for individuals insured in their health plans. Individuals receive plastic cards with magnetic strips that store information on encounters with the medical care system, diagnoses, and treatment. There is a provision for confidentiality of medical information, and access to the relevant information is available only to authorized health professionals. This information system also supports research, program evaluation, and planning. To avoid the fraudulent use of cards by non-registrants, the Northwest Territories, Ontario, Saskatchewan, and Quebec have introduced photo identification cards similar to the driver's license, and other provinces are in the process of adopting such a system.

In addition to such integrated systems of health information gathering, most provinces also emphasize the need for evidence-based decision making as a critical component in increasing the cost effectiveness of health services provision. Research institutes such as Ontario's Institute for Clinical Evaluation Sciences (ICES), Quebec's Conseil d'évaluation de la technologie de la santé and Manitoba's Centre for Health Policy and Evaluation play a critical role in health services research, clinical evaluation, and evidence-based policy recommendations.

6.8. HEALTH SERVICES DELIVERY REFORM

In part motivated by the ongoing fiscal constraints and the related pressure for increased cost effectiveness in health care, and in part by the desire to de-institutionalize health services delivery, many provinces are considering integrated delivery systems. As hospitals downsize, merge, or even close in an effort to cut costs, vertically integrated health systems — covering the entire spectrum of primary to tertiary care — have been proposed as an ideal service delivery solution. Integrated health delivery systems (IDS) are covered in greater detail in Chapter 14. Briefly, these vertically integrated systems usually involve placing a particular group or community on the roster of a central health services centre that either directly provides or contracts for the provision of a wide variety of health services. The service package usually includes primary care, secondary or specialist care, home care, long-term care, and health promotion and disease prevention services.

In spite of growing fiscal pressures, most Canadian provinces remain dedicated to the principles of universality as stated in the *Canada Health Act*, choosing not to pursue privatization of service financing as an option in their reform packages. Only the Alberta and Ontario governments supported increased privatization within health. Alberta temporarily allowed the existence of privately financed diagnostic centres, but later changed its stance when federal transfer funds for health were cut to the province. The conservative Ontario government also supported the theory of increased funding for certain health services that would form an alliance, but did not go as far as Alberta in proceeding with private-pay clinics. The future direction of health system development in Canada will continue to be hotly debated and carefully watched.

7.   SUMMARY

This chapter dealt with the types of health services provided by the federal and provincial governments.

At the time of Confederation, the federal government had relatively little jurisdiction and involvement in the health care of Canadians. In 1919, the Department of Health was established and its responsibilities "include all matters relating to the promotion or preservation of health, social security and social welfare of the people of Canada over which the Parliament of Canada has jurisdiction". In 1945, Health and Welfare Canada was created with two primary tasks: to promote, preserve, and restore the health of Canadians, and to provide social security and social welfare to Canadians. In 1993, the Welfare Department of the Ministry was separated. The federal ministry of health is now known as Health Canada and is composed of five branches: the Health Promotion and Programs Branch; the Health Protection Branch; the Medical Services Branch; the Policy and Consultation Branch; and the Corporate Services Branch.

Three branches are of particular relevance to readers. The *Health Promotion and Programs Branch* provides financial and technical support to the provinces and territories for insured health care services and certain extended health care services, as well as promotes the adoption and maintenance of healthy lifestyles and fosters public research. This branch is made up of five units: health insurance, extramural research programs, health services, health promotion, and fitness. The *Health Protection Branch* protects the public against unsafe foods, drugs, cosmetics, medical devices, radiation-emitting devices, harmful microbes, technological and social environments as they relate to health, environmental pollutants and contaminants of all kinds, and fraudulent drugs and devices. This branch also monitors the occurrence and causes of communicable and non-communicable diseases, and establishes laboratory medicine standards. The *Medical Services Branch* is responsible for health care and public health services for Aboriginal peoples and all residents of the Yukon, as well as for quarantine, the health of civil servants, a national prosthetics service, emergency health services in the event of civil or natural disasters, and civil aviation medicine.

Health Canada has a number of other affiliated interdepartmental initiatives dealing with specific areas. For example, there is the National Advisory Council on Aging, the National AIDS Secretariat, the Blood Inquiry Secretariat and the National Forum on Health.

Income security and social services programs of the Ministry of Human Resources Development also influence health. They promote and strengthen the income security of Canadians, share in the cost of provincial and territorial social assistance, welfare services and rehabilitation programs, and assist in the development of social services to meet changing social needs.

As noted in earlier chapters, provincial governments have primary responsibility for all personal health matters such as disease prevention, treatment, and maintenance of health. Activities such as preventive health services, hospital services, treatment services for tuberculosis and other chronic diseases, and rehabilitation and care of people who are chronically ill and disabled are all under the jurisdiction of the provincial government.

The responsibilities of the provincial government can be classified as service financing, service delivery, and administrative services. Service delivery involves those services that, in most provinces, are under jurisdiction of the ministry of health with regard to budget, policies, and control. Examples include home care programs, public health services, and mental health services. Service financing, on the other hand, involves those services that are paid for either totally or partially by either government-run health insurance programs (for example, hospital and medical services provided by a physician) or by subsidizing the cost for services, drugs, or appliances. With these mechanisms, provinces exert pressure on professionals and institutions for setting standards for the services and controlling costs. Administrative services are those operational functions that government undertakes to plan, forecast, and evaluate the necessary services.

8.   REFERENCES

1.   Health Canada. A Question of Health: A Guide to the Federal Department of Health. Ottawa: Minister of Supply and Services Canada, 1994.
2.   Health and Welfare Canada. 1993-94 Estimates, Part III, Expenditure Plan. Ottawa: Minister of Supply and Services Canada, 1993.
3.   Health Protection Branch. Laboratory for Disease Control. Ottawa: Ministry of Supply and Services Canada, Health Canada, 1997.
4.   Human Resources Development Canada. Canada Assistance Plan. Ottawa: Ministry of Supply and Services Canada, 1995.
5.   Human Resources Development Canada. Canada Pension Plan: Review of Contributors. Ottawa: Ministry of Supply and Services, 1994.
6.   Health and Welfare Canada. The Child Benefit: A White Paper on Canada's New Integrated Child Tax Benefit. Ottawa: Ministry of Supply and Services Canada, 199.
7.   Health Canada. Tobacco Control: A Blueprint to Protect the Health of Canadians. Ottawa: Ministry of Supply and Services Canada, 1995.
8.   National Forum on Health. Report on Dialogue with Canadians. Ottawa: National Forum on Health, 1996.
9.   National Forum on Health. National Goals and the Federal Role in Health Care. Ottawa: National Forum on Health, 1995.
10.   National Forum on Health. What Determines Health? Ottawa: National Forum on Health, 1996.
11.   National Forum on Health. The Public and Private Financing of Canada's Health System. Ottawa: National Forum on Health, 1995.
12.   National Forum on Health. Summary Report: Evidence-Based Decision Making; A Dialogue on Health Information. Ottawa: National Forum on Health, 1995.
13.   National Forum on Health. Advancing the Dialogue on Health and Health Care: A Consultation Document. Ottawa: National Forum on Health, 1996.
14.   National Forum on Health. Canada Health Action: Building on the Legacy, Vol. 1: The Final Report of the National Forum on Health. Ottawa: Minister of Public Works and Government Services, 1997.
15.   Health Canada. Provincial Health System Reform in Canada. Ottawa: Ministry of Supply and Services Canada, 1995.
16.   Health Canada. Canada Health Act Annual Report: 1994-95. Ottawa: Ministry of Supply and Services Canada, 1996.
17.   Health System and Policy Division. Drug Costs in Canada. Ottawa: Health Canada, 1997.
18.   Main PA. Dental Public Health Programs in Canada 1995: Cross Canada Dental Check-up. Canadian Journal of Community Dentistry 1995;10(1):12-15.
19.   Canadian College of Health Service Executives. Health Reform Update, 1996-1997 (4th ed.). Ottawa: Canadian College of Health Service Executives, 1997.

Chapter

14

Funding, Expenditures, and Resources

Canadians are spending an increasing amount of their country's gross domestic product (GDP) on health care. GDP is a measure of the market value of all final goods and services produced in Canada by both Canadians and non-Canadians during a specified period. Gross national product, or GNP, considers production by Canadians only and hence these measures differ. For example, in 1960, Canada spent 5.3% of GDP on health care, whereas in 1996, it spent 9.5% of the GDP, or $75.2 billion. This translates to $2,511 per person spent on health care (1). It has been estimated that Canada's health care system spends $1 million every 6.9 minutes, or $206 million every day. Provinces are also allocating larger proportions of their total budgets to health every year, and this stretches their available resources.

The Canadian health system is one of the most expensive publicly financed health systems in the world (see Table 14.1). Due to increased competition for tighter resources in recent years, one of the major concerns of the federal and provincial governments has been how to restrain costs in the health care sector. Questions have been raised about the type of health resources, the effectiveness and efficiency of health resources utilization, the amount of health expenditures, and the need for an alternative delivery system. To answer these questions, one must know the characteristics, functions, and distribution of major health resources and the process and determinants of resource utilization, health expenditures, and the type of services produced.

In late 1980s and early 1990s most experts believed that the fundamental financial problems in the health care system were neither due to underfunding nor to overspending, but rather to poorly distributed and misdirected spending and ineffectively managed resources (2-4). However, in the late 1990s, with restructuring and financial cuts in health care, the balance may have reached equilibrium or perhaps even gone too far given Alberta's and Nova Scotia's recent announcements of increased funding in health care.

This chapter describes the financing of health services in Canada. Expenditure figures on health care are compared among the provinces and internationally and the process and determinants of resource utilization are discussed. This chapter

Table 14.1:   International Comparisons of Total Health Expenditures as a Percentage of Gross Domestic Product

Nation	Percentage				
	1960	1970	1980	1990	1995
Canada	5.5	7.2	7.4	9.1	9.6
France	4.2	5.8	7.6	8.9	9.9
Sweden	4.7	7.2	9.5	8.7	7.7
United Kingdom	3.9	4.5	5.8	6.1	6.9
United States	5.2	7.4	9.2	12.4	14.5

Sources: *Overview of International Comparisons of Health Care Expenditures*. Geneva: Organization for Economic Cooperation and Development, Health Data Bank, 1989. Schieber GJ and Poullier J-P, eds. *Health Care Systems in Transition: The Search for Efficiency*. Geneva: Organization for Economic Cooperation and Development, 1990, p12. Organization for Economic Cooperation and Development. OECD Health Data, CD Rom, Paris, 1997.

also describes the institutions and human health resources that account for much of health care expenditure in Canada and reviews current and anticipated initiatives directed toward achieving greater productivity for the enormous investment in the health sector.

1.   THE ORGANIZATION OF HEALTH CARE SYSTEM FINANCING: WHERE DOES THE MONEY COME FROM?

One of the most basic series of questions about the organization of any health care system relates to the financing of health services: Where does the money for health care come from? Where should it come from? How is it collected? What services and which groups of people are covered?

As discussed in the previous two chapters, Canada does not have a single "national health care system", but rather has a series of ten provincial and two territorial health systems all operating under the same founding principles and guidelines. Thus, although every province is autonomous in making its health finance decisions, there are certain generalities that apply to all. All of Canada has a predominantly publicly financed health system for hospitals and physician services, with universal coverage for all permanent residents regardless of their to ability to pay for care.

Figure 14.1 shows the many sources of funds for health care in Canada. Money is raised predominantly through provincial and federal taxes and is allocated, for the most part, from general provincial budgets. According to the *Canada Health Act*, each provincial health plan must cover all "medically necessary" health services delivered in hospital and by physicians. Provinces may choose to provide additional services such as children's or welfare recipients' dental services, and drugs and appliances for certain groups such as those over age 65 or welfare recipients. Extended health care services

Figure 14.1:   The Funding Structure of the Health System in Canada

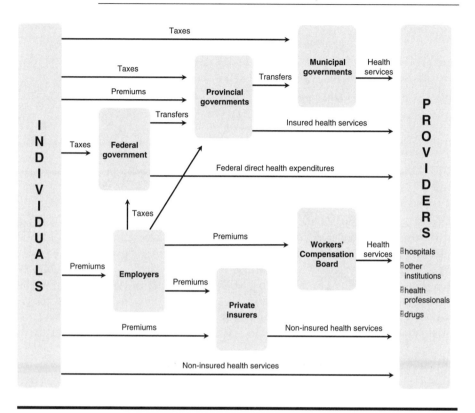

Source: Adapted from Health Canada.

and health care services offered by health care providers other than physicians may be covered at the discretion of each province or territory. Personal expenditures include dental and other services, such as those delivered by alternative health care providers not covered by government insurance and payments for extra services such as private hospital rooms. More recently, certain provinces have shifted costs to the private sector for post-accident rehabilitative care by charging personal automobile insurance policies for these fees. Non-insured health services and fees are covered either by private health insurance (voluntarily purchased on an individual basis or offered by an employee plan) or by the individuals. Treatment for work-related injuries and disease can be covered through the worker's compensation fund.

Public sector revenue (federal, provincial, and municipal government revenue generated from general taxes and borrowing) provides 69.9% of the money spent on health care (a few years ago, public spending used to be higher at 75%) and the remainder is paid by the individual either directly or through private health insurance (see

Table 14.2:   Percentage Distribution of Health Expenditures by Sector of Finance, Canada, 1996

Provincial expenditures*	64.4%
Federal direct	3.5%
Private expenditures	30.1%
Municipal expenditures	1.0%
Workers' compensation	0.8%
Other	0.2%

* includes federal funding from Canada health and social transfers

Source: *National Health Expenditures, 1996*. Canadian Institute for Health Information.

Table 14.2). This is much higher than the public share of health care costs in the United States, which is just under half (45.7%), but lower than the average figure of 75% public funding in other developed nations according to the Organization of Economic Cooperation and Development (OECD). Further, recent figures indicate that the public responsibility for funding health care in Canada is declining. In 1996, the total public sector share of health expenditures decreased by 0.5%, while the private sector increased by 5.5%. This marked the first public sector decrease in 20 years and reflects the current mood of government cost shifting that is leading to increased privatization of the Canadian health care system.

In Canada, the bulk of health care expenditures (64.4%) are financed from the general revenue by provincial governments. In turn, the federal government contributes to provincial revenue in the form of transfer payments, which are tax credits, and cash as agreed under the *Canada Health and Social Transfer Act*. Additionally, the federal government pays directly for 3.5% of the national health budget in the form of direct expenditures.

As described in Chapter 12, federal cash transfer payments to the provinces are diminishing, which has implications for the resources available to the provinces and the types of services they provide. The new transfer payment system — Canada Health and Social Transfer (CHST) — initially planned to cut the total amount of federal funds transferred to the provinces by $2.7 billion in the first year (1996/97) with an additional $1.8 billion cut in the second year. In the 1998 federal budget, however, the federal government promised that the CHST cash portion would be no less than $12.5 billion throughout the five-year agreement 1998/99 to 2002/03. This guarantee notwithstanding, the CHST federal block grant is designed to cover not only health services and postsecondary education (as the previous federal-provincial fiscal arrangements had done), but all social services as well. Because the CHST feeds directly into provincial budgets and allows each province to allocate whatever proportion it deems necessary for health, Health Canada and Statistics Canada no longer report statistics on proportions of provincial health expenditures financed through federal transfers.

Initially (as indicated in the historical overview in Chapter 12), the federal government split the costs of health care 50-50 with the provincial and territorial governments. Later, federal transfers were adjusted so that, up to 1996 the federal government paid for approximately one third of provincial health care costs in the form of federal transfers.

The provinces generate their share of the revenue for the health expenditures in the following manner (5):

- 72.5% of health care costs are paid by the public in the form of taxes;
- only Alberta and British Columbia charge individual premiums to those who request medicare benefits; Alberta earmarks money from the premiums for health care;
- Quebec, Manitoba, and Newfoundland levy payroll taxes on employers; Quebec charges a flat rate of 3.75% of every employer's payroll; Manitoba charges 2.25%; Newfoundland charges 1.5%, with smaller employers exempted. Payroll taxes tend to be controversial; they do not hit the poor as hard as flat-rate premiums, but they do not spread the net as wide, and the self-employed escape the tax altogether. Overall, however, payroll taxes do not generate a significant portion of health revenues and have recently been discontinued in Ontario.

Premiums and payroll taxes have only paid for about one tenth of health spending in Alberta and British Columbia and one quarter in Quebec in the past decade. General revenue is the predominant funding resource available for health care.

2.   HEALTH EXPENDITURES: HOW MUCH MONEY IS SPENT?

In 1996, Canada spent 9.5% of its GDP, or $75.2 billion, on health care. This is down slightly from its high point of 10.2% of GDP reached in 1992 and 1993. Table 14.3 shows that after many years of steady increases, health expenditures in Canada are currently slowly declining. Table 14.4 summarizes the most recent levels of health expenditures throughout Canada. The annual rate of increase overall in 1996 was 1.2%, which is down from 1.8% in 1994 and 1995, while substantially lower from the 8.6% increase experienced in 1991.

Statistics Canada, the chief source of such information, uses the following categories of health expenditures:

- *Institutional:* all types of hospitals and nursing homes;.
- *Professional:* services of physicians, dentists, chiropractors, naturopaths, osteopaths, optometrists, podiatrists, physiotherapists, private duty nurses, and Victorian Order of Nurses, but not professional services paid through institutions (e.g., nursing);

Table 14.3:   Trends in Health Expenditures in Canada, 1960-1996

	1960	1970	1980	1990	1996
Total expenditure (millions of dollars)	2,033	5,786	22,408	61,169	75,225
Per capita expenditure (dollars)	114	271	911	2,201	2,511
Percent of gross domestic product	5.5	7.2	7.2	9.1	9.5

These expenditures include both government and personal expenditures on health related goods and services.

Source: Canadian Institute for Health Information.

- *Drugs and appliances:* prescribed and over-the-counter drugs (except prescriptions dispensed in institutions), as well as eyeglasses, hearing aids, and other prostheses;
- *Other*: health services prepayment, administration of general public health activities, and research and construction of medical facilities.

The total health expenditure per capita in Canada has risen from $271 in 1970 to $2,511 in 1996 (in 1998 dollars). Over the last few years, less than half (34.2%) of Canadian health expenditures went to institutional care hospitals; homes for special care received, 10.0%; about a quarter (23.2%) was spent on professional services (physicians, 14.4%; dentists 6.4%; and other professionals, 2.4%), and about 14.5% on drugs and appliances (see Table 14.5). Thus the major portion (82.0%) was spent on personal health care, and the remainder on public and voluntary health agencies, research, and health insurance administration.

2.1. INSTITUTIONAL EXPENDITURES

Of the $34 billion spent on institutional care in 1994, more than three quarters (79%) was for general and allied special hospitals. On average, the per diem cost in acute care hospitals has been usually two to three times higher than that in chronic or long-term care hospitals. The estimated cost of one day's stay in a public hospital was $552 in 1992/93, of which about 73% paid staff costs (salaries, wages, and employee benefits, based on 16.8 staff hours per patient per day).

Almost all of the funding of Canada's 1,200 hospitals comes from provincial governments. The cost of running a hospital has risen roughly 8% per year over the past decade, although this rate of increase has significantly slowed since 1991. Due to increasing pressures across the country to control health care costs, public hospitals indicate a negative (-2.4%) average annual growth in operating expenses since 1991/92.

Table 14.4:   Provincial Health Expenditure Information, 1996

Province	1996 population (thousands)	Health expenditure as % of GDP	Health expenditure as % of provincial budget	Per capita health expenditure
Newfoundland	570.7	13.6	31.2	$2,340
Prince Edward Island	137.3	12.3	32.1	$2,435
Nova Scotia	942.8	11.4	31.9	$2,293
New Brunswick	762.5	11.8	31.3	$2,438
Quebec	7,389.1	9.8	29.0	$2,343
Ontario	11,252.4	9.1	36.8	$2,621
Manitoba	1,143.5	11.4	34.2	$2,652
Saskatchewan	1,022.5	9.8	35.0	$2,451
Alberta	2,789.5	7.4	31.1	$2,290
British Columbia	3,855.0	10.0	32.1	$2,685
Northwest Territories	66.6	14.9	16.9	$5,295
Yukon Territory	31.5	11.0	13.6	$3,381

Source: Canadian Institute for Health Information.

This has been largely due to hospital downsizing, restructuring, and re-engineering. Wages, salaries and benefits account for almost three quarters of the operating budgets of public hospitals, with 45% of this budgetary portion paying nurses. Canada has more than 264,000 working registered nurses, who earn between $27,475 and $52,000 per year (a total of 7.16 paid nursing hours per patient day).

Several factors have led to the traditionally increasing hospital costs:
* Binding arbitration of unsettled labour disputes;
* Increases in workers' compensation assessments, payroll health taxes, employment insurance, and Canada Pension Plan payments;
* New laws on environmental protection, pay equity, and occupational health and safety;
* New technology, drugs, and treatment methods (hospital drug costs alone have risen 10% to 14% per year);
* The cost of other supplies and services, which has risen faster than government financing.

As detailed in section 4.2 hospitals are treating more people on an outpatient basis in response to these increasing hospital costs. Between 1986/87 and 1994/95, the number of outpatient visits rose by 15%, while inpatient days decreased by 17%, which created significant financial advantages for Canadian hospitals. According to Statistics

Table 14.5:   Percentage Distribution of Health Expenditures by Category of Expenditure, 1996

Hospitals	34.2%
Physicians	14.4%
Drugs	14.4%
"Other" expenditures (e.g., home care, transportation, assistive devices)	10.7%
"Other" institutions (residential care for special needs groups, e.g., the elderly, disabled, mentally ill, addicted, disturbed children)	10.0%
"Other" professionals	8.8%
Public health	5.0%
Capital expenditures	2.5%

Source: *National Health Expenditures, 1996.* Canadian Institute for Health Information.

Canada's *Health Reports*, this shift from inpatient to outpatient care is one of the major contributing factors leading to the recent negative rate of growth of annual hospital operating expenditures between 1991/92 and 1993/94 (6).

2.2. PROFESSIONAL EXPENDITURES

In 1972, fee payments to physicians totalled $0.6 billion. Relatively high fee increases in some provinces, especially in British Columbia, Ontario, and Alberta in the early 1980s, caused significant changes in these figures. Physicians receive about 14.5¢ of every health care dollar in the form of fees; however, how they decide to treat patients significantly influences how the rest of the money is spent. For example, it is estimated that every doctor in Ontario costs the system about $500,000, one half in direct billings and the other half in drugs prescribed, laboratory tests ordered, and hospital admissions authorized.

In 1992, the 61,650 active civilian doctors in Canada billed an average of $188,000 each. More than 90% of doctors in private practice are paid on a fee-for-service basis. Government employees, community health centre staff, and most of Canada's 7,813 hospital interns and residents are salaried doctors.

In 1996, the expenditure for professional services by physicians, dentists, and other specialists amounted to about $17.5 billion (23.2% of total spending); this does not include professionals employed by institutions, such as nurses, physiotherapists, occupational therapists, social workers, and some physicians. Of that figure, physicians' services alone constituted approximately 62%, amounting to $10.9 billion. This includes gross fees for physicians in private practice only. Just under 9¢ of each health care dollar is spent on the services of dentists and other health care professionals such as chiropractors, optometrists, and physiotherapists. Almost all of this amount goes to dentists.

2.3. DRUGS, APPLIANCES, AND OTHER EXPENDITURES

Expenditures for drugs are the third largest category of health expenditures in Canada comprising 14.4% of total health expenditures. In 1996, $10.8 billion was spent on drugs and appliances, and half of that was for prescription drugs. Drugs and appliances claimed 14.5¢ of the health care dollar, up from 9¢ in 1975. The annual rate of increase of drug expenditures is 2.7%, making the drug category among the three fastest growing categories of health expenditures in 1996 (together with public health expenditures and "other" institutions). Furthermore, drug expenditures account for the largest category of private expenditures in Canada for health care, 36% of total private health expenditures.

British Columbia, Manitoba, and Saskatchewan provide subsidized prescription drug coverage to all of their residents subject to certain limitations (such as only certain drugs are covered); the other provinces usually pay only for certain groups, such as those over age 65, people with certain serious or chronic illnesses, and people on social assistance. Recently, however, small co-payments or user charges have been introduced even for these population groups. Efforts to prevent illness, mainly on the part of public health units and voluntary agencies, cost about 5% of total health expenditures. Other items (such as eyeglasses and the administrative costs of running private health insurance plans) accounted for about 11% of the health care dollar.

3.   DETERMINANTS OF RESOURCE UTILIZATION: HOW IS THE MONEY SPENT?

The utilization of resources is a very complex subject, so only the most salient features are described here. Resource utilization depends on several factors:
- Availability of resources, such as the ratio of health care professionals to population, hours of work per person, the type and nature of health care professional mix, and the number and type of hospital beds per 1,000 people;
- General characteristics of the community that affect the need for services such as age distribution, housing quality, economic development, and level of sanitation.
- Personal factors that affect the need for services, such as attitudes, age, sex, family size, marital status, health insurance coverage, education, income, and perceived need for care;
- Characteristics of the health care system, such as points of entry, accessibility of resources, cost, and barriers to care;
- Burden of illness or the need.

The impact of points of entry on the utilization is described on the following pages and in greater detail in Chapter 15. There are many entry points into the health

Figure 14.2:   The Points of Entry to the Health Care System

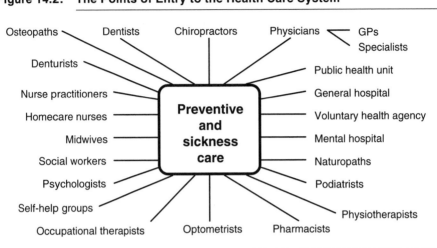

care system (see Figure 14.2). With provincial and private health insurance plans (which cover dental, drug, and private nursing), there are relatively few financial barriers at these entry points. The services of psychologists, social workers, dentists, denturists, and nurse practitioners in private practice are less commonly covered, except those in northern areas making these entry points more costly to the consumer, if not to government budgets. Most people however, receive their primary care through general/family practitioners and use specialized resources upon referral by those practitioners, who play a gatekeeper role.

It should be noted that current health care systems are heavily oriented to the treatment of illness. At present, there is little effective coordination of specialized care within and between hospitals, and arrangements for coordinating services between primary and specialized care are poorly developed in most parts of the country. People have direct access to primary or secondary care, depending on their proximity to and knowledge of resources and their attitudes toward the system. As most health care planners see it, there should be a linear progression by the individual to primary care to secondary care to tertiary care, as required (see Figure 14.3). However, this progression would be difficult to achieve in the present health care system unless its organization and payment system are drastically restructured, which is why several provinces are currently considering the creation of integrated service delivery systems.

Integrated delivery systems (IDS) are defined as "a network of organizations that provides or arranges to provide a coordinated continuum of services to a defined population and is willing to be held clinically and fiscally accountable for the outcomes and the health status of the population it services" (7). The continuum of both primary and specialized services provided in such care arrangements most often includes primary

Figure 14.3:   Patient Progress through System

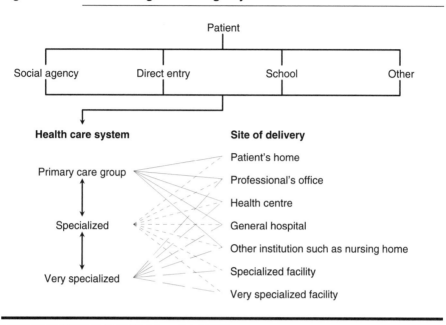

Source: *Report of the Health Planning Task Force (Ontario) 1974.*

care, health promotion and disease prevention programs, secondary care with links to tertiary care facilities, rehabilitation, palliative care, and long-term care, home care, and community support services (see also the description of comprehensive health organizations in Chapter 15). IDS can provide these services or purchase services through contracts with outside care providers — whichever is the most cost-effective use of existing resources. The system of payment for IDS varies, but most often requires a roster of a particular population group with physician remuneration for services based on a capitation formula. As illustrated in Figure 14.3, the physical site of service delivery in IDS may be the same for primary, specialized, and very specialized care. Certainly, most of these services, as well as their coordination, management, and financing, would occur in some single location. A recent Health Canada paper stated the *Canada Health Act* does not preclude rostering of individuals in a plan as long as a person has a choice to leave the group at specified time. This interpretation will pave the way for reform in primary health care.

The two major resources needed for the provision of health care are institutions and health care personnel. They are also the most expensive, accounting for 34.2% and 23.2% respectively of total health care expenditures in Canada in 1996 (see Table 14.5), although these figures are currently declining.

Table 14.6:   Number and Ratio of Active Health Human Resources, 1992

Health occupation	Total number	Ratio to population	Ratio in 1976
Audiologists & speech therapists	3,747	1 : 7,631	1 : 22,119
Chiropractors	3,748	1 : 7,629	1 : 13,623
Dentists	14,897	1 : 1,919	1 : 2,463
Dental assistants	2,091	1 : 13,675	1 : 7,909
Dental hygenists	10,529	1 : 2,716	1 : 11,962
Dieticians and nutritionists	6,397	1 : 4,470	1 : 8,726
Health records administrators	3,457	1 : 8,271	1 : 11,269
Health services executives	2,824	1 : 10,125	1 : 19,331
Technologists:			
Electroneurophysiology	293	1 : 97,588	1 : 69,965
Laboratory	19,367	1 : 1,476	1 : 1,415
Radiation	12,890	1 : 2,218	1 : 2,890
Respiratory	3,848	1 : 7,431	1 : 17,692
Nursing:			
Registered	234,128	1 : 122	1 : 168
Licensed nursing assistant	83,749	1 : 341	1 : 323
Occupational therapists	6,195	1 : 4,616	1 : 15,388
Opticians	4,352	1 : 6,570	1 : 10,056
Optometrists	2,734	1 : 10,458	1 : 13,128
Orderlies	17,763	1 : 1,574	1 : 1,554
Osteopaths	28	1 : 1,021,193	1 : 345,648
Pharmacists	18,969	1 : 1,507	1 : 1,658
Physicians	61,649	1 : 464	1 : 557
Physiotherapists	11,363	1 : 2,516	1 : 16,449
Public health inspectors	1,607	1 : 17,793	1 : 28,697

Source: *Health Personnel in Canada, 1990*, Ottawa. Ministry of Supply and Services, 1992.

3.1. TYPES OF SERVICES PRODUCED BY RESOURCE UTILIZATION

The ultimate aim of the health care industry is to produce good health. However, even though it is difficult to measure health, the measurement of sickness care has two dimensions.

- *Outcome measurement.* Improvement, no improvement, deterioration, or death constitute different measurable outcomes of sickness, although except for death, those may be subjective. Also, the outcome can result from factors other than health services. Hence, outcome measurement is not always possible, despite being preferred by many health care planners.

- *Utilization measurement.* It is easier, although ultimately less useful, to measure the type and amount of resources used rather than their effects on the patient. Utilization or process measurements are very commonly used, and considered to have a positive effect on the outcome, although there is no consistent evidence to support this hypothesis.

4.   HEALTH RESOURCES AND THEIR MEASUREMENT

4.1. INSTITUTIONAL RESOURCES

The most expensive health resources are the institutions, because they rely heavily on technology and human resources. The Federal-Provincial Task Force has classified institutions based on the type of care they provide: type 1 is residential care, type 2 is extended health care, type 3 is chronic care, type 4 is special rehabilitative care, and type 5 is acute care. Statistics Canada classifies hospitals according to the service provided:

- General hospitals that provide acute care in the community, which may have units for long-term care; if a general hospital is affiliated with the university, then it is called a teaching hospital;
- Allied special hospitals that provide chronic care, such as rehabilitation or extended care, or deal with special age groups (e.g., paediatrics) or specific conditions (e.g., cancer);
- Nursing homes that are organized residential facilities where some residents receive nursing care from full-time registered or licensed practical nurses, medications are supervised, and assistance is provided for three or more activities of daily living (e.g., bathing, dressing, walking, eating); and
- Mental institutions that include mental hospitals dealing with chronic long-term mental illness, psychiatric hospitals and psychiatric units in general hospitals dealing with short-term intensive psychiatric treatment, and special facilities for people who are emotionally or mentally challenged.

According to the most recent Statistics Canada figures, there has been a marked decline in the number of hospitals and hospital beds throughout Canada. Since 1986, the number of public hospitals in Canada fell by 14%, while their bed capacity fell by 11% (6). Nevertheless, in fiscal year 1996, hospitals accounted for 34.2% of all health care expenditures in Canada — the largest single component of the health budget — compared with 40.7% in 1986. In fiscal year 1994/95 (the last year for which complete hospital data are available at the time of writing), Canada had 901 general, allied, special, private, and governmental hospitals with a capacity of 120,774 staffed beds (the number of beds actually available, although the total number of beds approved was 156,547). Public hospitals accounted for 92% of all hospitals and 98% of the beds (8). Of the public hospitals, 73% of the approved beds were in general hospitals, 10% were in extended care hospitals, and the rest were distributed among psychiatric, paediatric, and rehabilitation hospitals. There were 41 separate mental institutions with 13,262 beds (1993 data).

Although there is no standard definition of "long-term care centre" in Canada, it usually includes homes for special care, nursing homes, homes for the aged, and community care facilities. In 1993, there were 6,148 long-term care centres with a total bed capacity of 238,386 (9). Most general and chronic hospitals and the majority of nursing homes are publicly owned, and most mental institutions are owned by provincial governments.

For every 1,000 Canadians in 1994/95, there were 4.1 beds in institutions (2.8 beds for short-term care or shared short-/long-term care beds, and 1.3 beds exclusively for long-term care) and 8.6 beds in homes for special care (including homes for seniors, people who are physically challenged, and people who are developmentally delayed). These bed capacities are among the highest in western nations but continue to fall each year as fiscal pressures on hospitals continue.

Of course, interprovincial variations exist within each category, due mainly to the fact that the population is widely dispersed rather than different morbidity patterns in population. For example, the small nursing stations in remote and rural areas each have a few beds, so there are more beds per 1,000 population even though the number of actual bed days per patient is less than the Canadian average. Alberta and Ontario have the lowest bed capacity for general and speciality hospital beds (non-residential care), Quebec the highest. Alberta and Prince Edward Island have the lowest residential bed capacity, while British Columbia and Quebec have the highest (8). As the policy of fiscal restraint continues in Canada, further closures of hospital beds will shrink the bed capacities even more in future years.

For mental institutions, the rated bed capacity in 1993/94 for Canada was 0.6 per 1,000 persons; the rates in New Brunswick and Quebec are significantly higher, and Saskatchewan, Nova Scotia, Alberta, and British Columbia are somewhat lower. The de-institutionalization of mental patients, which means a shift to community-based living, has resulted in a decline in bed capacity.

For special care facilities, the rated bed capacity was 8.6 per 1,000 population in Canada in 1993. In addition to providing care for people with special needs, these include nursing homes, and facilities with a minimum of four beds that provide nursing, custodial, or counselling services but not active treatment. Capacity rates vary widely among the provinces, from 11.9 beds per 1,000 population in Saskatchewan and 16.9 in Prince Edward Island to 5.4 in Quebec. Newfoundland, Yukon, and the Northwest Territories all have rates below the Canadian average, possibly because of the age structures of their population. However, federal-provincial financial arrangements prior to 1977 did not include extended care; the newer financing arrangements include a per capita grant for extended care as defined in the 1977 agreement, which has partially reduced the disparity.

4.2. UTILIZATION MEASUREMENTS FOR INSTITUTIONAL CARE

In the 1994/95 fiscal year, in those Canadian general and allied special hospitals that report this statistic, the number of inpatient hospitalization days (or patient days, as they are commonly called) reached 43 million. This is a 17% decline since 1986/87, and represents a rate of fewer than 1,500 days per 1,000 population. The average length of hospital stay for 1994/95 was 11.1 days including chronic care and long-term psychiatric cases, or 7.0 days if acute care only is considered. The average length of stay for hospital care was the shortest in British Columbia and Alberta (6.5 days), while Quebec had the longest average length of stay (9 days). Although provincial variations continue to exist, due to increasing pressures to use hospital resources more efficiently, the length of stay for inpatient care continues to decrease. By 1995, Ontario, for example, had reached an average length of stay of 9.7 days for all types of care, with an average of 3.1 days if acute care cases only are considered. While average length of stay for long-term care hospitalization (153 days) is much higher than for acute care, this too shows the same decreasing trends.

Hospital separation rates per 1,000 population ("separations" include discharges plus deaths) as another indication of hospital utilization. These rates also varied among the provinces. In 1992/93, the national rate was 128 per 1,000, ranging from 112.7 in British Columbia to 190.5 in Saskatchewan. There was a definite downward trend in hospital admissions per 1,000 population from 1974 to 1993 (from 165 to 128). More than 15.9 million patient days were spent caring for people in psychiatric and general hospitals in 1993/94, but many of these patient days were attributed to people with a very long duration of stay.

Another measurement of hospital utilization is the number of visits to emergency and ambulatory care units. During the 1993/94 fiscal year for example, there were 15.9 million emergency care visits in all types of hospitals in Canada; general and special ambulatory clinics received 17.7 million visits throughout Canada. Additionally, there were just over 1.8 million hospital separations involving surgical procedures on a day care basis. While the number of visits to emergency rooms has remained virtually unchanged in the past eight years, the number of outpatient visits for day surgery, visits to speciality clinics, and visits to ambulatory day-and-night-care programs has increased 37%, 24%, and 46% respectively. The transfer of patients from inpatient units to care on an outpatient or ambulatory care basis reflects an important trend in recent years, designed to increase hospital cost efficiency and decrease bed occupancy rates. While inpatient days declined by 17% to 43 million between 1986/87 and 1993/94, outpatient visits increased by 15% for a total of 38 million visits. In 1993/94, there were 0.88 outpatient visits recorded for every inpatient day recorded across Canada (up from 0.64 in 1987). The ratio of the outpatient visits to inpatient days varied from province to province, with the highest ratio recorded in the Northwest Territories (1.83 outpatient visits per inpatient day) and Alberta (1.25). The lowest ratio was recorded in British Columbia (0.5 outpatient visits per inpatient day).

4.3. HUMAN HEALTH RESOURCES

Human health resources consist of those individuals who provide direct health services (such as nurses, physicians, dentists, chiropractors, and respiratory technicians) and those who provide ancillary and support services (such as maintenance and repair, housekeeping, food services, and administration).

4.4. DISTRIBUTION OF HUMAN HEALTH RESOURCES

The health care sector is considered the third largest industry in the country, employing more than 800,000 Canadians. About 60% of these directly provide health services, and 40% are in ancillary jobs. About 80% of all health care employees work in institutions.

The most up-to-date data on health care personnel in Canada are kept on physicians, nurses and physiotherapists, and data from 1992 *Health Personnel in Canada* listed 557,080 individuals providing direct health services to Canadians (10). Of these, 57.1% (318,093) were nurses and nursing assistants, 11.1% (61,835) were physicians, 5.9% were health technologists, 5.0% worked in dentistry and allied occupations, and 3.4% were in pharmacy. Since 1992, the number of physicians and nurses has decreased, falling to 55,006 and 232,869 respectively. These numbers reflect current trends in downsizing. Since World War II, the traditional health care professions of physicians, nurses, and dentists have expanded to include over 150 categories of health care occupations. Most are extensions of established health care professions (e.g., nurses' aids, licensed practical nurses, technicians, nurse practitioners, dental hygienists, dental technicians). Others have developed from some special body of knowledge (e.g., clinical psychologists). As these new occupations evolved, many of their practitioners tried to achieve independent status as self-regulatory professions. Most provincial governments are now beginning to regulate and license them (see Chapter 16).

Human health resources are unevenly distributed and mainly concentrated in large urban centres and in wealthy provinces such as Ontario, Quebec, and British Columbia. Over the past few decades they have significantly increased in number, thus reducing their ratio to the population in most categories (see Table 14.6). This trend is now stabilizing, or slowly being reversed (as is the case with physicians and nurses) (11).

4.4.1. Nurses

Registered nurses represent just under 50% of all health human resources in Canada. In 1995, of the total 263,683 nurses registered in Canada, 89.1% were actively employed in nursing. There was one active nurse per 128 population. Most (66%) worked in hospitals (including psychiatric hospitals), while 6% worked in community health settings, 11% in nursing homes, 2.8% worked in educational institutions, and the remainder worked in other settings such as home care, rehabilitation centres or in private-duty nursing. Part-time nurses constituted a growing proportion of the nursing workforce in all health care sectors. In 1995, part-time nurses accounted for over one third of all actively employed registered nurses, and there was one licensed nursing assistant per 341 population (12, 13)

4.4.2. Physicians

In 1995, Canada had 61,649 active civilian physicians, of whom 7,813 (12.7%) were interns and residents. Of the remainder (55,006), 52.0% were general practitioners and 48.0% were specialists. The physician-to-population ratio was 1:542; according to the World Health Organization, the optimum ratio is 1:655. The national average in 1995 was one general practitioner per 1,042 population and one specialist per 1,130 population: Nova Scotia, Quebec, and Ontario were above the national average while the Yukon and Northwest Territories, Alberta, Saskatchewan, and the Atlantic provinces (with the exception of Nova Scotia) had relatively low ratios, primarily due to the small numbers of specialists in those provinces. However, Quebec had a relatively high proportion of specialists (50.3%) and was the only province where that figure exceeded 50%. Quebec and Ontario had the largest numbers of interns and residents, and Prince Edward Island and New Brunswick the smallest. Many provinces are now concerned about this high physician-to-population ratio and are taking steps to curtail the number of physicians.

4.5. UTILIZATION MEASUREMENTS FOR PROFESSIONAL SERVICES

The most detailed information is available for physicians because physicians are generally paid directly through provincial health insurance per item. For 1993/94, there were approximately 350 million medical consultations and visits in all ten provinces, an average of about 12 per person. The total amount of money spent on physician services in Canada in 1996 was less than $10.8 billion, or $362 per capita. This is lower (-1.0%) than in 1991. In Ontario, in 1994/95, for example, payments for professional fees-for-service amounted to $5 billion, with an average of 13 claims per insured person at a cost of $470 per capita. Of this amount, 90% went to physicians and the rest to other private-practice professionals, including chiropractors, optometrists, physiotherapists, dentists, chiropodists, and osteopaths, as well as to some professional services with special payment arrangements. Also covered were payments for out-of-province care, health centres, and sexually transmitted disease clinics. These figures may be compared with total payments of $541 million in 1972/73, an average of 5.10 claims per insured person, of which 94% were for medical services; and total payments of $742 million in 1975/76, an average of 6.14 claims per insured person and 95% for physician services. Thus the number of services per capita has steadily increased, as has the cost of these services. The factors affecting this trend may be driven by consumers or providers, or both.

Ontario's physician billing data according to the Ontario Health Insurance Plan (OHIP) illustrate some of the factors that results in rising expenditures. First, there has been an overall increase in total physician billings from $1.06 billion in 1980/81 to $4.1 billion in 1994/95. Due to government policies of "clawing back" physician earnings that exceed a specified amount in any given year, only $3.8 billion of this amount was actually paid to physicians. Nevertheless, this figure amounts to a 258.1% increase in OHIP billings over 15 years (or an average increase of 10.1% annually). Part of the increase is due to physician factors, such as an increase in the number of physicians working in Ontario, while a smaller portion is due to an increase in the province's population. From 1980/81 to 1994/95, the number of physicians billing OHIP increased by 56.3% (or 3.3% annually). In that same period, the number of people living in Ontario increased by 25.1% (1.6% annually). However, it is important to remember that within the increase in Ontario's overall population, there was a 51.6% increase in the number of people age 65 and over — that group of people who require more frequent and more costly medical care. Thus, the combination of increased numbers of physicians (increased supply) and increased numbers of people, especially of the elderly (increased demand) has greatly increased utilization. One may speculate about the extent to which this increase is also caused by increased needs or expectations of the consumer versus physician-generated factors, such as extra recalls and procedures. Also of great importance is whether better health resulted from this increase. Current provincial policies undertaken to alleviate some of these physician-related cost increases are covered in a later section of this chapter.

5.   CONTROLLING HEALTH CARE COSTS

Two of the major problems facing the Canadian economy in general and the health care system in particular are the amount and type of resources used to produce "health" and "sickness care."

In 1996, Canada spent 9.5% of its GDP on health care, which is a 180% increase from 1960 (but the fourth annual decrease in overall GDP spent on health since 1990). The first significant rise was in the late 1960s, following the introduction of universal health insurance. By the early 1970s, the federal and provincial governments became alarmed by this rapid rise and set up a task force on the cost of health services, which delivered its report in 1970. Attempts to control the level of health expenditure met with temporary success in the 1970s. The proportion of GDP declined initially and then levelled off from 1973 to 1980 in the range of 7.4% to 7.5%, although both the actual dollars and per capita dollars spent had risen. Since 1981, it has been rising again.

To put the current figure in an international perspective, it is useful to compare Canada's health care expenditures with that of other countries (see Table 14.1) The trend for health care expenditures indicates that the percentage spent on health continued to increase until 1992, when it stabilized and began slowly decreasing. While Canada spent 9.6% of its GDP on health care in 1995, the United Kingdom spent 6.9% and the United States, 14.5%.

Many factors contribute to these international variations in health care expenditures. As described in Chapter 12, these health care systems differ widely in their sources of funding, including the balance of private and public funding. They also vary in the degree and form of state planning, the remuneration of health care professionals (particularly physicians), and the nature of services provided. Thus international comparisons are of questionable significance since they tell us what nations spent, but little, if anything, about how they spent it — the mix of services, possible duplication of facilities, physician-to-population ratios, health care needs, or system inefficiencies. There is no evidence that Americans, for example, are healthier because their country spends a higher share of GDP on health care.

One significant difference between the health care system in the U.S. and in Canada is the administrative cost. In the U.S., which has voluntary medical and hospital insurance systems, 12.5% of spending goes to administrative overhead, whereas Canadian administrative costs are less than 3%. Furthermore, there are savings in Canadian hospital administrative costs because there is no need to price and itemize every service, bandage, and pill on the patient's bill. The savings in accounting, nurses' time, and paperwork are large.

Moreover, there are savings in the more rational distribution of high technology such as MRI scanners, which hospitals in the U.S. acquire for competitive reasons and then frequently under-utilize. The Canadian single-payer system — the provincial government — pays for hospital and physicians, covering 69% of the total cost of health care in Canada. Provincial governments are directly responsible for the overall allocation and coordination of resources to the health services sector. This avoids the fragmentation of decision making and wasteful competition for resources that can occur when independent non-profit or fee-for-service providers seek financing from a variety of private and public sources. Although Canadians are faced with their own set of health system challenges, the single-payer financing system, together with universal coverage for all Canadians has proven more effective than the U.S. market system of health in controlling overall health expenditures but less effective than in some European countries.

5.1. COST-CONTAINMENT STRATEGIES FOR INSTITUTIONAL RESOURCES

5.1.1. Rationalization

Rationalization of health services may involve restructuring, realignment, downsizing, decentralization, and some institutional closures. These changes are undertaken to minimize duplication of services, provide appropriate levels and types of care, consolidate strengths, and create innovative structures and functional arrangements that make more effective use of resources and contain costs. Many analysts maintain that the central problem of health services in Canada is that hospitals and other medical institutions have acted in the interests of the health care providers instead of the communities they serve.

Rationalization usually involves major transformations of the health care system. Although it occurs in every province, Alberta is a particularly good example

(14). Alberta began to restructure its health care system toward the end of 1993, when the Minister of Health announced the Health Plan Coordination Project. True to the current emphasis on public participation, the plan was guided by a Steering Committee made up of representatives of government, health care providers, union leaders, business leaders, and members of the public. It was tailored to meet certain previously determined goals recommended by the Steering Committee and involved the following main components:

- Devolution of decision making and decentralization of service delivery to 16 Regional Health Authorities (RHAs);
- Restructuring and reorganization of the Ministry of Health moving away from service delivery toward more policy development and evaluation;
- Rationalization and increased cost effectiveness of acute care services through decreased lengths of stay in hospital, hospital closures, consolidations, and downsizing; the amalgamation of all hospital and community agency boards into RHAs; and the implementation of a clinical practice guidelines program;
- Rationalization and restructuring of mental health services through the creation of the Mental Health Board, which assumed the responsibilities for two provincial mental health hospitals, 52 community mental health clinics, and two extended care clinics;
- Reallocation of existing resources from acute care to community-based services (especially in long-term care and for early discharge patients) and to health promotion programs;
- The definition of "core health services" that must be available or reasonably accessible to all Albertans who require them, while increasing the public's role in financing health services through increased health premiums, increased cost sharing and de-listing certain previously funded services.

An additional key component of system rationalization, especially in the transitional period, is the ongoing monitoring and evaluation of health system effects on the population. As part of this evaluation, the province conducted the Alberta Health Survey to solicit public views on the changing health system in Alberta. In spite of the many changes taking place, the 1995 survey indicated high levels of satisfaction with the Alberta health system overall and high levels of satisfaction with care received personally in the previous 12 months, and only low numbers of respondents indicating difficulty in accessing needed medical care. However, since then there has been growing dissatisfaction with the cuts in health care services. The government of Alberta has responded by increasing funding for health care.

5.1.2. Funding of Acute Care Hospitals

Approximately one third (34.2%) of all health expenditures in Canada relate to acute hospital care. Although implementing global budgeting for funding acute care hospitals had some effect in controlling the costs in Canada in the 1970s and 1980s, it has been recommended that hospitals be funded on a "case mix" basis; that is, by the type and severity of diseases treated at the hospital. This is similar to Diagnostic Related Groups

(DRGs), which gained prominence in the 1980s in the U.S.: hospitals were reimbursed for the intensity of care needed according to the severity classification of illness. However, hospitals tended to classify patients into more severe diagnostic categories to gain more reimbursement (popularly known as "DRG creep") and cost containment could not be achieved. In spite of the continuing debate about the advantages and disadvantages of the case-mix funding system, the Ontario Ministry of Health adopted this method in 1996.

5.1.3. Ambulatory Care, Day Care, and Extended Care

The original federal-provincial funding arrangements specified in the *Hospital Insurance and Diagnostic Services Act* of 1957 encouraged expansion and utilization of acute care hospitals, for which federal funds were provided. Ambulatory care, day care, day surgery, health centres, rehabilitation services, extended care facilities, and home care cost less than acute care hospitals but their costs were not shared with the federal government. This imbalance was addressed by *Established Programs Financing* (EPF) in 1977 and the *Canada Health and Social Transfer Act* (CHST), which replaced EPF in 1996. EPF included a per capita grant for extended health care, designed to cover nursing homes and ambulatory care; while the CHST allows provinces to make this funding decision on their own. The flexibility of the two funding formulas allowed provinces to develop these services in anticipation of the growing needs associated with the "aging society" in Canada. Consequently, there has been a shift in spending toward extended health care. According to Health Canada, the total federal cash contribution to extended health care increased from $20.00 per capita in 1977/78 to $51.21 per capita in 1995/96; for public health services, it increased from 3.6% of total health care cash transfers in 1975 to 5.0% in 1996.

5.1.4. Preadmission and Discharge Planning

Hospital stays for surgery or for elective procedures can be shortened by outpatient laboratory tests and other work-up conducted prior to admission. After-care in a stepped-down environment where the patient is provided with less intense care and preparation-for-discharge care are effective in reducing hospital costs.

5.1.5. Home Care

Home care makes institutional beds available for acute care and costs considerably less than hospital care. Some researchers claim that home care of the elderly can result in savings of 50% to 75% of the costs of equivalent care in a hospital (15). The elderly are better able to adapt to a disability in their own home, and home care patients tend to comply more readily to treatment requirements. Home care also results in psychological benefits experienced by the patient and his or her family. Furthermore, patients who are treated in hospitals often experience confusion, disorientation, anxiety, and personality conflicts, all of which can hinder healing. A home care program can also be tailored to an individual's particular needs and home.

Cost Effectiveness

In the current climate of increased fiscal restraint, there has been considerable emphasis on home care as a cost-effective alternative to institutionalized health care. However, efforts to determine this cost effectiveness are impeded by what has been termed the "paradox of efficiency." One would expect home care to be efficient if it resulted in more available hospital beds and if the treatment cost less than it would in an institution. If these available beds were closed, it would cost less to the system. However, available beds are filled immediately by other patients, which increases the cost. As well, some home care clients may not have otherwise sought any other form of medical care, and thus health care problems may be discovered that would have otherwise gone untreated. As a result of these two consequences, the overall costs to the health care system may actually increase with the expansion of home care services, as more people end up being treated. Nonetheless, if utilization can be monitored for appropriateness and the generally higher rates of patient satisfaction maintained, more care in the home remains a desirable goal.

Consumer Choice

In institutional settings, the physician makes the decisions, whereas in the home the patient is in his or her own environment and services are rarely delivered by a physician. This has the benefit of encouraging the participation of the patient and family in decision making, and may therefore improve the psychological health of the patient.

Risk and Liability

There is an increased risk to the home care patient in emergency situations since emergency services and technology are at a greater distance from the patient. Also, monitoring the home care patient is often less intensive than in an institutional facility. Thus there is a transition of a significant amount of responsibility from health care providers to the patient and family. In its report, the Federal/Provincial/Territorial Working Group on Home Care called this the downside of the power shift mentioned above: "You cannot both empower clients and families, and retain traditional notions of risk and responsibility at the same time" (16).

Turf War

Although many would be pleased with the reduced or stabilized rates of institutionalization that increased home care may bring, intersectorial rivalries within the health care field may result. For example, those opposing closure of hospitals may resent the argument that hospital care is not needed because of the home care alternative.

Rights

People who would normally be treated in institutions are likely to demand the "right" to receive treatment at home. Thus, whereas home care is currently provided in situations where the treatment would generally be short term or low cost, home care may be claimed as a right by high-cost, long-term patients such as young people with disabilities.

Private versus Public Home Care

Every province has undertaken to reform its extended care and home care programs in the last five years. Most provinces have opted for a "one-stop" assessment and coordination centre to assess and monitor patient needs. Although funding for the component of home care services that involves professional services and homemaking remains generally public, many provincial policies have arranged for their service coordination centres to contract out service provision on the basis of quality and price. Contracts are awarded to a variety of non-governmental organizations — some nonprofit, some for-profit. Additionally, voluntary community support services (including such services as "Meals on Wheels," transportation services for people with disabilities, patient visiting services, and respite care) frequently impose co-payments or user fees to recover some of their costs. Thus, although it is hard to pinpoint exactly what portion of financing and delivery of home care remains in which sector, it is safe to say that increasing privatization in both the public and private sectors seems to be the path of the future. Furthermore, home care services are not part of the federally mandated package of "medically necessary" services that require public financing and administration under the *Canada Health Act.* Home care reformers are thus faced with two opposing trends: On the one hand, with decreasing lengths of stay in hospitals and increasing pressures to push care into the community and home, away from institutional care, everincreasing numbers of patients require care in the home. On the other hand, as fiscal constraints tighten, provinces may continue to de-list services not strictly required by the *Canada Health Act.* There is concern that the private sector, especially the for-profit agencies, will provide services that are less accessible, less accountable, and of lower quality than those provided directly by not-for-profit voluntary agencies (17). It also encourages elitism and a two-tiered system. Concern about increased public/private collaboration revolves around the issues of quality control, coordination, and accessibility. However, recent federal initiatives to examine how home care can be more accessible and comprehensive may result in more public funding.

Other Issues

Issues in the home care field include the growing range of complex services required for patients such as those with AIDS, the increasing demand for palliative care, the high costs of treating people with Alzheimer's disease and other dementia (both at home and in institutions), training health care workers in the delivery of home care, and the high costs of 24-hour, seven-days-per-week coverage.

5.1.6. Risk Management

Risk management is method of reducing an institution's potential for liability by identifying predictors of an extended or complicated hospital course or an adverse outcome (such as mortality). For example, monitoring a sample of patient charts for indicator conditions concurrent with the patients' hospitalization can highlight what interventions are needed to avert a poor outcome. Complaints about care must also be handled appropriately by the institution's administration.

5.2. COST-CONTAINMENT STRATEGIES FOR HUMAN HEALTH RESOURCES: PHYSICIANS

Another method for containing costs is to control health human resources, particularly the number of physicians and their remuneration, which emerged in the early 1990s as major issues of concern to provincial governments (18).

5.2.1. Physician Human Resources

In 1992, commissioned by the Conference of Deputy Ministers of Health, the Barer-Stoddard Report on Canadian physician resource planning was published (3, 19-24). This report drew on the input and views of major stakeholders, and was based on the assumption that cost control in the health care system is intimately linked to the supply, mix, and distribution of physicians and their remuneration. Although physicians generate most health care costs either directly or indirectly, the public interest may not be met by this distribution of resources (25). Barer and Stoddard proposed a national strategy for physician resource management, and their major relevant recommendations are discussed below. Interested readers are advised to read the complete report.

Graduates of Foreign Medical Schools (GOFMS). These account for 25% of the physician supply in Canada, including Canadians trained elsewhere, visa physicians (meaning they come from other countries and hold a visa permitting them to work in Canada) recruited specifically to meet special needs, and visa trainees for postgraduate programs. The report recommended that Canada reduce its reliance on GOFMS, limit immigration of physicians, require compliance of visa physicians with the terms of their contract, and use the supply of GOFMS creatively, such as for areas poorly supplied with physicians.

Overall Supply of Physicians. The overriding objective of physician resource policy should satisfy the health care needs of the population, given the resources that society is prepared to commit. Barer and Stoddard rejected the notion of the ideal physician-to-population ratio that has been used as a planning tool. Canada, however, is faced with an oversupply of physicians; since the early 1950s, the supply has increased faster than the population. The report recommended an immediate 10% reduction in the number of medical undergraduate students in Canadian universities.

Mix and Number of Residency Training Positions. The current mix of residency positions bears no relation to a mix that would best meet current and future physician needs. Instead, it reflects historical precedent and the prestige of sub-specialities. The report called for the development of a reasonable and acceptable approach to rationalizing the mix and location of residency positions. Restructuring the funding of academic centres and replacing institution-specific bargaining for residency positions are necessary, as is reducing the number of training positions to redistribute physicians more appropriately toward the primary care sector.

The Geographic Maldistribution of Physicians. Despite the overabundance of Canadian physicians, northern and rural areas are underserviced. Incentives to locate in underserviced areas include student-loan remission programs for residents agreeing to practise in designated rural areas for specific periods, as well as other financial incentives. The Ontario government has already attempted to redistribute physicians to areas designated as underserviced (primarily Northern Ontario) through tax-free grants or guaranteed incomes for the first four years of practice in a designated area. In British Columbia, a so-called "northern differential" exists, giving a higher fee schedule to those in more remote communities, based on a percentage added above the standard provincial fee schedule and graded according to degree of remoteness from the lower mainland. The Quebec government has taken a different approach. It pays a much lower fee schedule to new physicians in urban centres than those in outlying areas. Imposing quotas on billing numbers is another way to restrict the number of urban practitioners.

By the end of 1992 a number of provinces had limited the number of medical students, enforcing compliance of GOFMS with visa requirements, and attempting to reduce physician-generated costs by reducing the number of physicians. Responses of organized medicine were, in part, mixed. The Royal College of Physicians and Surgeons of Canada expressed concerns about the reduction in undergraduate medical students and the adjustment of speciality ratios; however, it recommended a moratorium on the recognition of new specialities. Most recently, provincial policies have been the basis of labour disputes in many provinces. Provincial ministries of health, in an ongoing effort to control health expenditures have proposed such policies as physician billing caps, controlling the number of new billing numbers issued, limiting the number of new practices allowed in urban or overserved areas, and reducing subsidies for malpractice insurance.

Clearly, an accurate assessment is needed to determine the appropriate number of physicians required to provide enough but not excess services. In addition, the problem of inappropriate distribution must be addressed both among specialities and in terms of geography.

5.2.2. Physician Remuneration

In addition to the costs related to number of physicians, there is the issue of physician remuneration itself (26). This has become an increasingly contentious issue in recent years. Physicians want to receive what they consider fair compensation for their services, which may lead to practices such as opting out, extra-billing, or balanced-billing. All involve a payment by the patient to the physician in addition to the amount paid by the provincial health plan. Under the *Canada Health Act* of 1984, provinces that allow extra-billing are penalized financially, and by 1987 all provinces had banned the practice. However, questions of fair compensation continue. Recently, both Alberta and British Columbia allowed some form of private payment to physicians — in British Columbia, it is in the form of extra billing, and in Alberta it is in the form of private diagnostic clinics. Both provinces discontinued these practices when the federal government, citing the terms of the *Canada Health Act*, took dollar-for-dollar deductions from their federal transfer payments for health. The issue of extra-billing may arise again; however, the *Canada Health and Social Transfer Act*, which guarantees a federal payment of $12.5 billion, will maintain the federal government's influence over provincial health insurance programs' fulfilment of the requirements of the act.

It has also been argued that the present fee-for-service system does not adequately compensate preventive services and encourages rapid patient turn-over, excessive patient recalls, and the performance of unnecessary procedures. Although a restructuring of fee schedules might correct this problem, those holding this view usually favour salaries for physicians as a better way align services with patient needs. Another alternative is payment by capitation. Some combination of these mechanisms is also feasible (27).

A growing trend is to adopt a team approach to health care, particularly in ambulatory settings such as community health centres, with the effective utilization of nurses, dietitians, social workers, and other professionals. These professionals might provide primary care in their field of expertise or work as part of a more comprehensive approach to health care, particularly in its preventive aspects, than is now provided in many primary care settings. There have been alternative models recommended, such as the health services organization model or the health maintenance organization (HMO) model. Quality of care might be improved or services could be reduced as has happened in some HMOs in U.S. Clearly, for economic benefit to occur these alternative approaches must reduce the need for, and use of, physicians' services, and not simply be "added on" to them. The alternative health care delivery models should explore the use of health care professionals other than physicians for example, using midwives for normal home and hospital deliveries.

5.2.3. Caps on Physician Incomes

Other strategies to reduce the open-ended provincial spending on physicians are to cap individual incomes at a certain level (as occurred in Ontario in 1992) or to cap or limit overall provincial payments for medical fees. This latter strategy may be accompanied by utilization adjustment, or the deduction from physician payments for increases in the use of medical services beyond specified levels for a period. In some provinces, when physician billing exceeds the limits, the provincial government institutes a "claw back" policy. In Ontario, organized medicine collaborated with government to limit billings and to impose penalties, and in British Columbia, similar initiatives resulted in a protest from organized medicine and a number of doctors, particularly in the rural areas, withdrew their services temporarily.

5.2.4. Other Measures to Contain Physician Remuneration

Other recommendations include restricting the billing privileges and prorating payments for new physicians. Joint management committees of organized medicine and government have been struck in some provinces, principally in Ontario, where the Ontario Medical Association agreed to the limits on physicians' billings on condition that it was recognized as the exclusive bargaining agent for physicians in that province. However, given this is a contentious subject, there may be confrontations as well as partnership strategies to find solutions.

5.3. INCREASING COST EFFECTIVENESS: CAN THE MONEY BE USED MORE EFFECTIVELY?

Recent concerns in health care also have to do with increasing cost effectiveness. Efforts have been made to establish the costs and effectiveness of an activity or to compare similar alternatives to determine the relative degree to which they will obtain the desired objectives or outcomes. The goal is to find an action or alternative that requires the least cost and produces a given level of effectiveness or that provides the greatest effectiveness for a given cost.

5.3.1. Practice Guidelines

Today, when there is a constant explosion of scientific and clinical information, clinical guidelines have become explicit and structured so that the evidence-based approaches to medical decision making is used. Guidelines are not enforced; rather, they are recommendations that may change professional norms, but they are explicit, so they can provide standards for optimum care and evaluating the quality of care. Thus, they have the potential to enhance quality of care (28), cost containment, and more appropriate utilization of resources.

However, the existence of guidelines does not ensure their implementation. Some people see them as an intrusion into the professionalism of health care providers. If they are marketed effectively, guidelines can change behaviour. They also require practical assistance, such as the availability of alternative tests or procedures. For example, guidelines for the utilization of cesarean sections were developed by the obstetric profession in Canada in response to major variations in rates for cesarean sections in different provinces. By 1989, the rate in Ontario had tripled since 1970 to 19.5 per 100 hospital deliveries, which was far higher than that in Manitoba. Of these, 40% were performed because the woman had had a previous cesarean section. New standards were established that allowed for labour after cesarean section — vaginal birth after cesarean section or (VBAC). These standards did not, by themselves, result in changes in the rates of cesarean sections. A comparative intervention (29) in the U.S., however, which involved counselling and educating physicians and implementing a peer-review process to promote the guidelines, did reduce the number of cesarean sections. Cesarean sections became more frequent among women aged over 35 and in dystocia/breech deliveries. The rate of VBACs increased from 4% to 33% and the cesarean section rate went down. This was considered a more appropriate utilization of surgery and likely contributed to cost containment.

Increasing public interest in the outcome of medical care, the need for cost containment, and the suspicion that some medical care may be unnecessary or inappropriate are all likely to result in a shift toward the supervision of quality of care and the identification of optimal practice patterns. It is considered that "sensible, flexible guidelines produced by the appropriate panels will help improve practice" (30). Recently, government and organized medicine have become interested in the cost-containment potential of guidelines. For example, Ontario's Institute for Clinical Evaluative Sciences was established by the Ministry of Health and the Ontario Medical Association partly to undertake research into practice "styles", that is, the individual characteristic approaches of physicians to investigating and managing problems based on factors other than rational scientific evidence.

5.3.2. Technology Assessment

Technology (some of it very expensive) has made tremendous advances in health care in recent times. Technology assessment has been developed to examine the efficacy and safety of a technology, its appropriate clinical use, the relative risks and benefits, and the ethical and social implications. However, no systematic process for the identification and acquisition of new technology exists in Canada. Interprovincial differences in priorities and disparities in wealth make it difficult to establish uniform approaches to health technology. The Federal Health Protection Branch of Health Canada administers the *Food and Drugs Act,* which regulates a limited number of medical devices as well as medications. These devices include implantables, condoms, AIDS tests, menstrual tampons, and contact lenses. The Act does not cover devices used externally or most other technology that is introduced independently by the provinces. The Coordinating Office for Health Care Technology Assessment was introduced following proposals by Feeny and Stoddard (31) and undertakes technology assessments on request.

A fundamental concept which provides the rationale for technology assessment, is the diffusion of technology. As new technology emerges, it is usually taken up enthusiastically, followed by a period of reassessment during which limitations or adverse effects come to light. The technology then becomes incorporated into the practices of health care professionals and institutionalized, even if, as usual, the initial glowing promise is not fully realized. Unless this cycle is interrupted, such as by an assessment of the cost effectiveness, enormously expensive technology can become the standard of practice without evidence of its efficiency.

The Technology Assessment Iterative Loop (32) provides a model for informed decision making as a result of technology assessment. Its seven steps are the following:

1) Identify technologies with the greatest potential for reducing the burden of illness by primary, secondary, or tertiary prevention or by levels of care;
2) Establish efficacy; i.e., therapeutic potential under ideal circumstances;
3) Establish procedures for screening and diagnosis, i.e., accurate detection of those in need;
4) Determine community effectiveness (see also Chapter 3);
5) Assess efficiency (see also Chapter 3);
6) Develop procedures for synthesis and implementation;
7) Monitor and reassess the process.

Technology assessment may use cost-utility ratios, whereby the social value of the technology is incorporated into the assessment for comparison of competing technologies. The incremental costs of technologies are compared in order to achieve, for example, an additional quality-adjusted life year (QALY) (33). It has been recommended that the use of health technology be based on defined population needs.

5.3.3. Quality Assurance and Total Quality Management

Quality assurance (QA) is a management system that assures the quality of health care provided by workers and received by patients. Care should be correctly given, reliable, and empathetic. Quality assurance is a method of constantly improving standards and the frequency of attaining them. It is defined by the Canadian Council on Health Service Accreditation (CCHSA), a national agency that accredits health care facilities of all descriptions across Canada. The CCHSA uses the following five-stage process: the establishment of functional goals, the implementation of procedures to achieve those goals, the regular assessment of performance relative to the goals, the proposal of solutions to close the gap between performance and goal, and the documentation and reporting of this assessment activity.

For QA to work, institutions must encourage both the continuous assessment of quality and the communication of problems and attainment of desired changes through the management structure (34). A number of approaches have been developed specifically for the hospital sector, such as the Medical Audit Committee, which compares care for a specific disease with the standards of care set for that disease. Another example is the Tissue Committee, which reviews all tissue removed during surgery and compares it with the pre-operative diagnosis. The third example is the Health Record Committee, which reviews selected patient records for completeness. The Canadian Institute for Health Information also provides large sets of data for comparisons between institutions of similar size.

Although institutions have quality assurance programs, there is rarely an organized review of the community-based practices of health care professionals. Licensing or regulating bodies usually deal with patient complaints; however, recent legislations in a number of provinces now require them also to monitor the quality of care provided by their constituents. Increasingly, health care professions and institutions are required to be accountable to the public and the government for the resources they use and how they practise.

Total quality management (TQM) is a management philosophy that provides a framework for health care to improve quality while controlling costs. In TQM, management focuses on the system rather than the individual, so decisions are made to support quality and remove barriers to quality inherent in the bureaucratic, hierarchical system. Participation and teamwork are vital. Because TQM is based on a continuous feed-forward process called continuous quality improvement (CQI), it differs from quality assurance, which tends to depend on retrospective recognition of "outliers" in patterns of care. However, TQM has not yet been widely implemented in the health care system in Canada, although a number of initiatives for implementation have commenced. It complements quality assurance in that it provides a management system for rectifying identified difficulties. This aspect is frequently missing from quality assurance activities, which tend to emphasize data collection. QA also focuses on individuals, often in relation to their peers, and is thus less powerful than total quality management, which examines issues affecting the performance of the organization as a whole.

5.3.4. Utilization Review and Management

Utilization review compares the volume and intensity of how services are used. Large differences exist in the rates of use of medical services among geographic regions or practitioners, yet there are no discernible differences in health outcomes. However, establishing ideal "rates" is problematic. Big variations in the rates of medical or hospital services among geographic regions are called small-area variations (SAV), which are adjusted for age, sex, and other variables. SAV findings question the assumption that all the services in the regions with higher rates are medically necessary (35).

Utilization review and management monitor the utilization of services, analyse variations, and assess interventions in order to reduce the inappropriate use of services and to provide feedback and education (36). This process may be hospital-based or, less frequently, community-based.

5.4. RATIONING IN HEALTH CARE

When resources for health care and services are finite and limited, rationing is one option that may result in equitably distributed health care. An example of explicit rationing is the proposed Oregon Health Care Plan in the United States.

5.4.1. Oregon's Basic Health Care Act

In 1989, the Oregon Legislature passed the *Basic Health-Care Act* (37), which called for broadening the extension of medicare coverage to all Oregonians living below the poverty level and for reducing the number of benefits covered. Seventeen per cent of the state's population was not covered by health care insurance, but under the new legislation some coverage would be provided to people who are single, childless, poor or working poor. In order to pay the costs of the extended medicaid coverage, the state legislated the rationalization of health care services. Based on cost, social value, and the effectiveness of procedures, the state ranked 709 condition/treatment pairs. Services were divided into three types:

- *Essential:* life-preserving services, maternal care, preventive care for children and adults, reproductive services, and comfort care for terminally ill patients. These types of services are considered effective, contribute to the quality of life, give good value for the money, and demonstrate community compassion for the terminally ill.
- *Very important:* treatment for non-fatal conditions where full or partial recovery is expected, or where the quality of life is expected to improve through treatment.
- *Valuable to certain individuals:* non-fatal conditions that are not responsive to treatment, infertility, and conditions in which treatment would not significantly improve the quality of life.

Those services deemed valuable to certain individuals may not be covered by the standard benefit package. Thus the central issue in the proposed Oregon health care funding changed from *who* is covered to *what* is funded. It must be noted that while the

Oregon plan proposed limiting the types of services provided by the standard benefit package, it exceeded medicare coverage by providing unlimited hospitalization. The standard package also included prescription drugs, dental services, physical and occupational therapy, and other services that the federal guidelines did not cover.

The Oregon plan was vetoed by President George Bush in 1992, claiming violation of the *Americans with the Disabilities Act,* but later approved by President Bill Clinton in March 1993. Implementation of the program began in 1994. Four years later, the results of Oregon's experiment were mixed. An increasing number of Oregon residents are now covered by a health plan, and the plan has met with widespread approval from both consumers and physicians, but the plan is starting to run into fiscal difficulties. The Oregon plan initially targeted 745 condition/treatment pairs to be included in its package; so far the government has been able to only pay for the top-rated 581 pairs. In addition, although an increasing number of Oregon residents have signed onto the Oregon health plan, an equal number are losing their workplace insurance packages every year as small businesses continue to drop health insurance benefit packages for their workers. The fiscal pressures of insuring these increasing numbers of residents are becoming substantial.

Critics claim that the reform plan failed to ensure universality of coverage. They also maintain that due to the continued availability of a large number of private health insurance schemes to certain consumers, physicians continue to discriminate against the lower-paying Oregon health plan patients and provide them with lower quality care. The plan has been also criticized for its consultation process, which only involved middle class and professionals and failed to consult poor and unfranchised individuals, for whom the plan was devised. In defence of the Oregon plan, the program's director claims that the amount of charity care in hospitals for uninsured patients, the number of emergency room visits, and the per capita costs of providing health care to Oregon residents have all decreased (38).

Other issues regarding the Oregon plan relate to the principle of rationing health care. Critics of the plan claim that prioritizing services inevitably means that future budget cuts will force upward the line below which services will not be funded. However, proponents argue that rationing already implicitly occurs whenever decisions are made to spend money on one service or set of services, because health care resources are not infinite. Recently, almost every Canadian province has undertaken a more explicit form of health rationing in the form of "de-listing", whereby services are removed from the list of those covered by their health insurance plans. In these cases, the costs for services are shifted to the private sector in the form of user fees or covered by industry through negotiated health and welfare benefits (4, 39). What distinguishes the Oregon system of rationing from others, however, is the process used to arrive at the list of priorities. The communities to be affected, including health care workers and consumers, were surveyed about what types of services they valued most. The responses from these surveys typically ranked quality of life, disease prevention, and cost effectiveness high on the list of values. Scientific analyses of the effectiveness and costs of procedures and treatments were combined with the input from the community, and the condition/treatment pairs were ranked accordingly. Unlike Canada's hidden rationing and politically determined procedures for assigning priority to funding health care services, the Oregon plan offers Oregonians an open, publicly determined procedure for providing basic health care coverage (40).

6. SUMMARY

One of the most basic series of questions about the organization of any health care system concerns the financing of health services: Where does the money for health care come from? Where should it come from? How is it collected? What services and which groups of people are covered by the various methods of health care financing?

Canada has a predominantly publicly financed health system with universal coverage for all permanent residents, without regard to their ability to pay for care. Most money for health care is raised through provincial and federal taxes and is allocated, for the most part, from general provincial budgets. According to the *Canada Health Act*, each provincial health plan must cover all "medically necessary" health services, which currently includes all services delivered in hospital and all services delivered by physicians. Extended health care services and health care services offered by providers other than physicians may be covered at the discretion of each province or territory. Personal expenditures (30% of all health care expenditures) include dental and other services not covered by government insurance, drugs, and medical equipment for the bulk of the population, and payments for extra services such as charges for private hospital rooms. Treatment for work-related injuries and disease is covered through worker's compensation funds.

In 1996, Canada spent $75.2 billion on health care (which represents 9.5% of the GDP). Due to concerns about the high costs of health care, the rate of growth of health care expenditures has levelled off and is beginning to slowly decrease. Health expenditures are categorized as institutional, professional, drugs and appliances, and other. Over the last few years, just under half (44.2%) of Canadian health expenditures was spent for institutional care, about one quarter on professional services, and 14.4% for drugs and appliances. The total health expenditure per capita in Canada rose from $271 in 1970 to $2,511 in 1996. These rapidly rising costs in health care, particularly in the acute care sector, and expanding high-cost technology are straining Canada's resources. The potential demands for health services are unlimited, so clearly they cannot all be met. In a system of universally accessible services, demand alone cannot be allowed to determine provision of services. This raises many difficult issues.

Resource utilization depends on several factors: resources ratio, which is the availability of resources; general characteristics of the community or population (such as age distribution, housing quality, level of sanitation, etc.); personal factors affecting usage of services such as attitudes, age, sex, family size, etc.; and system characteristics, including points of entry in the health care system, accessibility of resources, cost, and barriers to care. The present system allows patients direct access to primary or secondary care depending on their proximity to and knowledge about resources and their attitudes toward the system. The ideal, however, is the patient's linear progression from primary to secondary to tertiary care resources as required.

The ultimate aim of the health care industry is to produce good health. Expenditure on health care currently focuses on treating sickness rather than prevention. Measurement of sickness care has two dimensions: *outcome measurement* (e.g., improvement, no improvement, deterioration or death) and *utilization measurement*.

Institutions are the most expensive element of health care as they rely on both technology and human resources. In 1994/95, Canada had 978 general, allied, special, private, and public hospitals. Public hospitals accounted for 92% of all hospitals and 98% of the beds. There were 41 separate mental institutions with 13,262 beds. Utilization of institutional care is measured by hospitalization days, hospital separation rates, and the number of visits to emergency and ambulatory care units.

Human health resources consist of individuals who provide direct health services such as nurses, physicians, dentists, chiropractors, respiratory technicians, and those who are indirectly involved in health sectors. The health care industry is the third largest industry in the country, employing about 834,000 Canadians of whom 80% work in health institutions. Thanks to technical advances, there are over 150 categories of health occupations. They have been developed either as extensions of established health care professions or alongside some special body of knowledge. Human health resources are unevenly distributed, because the main concentration is in large urban centres and traditionally wealthy provinces.

The following are current approaches to increasing efficient utilization of resources:
- With respect to *institutional resources*:
  - Rationalization of health care services involving restructuring, realignment, some closures, and decentralization of institutions;
  - Increased ambulatory/day care/extended care;
  - Preadmission planning and discharge planning, which shorten hospital stays;
  - Risk management, which reduces an institution's potential liability by identifying predictors of either an extended or complicated hospital course or adverse outcome.
- With respect to *human health resources* (specifically physicians):
  - Management of physician human resources, including linking cost control in the health care system to the supply, mix, and distribution of physician human resources and their remuneration. Proposed strategies address graduates of foreign medical schools, oversupply of physicians, mix and number of residency training positions, and the geographic maldistribution of physicians;
  - Management of physician remuneration, particularly the rights of physicians to receive what they regard as fair compensation for their services and team approach to health care;
  - Caps on physician incomes.

- *Clinical practice guidelines*, which use clinical judgement and decision making to enhance the quality of care and facilitate cost containment and appropriate utilization of resources.
- *Technology assessment*, a process that examines the efficacy and safety of a technology, its appropriate clinical use, its relative risks and benefits, and its ethical and social implications.
- *Quality assurance*, a five-stage process for establishing functional goals, implementing procedures to achieve these goals, regularly assessing performance, closing the gap between performance and goal, and documenting and reporting this assessment activity.
- *Utilization review and management*, which involves monitoring the utilization of services, analyzing variations, assessing interventions to reduce inappropriate use of services, collecting feedback, and providing education. Utilization review is based on total quality management, a management philosophy for improving health care quality while controlling costs.
- *Health care rationing*, one option for equitably distributing health care when resources and services are finite and limited.

7. REFERENCES

1.   Health System and Policy Division. National Health Expenditures in Canada, 1975-1996. Ottawa: Health Canada, 1997.
2.   Armstrong P, Armstrong H. Wasting Away: The Undermining of Canadian Health Care. Toronto: Oxford University Press, 1996.
3.   Barer M, Stoddard G. Toward Integrated Medical Resource Policies for Canada: 1. Background, Process and Perceived Problems. Canadian Medical Association Journal 1992;146(3):337-351.
4.   Deber R, Wiilliams P, Duvlako K, Baranak P. Report to the Task Force on the Funding and Delivery of Medical Care in Ontario: The Public-Private Mix in Health Care. Toronto: Department of Health Administration, University of Toronto, 1995.
5.   Health Canada. Canada Health Act: Annual Report. Ottawa: Health Canada, Health Policy Directorate, 1994.
6.   Tully P, Saint-Pierre E. Downsizing Canada's Hospitals, 1986-87 to 1994-95. Health Reports 1997;8(4):33-9.
7.   Shortell SM. Health Care Management: Organization, Design and Behavior. (3rd ed.) Albany, New York: Delmar Publishers, 1994.
8.   Statistics Canada, Health Statistics Division. Hospital Statistics: Preliminary Annual Report, 1994-1995. Ottawa: Ministry of Industry, Science and Technology, 1996.
9.   Statistics Canada, Health Statistics Division. List of Residential Care Facilities, 1993. Ottawa: Ministry of Industry, Science and Technology, 1994.
10. Minister of National Health and Welfare. Health Personnel in Canada 1992. Ottawa: Ministry of Supply and Services, 1994.
11. Canadian Institute for Health Information. Health Human Resources: National Information. Ottawa: 1995.

12. Statistics Canada, Health Statistics Division. Nursing in Canada, 1993. Ottawa: Ministry of Industry, Science and Technology, 1994.
13. Statistics Canada. Data Releases: Registered Nurses, 1994. Health Reports 1994;6(3):389-390.
14. Alberta Health. Annual Report: 1994-1995. Edmonton: 1996.
15. Home-Based Care, the Elderly, the Family and the Welfare State: An International Comparison. Ottawa: University of Ottawa Press, 1993.
16. Federal/Provincial/Territorial Working Group on Home Care. Report on Home Care. Ottawa: Ministry of Supply and Services, Health and Welfare Canada, 1990.
17. Nahmiash D, Reis M. An Exploratory Study of Private Home Care Services in Canada. Ottawa: Health and Welfare Canada, 1992.
18. Barer ML, Lomas J, Sanmartin C. Re-minding our Ps and Qs: Medical Cost Controls in Canada. Health Affairs 1996;15(2):216-234.
19. Barer M, Stoddard G. Toward Integrated Medical Resource Policies for Canada: 3. Analytic Framework for Policy Development. Canadian Medical Association Journal 1992;146(7):1169-1174.
20. Barer M, Stoddard G. Toward Integrated Medical Resource Policies for Canada: 2. Promoting Change: General Themes. Canadian Medical Association Journal 1992;146(6):697-700.
21. Barer M, Stoddard G. Toward Integrated Medical Resource Policies for Canada: 6. Remuneration of Physicians and Global Expenditure Policy. Canadian Medical Association Journal 1992;147(1):33-38.
22. Barer M, Stoddard G. Toward Integrated Medical Resource Policies for Canada: 4. Graduates of Foreign Medical Schools. Canadian Medical Association Journal 1992;146(9):1549-1554.
23. Barer M, Stoddard G. Toward Integrated Medical Resource Policies for Canada: 7. Undergraduate Medical Training. Canadian Medical Association Journal 1992;147(3):305-312.
24. Barer M, Stoddard G. Toward Integrated Medical Resource Policies for Canada: 5. The Roles and Funding of Academic Medical Centres. Canadian Medical Association Journal 1992;146(11):1919-1924.
25. Lomas J, Barer M. And Who Shall Represent the Public Interest? The Legacy of Canadian Health Manpower Policy. In Evans R, Stoddard G, eds. Medicare at Maturity. Calgary: University of Calgary Press, 1986:221-286.
26. Hall EM. Canada's National-Provincial Health Program for the 1980's: A Commitment for Renewal. Ottawa: Health and Welfare Canada, Special Commissioner, 1980.
27. Advisory Committee on Health Services. A Model for the Reorganization of Primary Care and the Introduction of Population-Based Funding. Prepared for the Federal/Territorial/Provincial Conference of Deputy Ministers, September 1995. Ottawa: Federal/Provincial Liaison, Health Canada, 1995.
28. Health Services Research Group. Standards, Guidelines, and Clinical Policies. Canadian Medical Association Journal 1992;146(6):833-837.
29. Myers S, Gleicher N. A Successful Program to Lower Cesarean Section Rates. New England Journal of Medicine 1988;319(23):1511-1588.
30. Linton A, Peachy D. Guidelines for Medical Practice: 1. The Reasons Why. Canadian Medical Association Journal 1990;143(6):485-490.
31. Feeney D, Stoddart G. Toward Improved Health Technology Policy in Canada: A Proposal for the National Health Technology Assessment Council. Canadian Public Policy 1988;14(3):254-265.

32. Feeney D, Guyatt G, Tugwell P. Health Care Technology: Effectiveness, Efficiency and Public Policy. Montreal: Institute for Research on Public Policy, 1986.

33. Goel V, Deber R, Detsky A. Non-ionic Contrast Media: Economic Analysis and Health Policy Development. Canadian Medical Association Journal 1989;140(4):389-395.

34. Wilson CRM. Hospital-Wide Quality Assurance: Models for Implementation and Development. Toronto: WB Saunders, 1987.

35. Health Services Research Group. Small Area Variations: What Are They and What Do They Mean? Canadian Medical Association Journal 1992;146(4):467-470.

36. Anderson G, Sheps S, Cardiff K. Hospital-Based Utilization Management: A Cross-Canada Survey. Canadian Medical Association Journal 1990;143(10):1025-1030.

37. McPherson A. The Oregon Plan: Rationing in a Rational Society. Canadian Medical Association Journal 1991;145(11):1444-1445.

38. Fiscus J. A Check-up on Oregon's Grand Medicare Experiment: After Two Years, It's Working. Medical Post 1996 :14.

39. Health Canada. Provincial Health System Reform in Canada. Ottawa: Ministry of Supply and Services Canada, 1995.

40. Emson H. Down the Oregon Trail: The Way for Canada? Canadian Medical Association Journal 1991;145(11):1441-1443.

Chapter

15

Community Health Services

1. OVERVIEW OF COMMUNITY HEALTH SERVICES

When illness, suffering, or symptoms occur, an individual usually relies on informal support, sometimes for prolonged periods. When this support is exhausted, the individual turns to local community-based health services, which can include primary care, secondary care, hospital care, home care, public health services, and private nursing homes. Community health services may also deal with specific groups of people, e.g. Aboriginal peoples, battered women, and people with Alzheimer's disease.

Government health insurance plans cover basic hospital and medical services in all the provinces, but there are variations in the coverage of extended health services, whether in the home or in the community, paid by provincial or private insurance or by the individual. Affluent provinces provide a larger range of services financed through public revenue.

This chapter discusses basic health services; however, many other services related to health promotion, disease prevention, and health maintenance are discussed, as are support services (such as social, educational, and vocational services) for those who are chronically or acutely ill.

1.1. PRIMARY HEALTH CARE SERVICES

At this point, it is appropriate to define some commonly used terms. **Primary health care** (or first-contact care) includes services provided at the first contact between the patient and the health care professional. It is generally provided by physicians, dentists, chiropractors, pharmacists, nurse practitioners, midwives, optometrists, dietitians, and others. Services include treatment, promotion and maintenance of health, follow-up care, and the complete continuing care of the individual (including referral when required). Therefore, primary health care providers perform three essential functions beyond treating the patients (1):

- *Guardian.* The primary care provider and patient and his or her family enter into a relationship in which continuity is implicit. As a result of the increasing complexity of the Canadian health care system, there is an increasing need for someone (perhaps a team) to accept responsibility for the ongoing care of the person or family.
- *Gatekeeper.* The primary care provider has a dual role as a guide or information resource and as the appropriate source for referral elsewhere in the health care system.
- *Chronicler.* The primary care provider acts as a chronicler or recorder of the patient's health-related interactions with the system and its providers.

1.2. SECONDARY AND TERTIARY HEALTH CARE

Secondary health care is usually delivered by people with specialized training. Patients normally enter secondary care after referral from primary care providers because their health problems require specialized skills and facilities not available in the primary care sector. Problems seen in secondary care include serious cardiovascular disorders, accidental injuries, burns, fractures, cancers, behavioural disorders, and paediatric, medical and obstetric problems. These conditions usually require specialized care provided by specialists in a community or general hospital. Unusual inherited disorders, certain forms of cancer, complicated pregnancies, rare and complicated cardiovascular disorders, catastrophic trauma, and complex immunological disorders need treatment by further referral to **tertiary health care** centres, which have very specialized facilities and professional skills and are usually found only in university teaching hospitals. Extremely complex situations, such as heart, lung, kidney, liver, bone marrow transplant, and unusual procedures such as separation of Siamese twins require services of **quaternary care** which is always associated with the teaching hospitals.

2.   PROVISION OF MEDICAL SERVICES

The major component of primary health care in Canada is **primary medical care**, usually provided in the community by general or family practitioners and, to a lesser extent, by nurse practitioners, paediatricians, internists, obstetricians, gynaecologists, and midwives. This is not the case in the United States where primary medical care is provided predominantly by specialists. A small proportion of the Canadian population seeks their primary medical care through community health centres, walk-in clinics or hospital emergency rooms. More than 90% of the Canadian population can identify their primary medical care provider. The major part of **secondary medical care** is also provided in the community setting, and **tertiary medical care** is mainly provided by physicians and others practising in the hospital setting, usually in teaching centres.

Walk-In Clinics

Since 1984, when walk-in clinics first appeared, there has been a growing interest in the medical care they provide. Although there is no universally accepted definition of a walk-in clinic, it is usually a freestanding group practice that offers extended hours for services (weekend and evening hours) and usually does not require an appointment. Walk-in clinics are usually located in urban or suburban centres with large proportions of young families.

Although they are convenient for consumers, there has been a growing concern in the medical community that walk-in clinics may provide lower quality care due to lack of physician and care continuity, or because they are more often staffed by recent medical school graduates or physicians who might have less than adequate training. There is also concern that walk-in clinics may increase the overall cost of medical care by duplicating services that should be provided by a family practitioner. In fact, there is some anecdotal evidence that people who see physicians at walk-in clinics after hours see their family practitioner for the same problem during working hours the next day. However, in spite of these concerns, there has been very little systematic evaluation of walk-in clinics conducted (2).

Physician Remuneration

As discussed in Chapter 14, Canadian physicians receive remuneration for their services by different methods, namely fee-for-service basis, by sessional payment, or by salary. The majority bill for most of their services through provincial health insurance plans (i.e., fee-for-service). According to 1994/1995 estimates from the Canadian Institute for Health Information, 85% of physicians in Canada receive payment on a fee-for-service basis only which is a "volume-driven" mode of payment. The remaining 15% receive some type of combination of fee-for-service, salary and sessional payments (3). Those who receive **sessional payments** receive a lump sum for the time they make their services available; for an example, psychiatrist works a half day in a mental health clinic and receives a flat rate for this service. Provider organizations, such as health services organizations (HSOs) in Canada and the managed care organizations in the U.S., follow the capitation space system used by funding organizations. In the capitation system, an organization receives a fixed amount per patient for all services rendered and, in turn, purchases physicians' services by salary or fee-for-service. Some consider the **capitation** or the **salary** system to be conducive to a holistic approach to health care, so the physician is more likely to pay attention to all determinants of health and practise disease prevention and health promotion. The capitation system for primary care physicians is used in the United Kingdom and is usually found in health maintenance organization in the U.S. and HSOs in Ontario. Traditionally, salaries and sessional payments are more often used in rural regions or under-served areas of the provinces (4). However, the capitation system is currently drawing increased interest as part of provincial health reforms and endeavours to control health expenditures on physician services.

2.1. ORGANIZATION OF MEDICAL PRACTICES (5)

Most physicians in Canada practise medicine either as solo practitioners (over half), in shared practices, or in group practices. Generally, a **shared practice** is distinguished from a group practice by the extent of patient-sharing among the participating physicians that is involved. **Group practices** usually involve income distribution, formal contracts, shared patient records, shared practitioner responsibilities, and possible provision of care in each other's absence. Shared practices are usually limited to two or more physicians who have completely separate practices but share office space, rent, and secretarial services. Most group practices (80%) consist of physicians in the same discipline, such as family practitioners, while a smaller proportion consist of specialists from different disciplines. Most practitioners have their offices in the community. In urban centres with medical schools, practices of full-time teachers are located in the university hospitals. These physicians are called geographic full-time practitioners.

2.1.1. Alternate Delivery Models

Most primary health care is delivered in physicians' offices on a fee-for-service basis. The fee schedule offers physicians the incentive to provide more expensive and less time-consuming services. Many preventive services that incorporate counselling take a longer time, provide less remuneration, and are often neglected.

With an emerging emphasis on cost containment, disease prevention, and health promotion, governments and physicians are looking for alternate models for health care financing and delivery to enable them to be less volume driven and put a cap on health care costs. However, as yet, such models of health care comprise only a small proportion of the health services delivery system. The following three sections present examples of alternative delivery models (5, 6).

Community Health Centre

A community health centre (CHC) has a voluntary board composed of members from the community. It receives an annual budget from the provincial government for specific health programs, and it provides a wide range of services such as medical, dental, social, and nursing by a multidisciplinary staff all under one roof. All the professionals, including physicians, are on salary. In all provinces except Quebec, many of these centres are located in under-served areas or serve groups that are often not well served, such as the poor, the elderly, Aboriginal peoples, and immigrant groups.

In Quebec, these centres are part of the regionalized health and social service system, and are called local community service centres (centres locaux des services communautaires, or CLSCs), of which there are approximately 146. CLSCs integrate health and social services and emphasize prevention, health promotion, and provision of other personal services, including occupational health services, at one location; they are also required to provide services for extended hours in the evenings and weekends. Outside Quebec, CHC programs are most extensive in Ontario where, as of 1993, there were 47; CHCs have also been established in Nova Scotia (four), New Brunswick (four), Manitoba (14), Saskatchewan (five), Alberta (two), and British Columbia (four).

Health Services Organizations in Ontario

Health services organizations are a form of group practice with two or more physicians. Instead of fee-for-service, physicians receive remuneration on a fixed per capita rate. These payments are based on the current provincial average costs of physician utilization under fee-for-service for different age and sex groups. In this form of practice, patients enrol voluntarily to receive services from the group for a defined period of time. The HSO is penalized financially when patients on its roster receive services outside the HSO for which it receives funding. Unlike health maintenance organizations in the U.S., this penalty is incurred by the HSO; in the U.S., it is the patient who must pay. At present, there are 88 HSOs in Ontario, serving approximately 5% of the province's population and employing 2% of its physicians.

Comprehensive Health Organization

The comprehensive health organization (CHO) is as a non-profit corporation that purchases or provides a wide range of ambulatory, inpatient, preventive, and social services to groups of local residents who choose to become members. Sometimes called integrated delivery systems (IDS, described in the previous chapter), CHOs have been proposed as part of health services delivery reform in most provinces. In general, they would provide a much more comprehensive range of services than either CHCs or HSOs because they offer medical, hospital, home care, and other support services with a single unified management. This system would also provide a comprehensive approach to health that includes disease prevention and health promotion. Institutional care would be replaced, where possible, with ambulatory and community-based care. CHOs would have a voluntary board, at least half made up of CHO members, and would be similar in some ways to HMOs in the U.S. CHOs would be funded by provincial health insurance plans via a regional health authority on a capitation basis; physicians would be paid by the CHO in a manner mutually agreed upon (fee-for-service, capitation, or salary). In large or medium urban communities, CHOs would serve defined population of 15,000 people and more. At present, there are very few functioning CHOs in Canada.

3.   SERVICES OF OTHER HEALTH CARE PROFESSIONALS

Among the many other health care professionals who provide primary health care in their speciality are those described here.

3.1. NURSES

Some nurses work together with a physician and provide primary health care with the physician's supervision, while others work independently in community health centres or occupational health services, or in remote areas where no physicians are available. They are generally paid by salary. Although there has been increasing recognition of nurse practitioners in Canada recently, not every province recognizes the speciality. Currently, only Ontario, Newfoundland, and Alberta have training programs for nurse practitioners, and only Alberta, Ontario, British Columbia and Newfoundland use nurse practitioners for service delivery. Nurse practitioners are nurses who are trained to provide primary care and are allowed to dispense certain drugs.

3.2. DENTISTS

Primary dental services are provided mainly in the offices of dentists with the support of dental hygienists. To some extent, local public health units or government-sponsored clinics also provide primary dental health services, usually to particular at-risk groups such as seniors or immigrant children. More specialized dental care can be provided by dental surgeons in hospital. Dentists are paid mainly by fee-for-service through private insurance or by the individual. Provincial health insurance plans in the Maritime provinces and Quebec cover routine dental care for children, Saskatchewan Health covers dental education for children, and Alberta covers dental care for seniors, widows, and widowers. Services provided by dental surgeons in hospital are covered by all provincial insurance plans (7).

3.3. CHIROPRACTORS

Chiropractors usually specialize in the manipulation of joints and muscles in order to correct musculoskeletal and other disorders. Chiropractic services are mainly provided in offices and, to a limited extent, in clinics organized by workers' compensation boards. Chiropractors are usually paid on a fee-for-service basis, through private insurance, or out-of-pocket by individuals, and partially by provincial government health insurance plans in British Columbia, Alberta, Saskatchewan, Manitoba, and Ontario (7).

3.4. PODIATRISTS

The podiatrist usually deals with foot problems. Like chiropractors, most work in private offices, although some work in either public health units or general hospitals. Their payment mechanism is also similar to that of chiropractors. The provincial insurance plans of British Columbia, Alberta, Saskatchewan, and Ontario cover part of the cost of services provided by podiatrists (7).

3.5. OPTOMETRISTS

The optometrist usually deals with refractory errors and minor ailments of the eye. They usually work in private offices or with optical dispensing outlets. Most optometrists are paid on a fee-for-service basis with a variety of payment mechanisms, depending on who is receiving services. Newfoundland and Prince Edward Island are the only provinces in Canada that do not cover any services provided by optometrists. Other provinces, such as British Columbia, Saskatchewan, Manitoba, and Ontario, cover some costs through their provincial insurance plans. Alberta and Nova Scotia cover optometrists' services to children and the elderly, and Quebec covers services to the poor and to "certain groups". The balance of the costs is covered by private insurance companies or directly by consumers (7).

3.6. MIDWIVES

Midwives usually deal with normal pregnancy, labour, delivery and post partum care. Since 1993 a few Canadian provinces — British Columbia, Alberta, Manitoba, Ontario, and Quebec — recognized midwifery as a licensed health care profession; New Brunswick is currently considering the role of midwifery as part of its Obstetrical Services Review. Midwives usually work in small group practices and are generally paid a yearly salary or on a per-case basis. Their main source of income used to be charges to individual users of their services; however, funding mechanisms through government health insurance plans are being worked out in the provinces that recognize midwifery. For example, since 1994, the Ontario Ministry of Health has covered all of the costs of midwifery services in the province (8-10).

3.7. PHARMACISTS

Pharmacists mostly provide their services through privately owned and operated drug stores, and receive a dispensing fee for filled prescriptions as part of their remuneration. Non-owner and institution-based pharmacists such as those working in hospitals are usually paid by salary.

3.8. OTHERS

Physiotherapists, occupational therapists, speech pathologists, audiologists, social workers, nutritionists and clinical psychologists are usually employed by hospitals, home care, and public health units. A number of them are in private practice and the costs of their services are covered by individuals out-of-pocket or by private health insurance.

3.9. ALTERNATIVE HEALTH CARE PROVIDERS

Increasingly, significant numbers of Canadians (approximately 15%) seek the services of alternative health care providers, which includes reflexologists, naturopaths, homeopaths, and traditional healers. These practitioners usually work in solo practices and are paid out-of-pocket by those individuals seeking such services (11).

As one can see, there is a range of primary health care services provided by different professionals. The entry point into the primary health care system depends upon various factors, such as the economic status and education of consumers, their health beliefs, type of health insurance, and the availability and accessibility of services and professionals.

4. HEALTH CARE INSTITUTIONS

Major institutions include allied special hospitals, chronic care hospitals, and nursing homes. In Quebec, the organization and activities of health care institutions is regulated by the *Act Respecting Health Services and Social Services and Amending Various Legislation* (passed in 1991). According to this act, Quebec differentiates between a "centre" and an "institution": A centre is a place where health and social services are dispensed and can include general and specialized hospitals, psychiatric hospitals, local community service centres, residential and long-term care centres, and certain categories of rehabilitative care centres. An "institution" (*établissement*), is an organization responsible for service activities pertaining to the mission of one or more centres and is, in effect, an umbrella organization that ensures the provision of a continuous spectrum of accessible and high-quality health or social services, as well as the reduction of the health and welfare problems of its particular population group. An institution is frequently responsible for the management of several centres with differing missions thus allowing for better integration and coordination of care, while centres are directly involved in service delivery (12). Many provinces are trying to emulate this concept of health care delivery through their regional health authorities.

4.1. HOSPITALS

4.1.1. Characteristics and Functions

The first hospital in Canada, Hôtel Dieu de Précieux Sang, was established in Quebec City in 1639. Prior to 1850, hospitals were perceived as dirty, infested, crowded, and unpleasant places, staffed by heartless and ignorant attendants, to which people would go only as a last resort. At the time, the overall mortality rate was high (20%). Florence Nightingale, Joseph Lister, and others revolutionized hospital care by introducing antisepsis, asepsis, good food, and proper nursing. This reduced mortality from

20% to 2%. By the beginning of the 20th century, people were choosing to go to hospitals to be cured.

Today, hospitals are the major centre for health care activities. Hospitals are institutions that primarily take care of sick people by providing inpatient services, services for many ambulatory patients in outpatient clinics and emergency rooms, and rehabilitation services. In certain cases, they also provide limited public health and home care services. Some large hospitals act as teaching resources for the education of physicians, nurses, and other allied health care professionals. Many teaching hospitals are also engaged in research activities. In recent years, there has been a trend to broaden the hospital's role to include disease prevention and health promotion.

Traditionally, most hospitals are paid by the provincial government. Payment methods include:

- **Global budget** — a prepaid sum covers all costs of services provided on a line-by-line basis, with payments allocated on individual items of expenditures;
- **Per diem** — a fee paid for each day the patient receives care in the institution. The average per diem cost is entirely artificial and the true cost of care for each day is generally unknown and highly variable (expensive at the beginning of the stay, cheaper at the end):
- **Per case** — a fee paid for each case, usually based on the diagnosis, using diagnostic related groups or case-mix basis that may be adjusted for severity.

Although these payment methods remain in place, the procedures for funding hospitals have changed with the advent of regionalized health authorities (RHAs) in all provinces except Ontario. Provincial governments transfer a lump sum of money to RHAs in funding envelopes that cover the costs of providing health care to their population, with the exception of money needed to cover physicians' services. The regional boards decide how much money is allocated to institutional care and how hospitals in their region are reimbursed. In New Brunswick, the eight regional hospital corporations receive a global budget from the province that they administer to cover hospital costs in their region and the costs of physician services. Generally, provincial ministries of health make special arrangements for the financing of highly specialized tertiary and quaternary hospitals, which provide services to the entire provincial population regardless of region of residence.

4.1.2. Organization of Hospitals

Hospitals, under legislation such as Ontario's *Public Hospitals Act,* are governed by a voluntary board of trustees. There are various forms of hospital boards which are constantly evolving; some boards are being phased out. Generally speaking, most board members are not professionals in the health care field and are either elected or appointed. Recently, physicians practising in the hospital and other hospital employees have also been represented on some hospital boards. In addition, some hospital administrators now also sit on hospital boards as voting members, sometimes as office holders. Under provincial legislation, the board is responsible for the governance of the hospital, subject to compliance with the terms, of the legislation. The board acts as the agent for the public in assuring proper financial operations and quality of care.

With the advent of regionalization in health (discussed in Chapter 13), the functions of most hospital boards have been taken over by regional health boards (RHBs) and the legislation has been amended accordingly. In Nova Scotia, Prince Edward Island, and British Columbia, RHBs have replaced all hospital boards (13). In Alberta, all hospital boards have been replaced except Catholic hospital boards, and Saskatchewan and Quebec have amalgamated at least some (if not all) hospital, community health centre, and long-term care facility boards. New Brunswick and Newfoundland have each created eight regional hospital/institutional boards that oversee the administration and delivery of services by hospitals and physicians in their respective provinces (14). Ontario has not regionalized its health services organization, and retains fully functioning hospital boards.

Almost all traditional hospital boards have a chief executive officer (CEO), president, or administrator in charge of daily operations and executing policies formulated by the board, and to whom all personnel report. The administrator may be supported by one or more assistant administrators, each controlling a functional area (e.g., medical director, and directors of nursing, plant and engineering, finances, and human resources). In Quebec, where health care institutions can oversee the work of several different health centres, the CEO and the senior management staff are responsible for the administration and operation of all of the centres operated by the institution. The CEO and the board are assisted by a management staff (including a director of professional services), a council of physicians, dentists, and pharmacists, a council of nurses, and a multidisciplinary council.

Legislation requires that the board establish a professional or medical advisory committee (PAC or MAC). In many hospitals, the PAC is responsible for advising on capital purchases of medical equipment, regulation of the professional staff, and similar matters. It is usually chaired by the chief of staff and consists of chiefs of different medical disciplines, chiefs of other health care professional services, and a member from the board.

The work of a hospital is usually organized according to either functions or divisions (15). A functionally organized hospital is divided into departments according to the number of functions performed. This usually involves vertically hierarchical reporting and decision making, and is well suited to small organizations with few goals and uncomplicated environments, such as a small community hospital or nursing home. The traditional functional organization of a hospital is illustrated in Figure 15.1 which is an organizational chart that covers the whole range of services a hospital may provide, although not all hospitals provide all the services listed. A hospital's size and teaching status determine the complexity of services available. Large teaching hospitals provide the widest range of services.

Larger hospitals with multiple stakeholder interactions — frequently teaching hospitals and academic health centres — are organized by division or programs. This type of hospital organization involves the creation of smaller, semi-autonomous units organized according to traditional medical specialities. Each sub-unit has its own

Figure 15.1:   Functional Organization of a Hospital

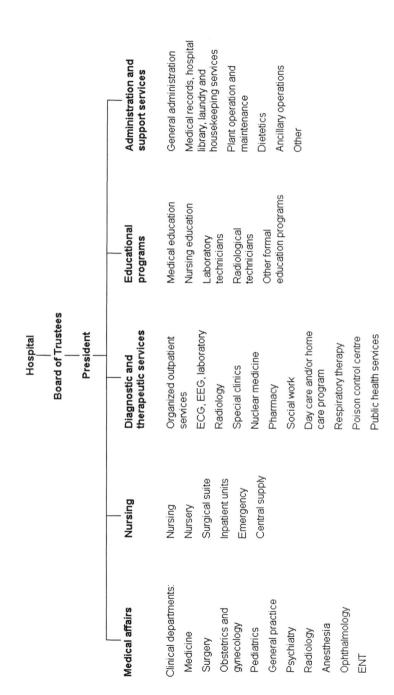

management team composed of medical, nursing, and administrative representatives, and usually has complete authority for the operation of the unit. Although divisional structures are much better at dealing with the multiple tasks required of an academic teaching hospital, and usually increase turn-around time for decision making, they run into problems of coordination, competitiveness among units, and, at times, goals incompatible with the goals and objectives of the larger corporate structure.

Organizational measures undertaken to integrate all hospital units (regardless of functional or divisional organization) include matrix designs that create dual reporting structures by function and by medical division (e.g., a nurse working in a cardiac unit is responsible to both the director of the cardiac unit, and to the director of nursing), and parallel structures such as special problem-solving teams or task forces.

More recently, in an effort to improve quality of care, responsiveness to patient needs, and accountability, many hospitals have adopted an organizational structure of program management. Program management is "a Canadian health care term that is synonymous with product line management in the private sector and in hospitals in the United States" (16). In this structure, the hospital is a portfolio of separate businesses with decision making pushed down the organization to teams of managers who are fully responsible for their programs. Programs have 100 to 150 beds each and can be defined according to population group (e.g., gender, ethnicity, age, geography), by disease or health problem (e.g., AIDS, cancer, heart disease), by patient need (e.g., rehabilitation, continuing care), by type of service (e.g., outpatients, home care), or by medical speciality (e.g., medicine, surgery). Most importantly, programs are multidisciplinary, self-contained units that are each unique or special in some way, with the capacity to become centres of excellence. This method of organizing hospitals has developed in the last few years and is currently being evaluated for effectiveness.

In recent years, communities have been concerned about the organization, governance, accountability, and functions of public hospitals. Many provinces have chosen regionalization as a response. As indicated above, the regionalization of responsibilities for health care has been undertaken to improve accountability and responsiveness to community needs. For the most part, regional health boards or regional institutional boards (in the case of New Brunswick and Newfoundland) have replaced individual hospital boards. Because RHB members are usually elected and include representatives from local communities, it is hoped that the RHBs will address some of these community concerns. Indeed, regionalization and devolution are so popular across Canada because they address these very concerns. Although there is a great deal of interest in the effectiveness of regionalized governance structures (17), however, systematic evaluation has so far been limited.

4.1.3. Organization of Staff in Hospitals (18)

Physicians play a pivotal role in terms of hospital utilization. They admit patients, determine what tests and treatments are needed, and how long patients stay. In most Canadian hospitals, physicians are not employees but users of hospital facilities on behalf of their patients. Physicians have "privileges" at a certain hospital but are not paid by the hospital. However, this is not the case for some radiologists, pathologists, and a few other specialists such as emergency room physicians.

Typically, a physician requests the privilege of admitting patients to a general hospital, and expects to be responsible not only for their care but also for patients referred by other doctors. The hospital's board screens the physician's qualifications and confirms its need for another physician. Admitting privileges are granted according to an impact analysis, which considers the potential number of patients who would be attracted to the hospital by the physician's specialized skills, the effect on hospital resources caused by the physician's activities, the ability of the physician's reputation to enhance the hospital's prestige, and the number of physicians providing the same or similar services. The board may reject the application or grant full or partial privileges, perhaps with some conditions (e.g., a general practitioner may not be allowed to do major surgery). Physicians usually complete a probationary period of an average of 12 months before receiving full hospital privileges; appointments are usually made for one year. Once physicians become members of the medical staff they undertake certain responsibilities to the hospital, in addition to the right and responsibility of looking after any patients they admit. Medical staff members may be required to provide service in the emergency room in rotation, serve on committees, maintain and give final approval to hospital medical records, and attend staff meetings; they must abide by the rules and regulations passed by the medical advisory committee or hospital board.

The medical staff is expected to be self-governing and self-disciplining through peer review and a wide variety of devices that have developed between medical staff and boards and, in some cases, governments. The most common devices are organizational. For example, it is assumed that every hospital should have a chief of staff, usually a respected senior doctor, for each medical and surgical discipline. This individual is responsible for ensuring the quality of care delivered. Formerly, the chiefs of staff exercised their influence by example or persuasion, but recent legislation in some jurisdictions gives them authority to relieve a physician of a case if it is obvious that the physician is not giving adequate or proper care to the patients.

In addition, it is common practice for hospitals to set up a series of committees charged with responsibility for monitoring the hospital's functioning. Some of these are the admission and discharge (or utilization) committee, the medical records committee, and the tissue committee. Sophisticated data processors can automatically examine performance in terms of established norms (e.g., how many cases admitted with a diagnosis of pneumonia had appropriate bacteriological work done? How many had antibiotic sensitivity tests?). For most provinces, this type of analysis for monitoring is done on a collective basis by the Canadian Institute for Health Information.

5.   PUBLIC HEALTH SERVICES

Since 1961, there has been a rapid growth in public health services at the provincial and local levels of government; however, with fiscal constraints, these services may now be curtailed. Currently, public health services are, for the most part, a responsibility of regional boards with funding for services allocated from regional envelopes. All provincial governments maintain departments responsible for public health matters and divide geographical regions into health units. Because metropolitan areas have a high population density, they have their own health units. Health units are semi-autonomous, form liaisons with local hospitals, medical practitioners, and voluntary health agencies, and have their own buildings and staff, except in Quebec. The province of Quebec has been divided into 18 regional boards of health and social services (Régies régionales de la santé et des services sociaux), each with a director of public health responsible for the assessment of the health needs of the population and development of the most effective preventive interventions, surveillance, and control of communicable and noncommunicable diseases, dealing with real or perceived public health emergencies, and developing an expertise in health promotion and disease prevention. The public health director works closely with the CLSCs and other regional health and social services agencies. Most health units are now under the direction of regional health boards that determine the overall direction of programs and policies, as well as the amount of public health services funding. Despite the rhetoric of increased emphasis on disease prevention and health promotion, less than 5% of total health care funding is devoted to local health units. The major portion of funding for local health units comes from the provincial government (through regional funding envelopes) with some funding from local governments. However, in Alberta, total funding comes from the provincial government, and in Ontario, the total funding of public health services comes from local governments. With these financial arrangements, local governments retain autonomy in policy and program planning while following provincial guidelines. The lack of uniformity in services provided across the province is compensated by assessment and fulfilment of local needs.

5.1. FUNCTIONS OF PUBLIC HEALTH UNITS

The mandate of the local health units stem from the public health acts or regulations passed by the provincial legislature. For example, the document *Mandatory Health Programs and Services Guidelines in Ontario* outlines standards for public health services in general and lists the goals and objectives for specific programs (19). Local governments also pass bylaws related to health if the province so authorizes (e.g., bylaws regulating noise levels and smoking in public places). The extent of services provided depends on the province's public health act and the number of qualified personnel employed by each agency in relation to the population. Many rural agencies do not have enough personnel and are unable to employ a full complement of public health staff. In addition to mandated activities, regional health authorities have expanded into many new health fields outside their traditional role especially in urban areas. Foremost among these are health promotion, mental health, services for people who are aged, disabled, and issues related to the physical environment.

5.1.1. Communicable Disease Control

The control of communicable disease continues to be a basic function of health units. Their duties include disease surveillance, the provision of consultation services to local physicians and hospitals, the supply of immunizing agents, health education, and special epidemiological surveys and studies. Health units are granted authority to control communicable disease by legislation and regulations; they are also responsible for the investigation and management of outbreaks such as food poisoning in nursing homes, measles in schools, and diarrhoea in day care centres. Most local health units operate sexually transmitted disease (STD) clinics, either by themselves or in conjunction with the local hospital; these clinics provide free diagnostic and treatment services at convenient hours. In some areas, these units pay private physicians to give free and anonymous treatment with the help of physicians practising in the community. Local health units are involved in case finding of STD and other communicable diseases, follow-up of contacts and health education programs for STDs. They also provide contraception and family planning services.

5.1.2. Maternal and Child Health, and Women's Health

In recent years, maternal and child health divisions in public health units in many provinces have been renamed and their functions expanded to focus more on family and women's health. They have different names in different provinces, but they have similar functions. Public health nurses employed by local health units carry out preventive health programs such as education and immunization of infants and children in clinics. The maternal and child health services may include classes for expectant parents, postnatal visits to all or high-risk new parents, advice on parenting, and visits to day care centres. Immunization of children is a statutory program in public health units in Alberta and Prince Edward Island, whereas immunization is shared by private physicians and health units in other provinces. Alberta also has comprehensive preschool surveillance programs (to monitor growth and development), which cover about 90% of children.

In many provinces, health care services for school children are provided by health units; however, in others, the local education authority or private practitioners may provide this service. The type of school health services varies considerably across Canada, and the provision of services by larger city departments may differ from that found in a rural health unit. Vision screening tests and immunization programs have become standard practice in most local areas, while audiometric screening is discretionary in some areas. The public health nurse provides continuity for the health surveillance of school children, and maintains contact with the parents and family doctor.

5.1.3. Health Promotion

Public health units increasingly emphasize health promotion, community development, and health advocacy. Health promotion as a separate discipline has been receiving growing recognition. Strategies include educational methods to improve knowledge and skills, encouragement of public participation in health practices conducive to healthy living, and public policies that create environments that support health. Many local health departments employ health promotion specialists. Their responsibility includes continually assessing the health needs of their community, coordinating local health promotion services, and consulting with personnel in the voluntary and civic organizations interested in health. Public health nursing is involved in implementing and planning health promotion strategies. Community development workers may help communities mobilize against a public health problem; for example, they can provide information on second-hand smoke and its effects on health, enabling citizens to bring about the necessary environmental changes through political or legislative processes. Nutrition consultants prepare reference and educational materials for professional health care personnel and for the public. Examples of health promotion programs include the heart health programs in most provinces, and the City of Toronto programs aimed at groups such as recent immigrants, refugees, visible minorities, and the homeless. Health promotion programs provide education in schools on smoking, alcohol, drugs, AIDS, sex, and nutrition. The extent of the diffusion of the innovative approach of health promotion in public health units has, however, not been evaluated. Academic health promotion units in many provinces have developed affiliations with public health units to promote basic research in the discipline of health promotion and its application.

5.1.4. Dental Health

Public health initiatives such as fluoridation of municipal water supplies and improved dental hygiene have successfully reduced dental caries in Canadian children. Public health now focuses on provision of dental treatment to underprivileged groups and the elderly. Dental health divisions of provincial ministries, in collaboration with local health units, have sponsored the provision of dental care for children in remote areas. There are travelling clinics staffed by provincial dental teams in Manitoba, Nova Scotia, Ontario, and Prince Edward Island that visit rural and remote areas. These clinics deliver a considerable amount of emergency care for all age groups. A program to subsidize dental expenses in communities that do not have a resident dentist has been developed in British Columbia; in rural Alberta, dentists who volunteer to supply services on a private practice basis for short periods are provided with dental equipment, office facilities, and living accommodation. In some provinces, the dental health division of the provincial health department administers school dental programs. This responsibility may be delegated either to the department of education or to the board of health, particularly in cities.

In all of these models, dentists or dental hygienists are employed to carry out functions such as case finding, education, prevention, and treatment. Such services are generally provided to preschool children or up to grade one or two. Treatment services are offered primarily to children from lower income groups.

5.1.5. Environmental Health

Public health inspectors hired by local health units protect the public from physical, chemical, and biological hazards. This is carried out through the inspection of food-handling premises such as restaurants, butcher shops, and bakeries. Public health inspectors are responsible for community sanitation such as the maintenance of sanitary supplies of potable water, milk, and food, disposal of wastes, and the quality of recreational water. They also respond to public complaints and emergency situations such as spills of toxic chemicals. In some of the larger cities, indoor air pollution monitoring is carried out by public health units. A number of health units have hired environmental specialists to conduct environmental risk assessments and provide consultation for their staff.

6.   HOME CARE

Most current health reform aims to strengthen and expand community-based and home-based care. This shift away from hospital-based care is motivated in part by fiscal constraints (home care is purportedly less expensive than institutional care) and in part by the belief that services provided in the home effectively meet the needs and preferences of patients, especially among the elderly. Only a small percentage of provincial health budgets is allocated to home care, but most provinces have increased these budgets in recent years.

6.1. HISTORY

Until early in this century, the rich were cared for at home and the poor, homeless, or indigent were treated in hospitals. With the emergence of provincial and national health insurance plans and the resulting expansion in the institutional sector, home care functions were transferred to hospitals and nursing homes. However, this pattern has gradually been reversing in the past 20 years. In most provinces, provision of home care services began with smaller, urban programs run by agencies such as the Victorian Order of Nurses (20). As a result of rising hospital costs and pressure on hospital facilities, home care programs were developed, mainly to relieve hospitals of the care of patients who only needed additional nursing services or physiotherapy. Comprehensive, government-oriented home care plans were developed by some provinces in the 1970s. In 1977, as a part of the Extended Program Financing services, legislation provided the first concrete financial support for home care programs (see Chapter Twelve). By the late 1990s, all provinces and territories have government home care directorates or divisions, although there is no common approach to funding and delivery. It still remains unclear whether the development and strengthening of home care programs is an effective cost-saving measure for provincial budgets, or whether it is currently an added cost to health systems, and transfer of cost to patients and their families.

6.2. TYPES OF HOME CARE

Different basic forms of home care are described below:

Maintenance and Preventive. Home support services (such as homemaker, transportation and meals-on-wheels programs) provide autonomy and mobility for those with assessed functional deficits. These services are not primarily medical, and may be provided along with medical treatment. Although many people can remain at home without the help of these services for some time, early use of the services can prevent health decline and institutionalization.

Long-Term Care Substitution or Chronic Care Services. These services are provided to people with significant functional deficits, usually resulting from one or more medical conditions, who require these services in order to remain in their homes. Chronic care services are designed for people with stable conditions, or to delay deterioration and thus institutionalization.

Acute Care Substitution. Acute home care is usually provided after hospitalization to people who are unable to travel to outpatient facilities, and it is provided on a short-term basis according to need. It is designed to reduce the length of hospital stay and to assist the recovery process. People usually receive acute home care from two or three days to a maximum of 90 days.

Extra-Mural Hospital or Hospital without Walls. This New Brunswick program is one of the most innovative programs. It is administered free of charge to a case-load equivalent to that of a 200-bed hospital. Services include a range of palliative and acute care services such as nursing, physiotherapy, intravenous medication, nutritional counselling, respiratory care oxygen therapy, and sick room equipment. Meals-on-wheels, homemaking, and other support services can be purchased by the patient, who must be formally admitted by an attending physician who directs the medical care plan and authorizes discharge. To be eligible, the patient must be acutely but not critically ill, and must require one or more professional services such as nursing, occupational therapy, or physiotherapy.

Palliative home care. Palliative home care is provided to terminally ill patients such as those with AIDS or cancer. The care is provided by a multidisciplinary team at home and is described in greater detail in section 7 of this chapter.

6.3. FUNDING AND DELIVERY

Most home care programs are characterized by two features: centralization of control of services within the program, and ongoing coordination of services to meet the changing needs of the patient. In some provinces, the provincial department of health plays an active role in the financing and administration of home care programs, while in other provinces, local agencies, municipalities, and hospitals assume the major responsibility for home care. There is also a substantial private sector component to home care with services financed directly by the patient or family. Between 1977 and 1996, when Established Program Financing was in effect, home care services became associated with local public health units in some provinces. Since the change over to the *Canada Health and Social Transfer Act* of 1996, federal transfers to the provinces no longer require a home care component in health budgets, nor do they allocate separate money for them. Home care services must now compete with all other provincial health, postsecondary education, and social services for their budgets.

At present, spending on home care programs accounts for just over $2 billion a year, or less than 4% of total public spending in the Canadian health system. Most provincial home care programs are funded by the government, but some charge user fees, often based on the ability to pay. For example, in British Columbia, all public home care programs are fully or partially funded by the Continuing Care Division of the Ministry of Health. Home care services such as case management, home nursing care and community rehabilitation are provided to those who qualify at no charge, while the homemaker services charge people according to income testing (21).

7. PALLIATIVE CARE

Medicine can be either curative or palliative, according to the philosophy of treatment. Curative medicine is usually considered as traditional medicine; its objective is to ensure a patient's health. Palliative medicine is defined as relieving without curing, based on an acceptance of the inevitable. Palliative care is a relatively new field in Canada, having emerged in 1974, and the demand is increasing (22). It is directed to those suffering from a terminal illness, who have different needs from those with acute illness, and focuses on the management of pain and other symptoms. It also addresses the psychological, emotional, and spiritual needs of patients and their families when curative care is no longer appropriate.

Palliative care should involve psychological support, assistance in interpersonal skills, coordinated service delivery, symptom control, bereavement counselling, independent living, legal and financial issues, matters of spirituality, lifestyle, culture, and religion (23, 24). It requires a multidisciplinary team approach, often supplemented by volunteers, and can be given in the home or in an institutional setting. Acute care facilities, which are geared to diagnosis and treatment, do not usually have the environment, skills, and flexibility needed to provide support to terminally ill patients and their families unless specialized facilities are available, such as designated palliative care beds and a palliative care team (25). In 1990, there were 345 palliative care programs in Canada, with 767 designated beds. Each province reported operational palliative care beds.

There are many types of palliative care programs available in Canada, and national standards do not exist. A recent decrease in the total number of palliative care programs prompted the formation of the Expert Panel on Palliative Care, made up of ten health care professionals from across Canada. In 1991, this panel made recommendations to the Cancer 2000 Task Force and extended its mandate to present a broad national vision for the palliative care community (26). The panel called for a radical restructuring of resources and priorities to make palliative care and the relief of suffering an essential fourth phase of those who are terminally ill and to ensure equitable resource allocation.

8. SERVICES FOR MENTAL ILLNESS

Among provincially operated health services, mental health services represent one of the largest administrative areas in terms of expenditure and employees. In every province, at least 88% (nationally, 96%) of the revenue for mental institutions comes from the provincial government or the provincial insurance plan. For the past four decades, the provision of mental health services has gradually shifted from institutions to community-based services. Depending on the nature and the severity of illness, services are now provided by mental institutions, psychiatric units of general hospitals, special hospitals, private hospitals, clinics, mental health care centres, prisons, halfway houses, sheltered workshops, and private practitioners such as psychiatrists, family physicians, clinical psychologists, and social workers.

Community mental health facilities are now extended beyond mental institutions to provide greater continuity of care, to deal with incipient breakdown, and to rehabilitate patients in the community. Psychiatric units in general hospitals contribute by integrating psychiatry with other medical care and making it available in the community. Hospital psychiatric units admit approximately 48% of total admissions to all kinds of mental institutions. Inpatient services in psychiatric units are paid for by all provincial hospital insurance plans. Some provinces have small regional psychiatric hospitals that facilitate patient access to treatment and complete integration of medical services. Day care centres that allow patients to be hospitalized during the day and return home at night exist across the country, as do community mental health clinics (some provincially operated, others municipally) and psychiatric outpatient services.

Specialized rehabilitation services assist former patients to function optimally and are operated by mental hospitals and community agencies. They include sheltered workshops that pay for work and provide training, and halfway houses where patients can live and continue to receive treatment while settling in a job. At present, there is a large gap in available community services for mental health patients because of shortages of affordable housing, jobs, recreational facilities, and mental health workers.

Facilities for people who are mentally challenged include day training schools or classes, summer camps, and sheltered workshops, as well as residential care in institutions and community group homes. These provide social, academic, and vocational training; some offer academic education, some support self-care, some teach manual skills, and some help find job placements in the community. Children with personality or behaviour disorders are treated at hospital units, community clinics, child guidance clinics, and other outpatient facilities.

At least 2% to 5% of adult Canadians are addicted to licit and illicit drugs and alcohol. Substance abuse and addiction are treated in hospitals, outpatient clinics, hostels, long-term residences, or special farms and facilities. Official and voluntary agencies conduct public education programs, treatment, rehabilitation, and research, including Alcoholics Anonymous, the Alcoholism Foundation of British Columbia, Quebec's l'Office de la prevention et du traitement de l'alcoolisme et des autres toxicomanies, the Addictions Foundation of Manitoba, and the Nova Scotia Alcoholism Research Foundation. Community treatment programs have been established by the Narcotic Addiction Foundation of British Columbia and the Addiction Research Foundation of Ontario, supported primarily by provincial funds. However, there are not enough available services for addiction.

9. SERVICES FOR CANCER PATIENTS

More than one in three Canadians will get cancer in his or her lifetime; most will be diagnosed in their middle and later years. Special provincial agencies for cancer control, usually run by the health ministry or a separate cancer institute, carry out cancer detection and treatment, public education, and professional training and research, in cooperation with local public health services, physicians, and voluntary Canadian Cancer Society branches (e.g., the Alberta Cancer Board, the British Columbia Cancer Agency). Although the provisions are not uniform, cancer programs in all provinces provide a range of free diagnostic and treatment services both to outpatients and to inpatients. Hospital insurance benefits for cancer patients include diagnostic radiology, laboratory tests, and radiotherapy. A number of provinces, including British Columbia, Ontario, Quebec, New Brunswick, and Nova Scotia, have organized screening programs for breast cancer for women.

The lack of uniform provision of services, however, results in differences in community cancer services between provinces and between communities. This can result in a lack of coordination of treatment and less than optimal dissemination of cancer treatment knowledge and information in the major centres. The recommendations of the National Conference on Community Cancer Programs called for a survey of existing cancer services in Canada and ongoing evaluation of the efficiency and quality of cancer care (27).

10. SERVICES FOR PERSONS WITH SPECIAL NEEDS

Social and support services are available in the community for people with special, multidisciplinary needs (such as seniors, or people with mental or physical challenges) and vary depending on the location of the community and the nature and type of disability. Overall, rural communities have sparse services, whereas metropolitan areas offer a full range of services. People with rare or very severe disabilities have fewer resources available for their care in the community. Medical and institutional care, such as long-term care in hospitals, extended care, rehabilitation care, and nursing home care, as well as many assistive devices for daily living, are available through either government insurance or subsidies and have been described in Chapter 13. Most communities have home care programs available for those with multiple needs. In addition, the provinces are increasingly establishing "one-stop" access centres (such as multiple service agencies) to evaluate, assess, coordinate, and provide (or contract for the provision of) a wide range of health, social and support services to seniors or people with disabilities. There are two types of voluntary agencies that deal specifically with people with mental or physical challenges: agencies that exclusively deal with people with a specific disease or problem (e.g., the Multiple Sclerosis Society); and agencies that deal with specific groups with a disability (e.g., the Easter Seal Society, which deals with children with physical disabilities). Depending on the special needs of each individual, many voluntary agencies also provide a range of services, such as meals-on-wheels, visiting homemaker services, travelling clinics, provision of appliances and equipment, and wheelchairs. At the social service level, there are income maintenance programs, recreational programs, vocational rehabilitation services, special transportation services, and independent living accommodations available for individuals so they can lead independent lives.

11. VOLUNTARY AGENCIES

Voluntary organizations play an important part in shaping our health, welfare, and educational systems. These are non-profit organizations led by boards of volunteers rather than under the direct control of the government. Their primary or major objectives are the promotion of health, the prevention of illness or disability, and the identification, treatment, or rehabilitation of people with a disease or disability. Voluntary organizations differ in the nature of their membership: some are organized by citizens to provide service to others and are designated as citizen-member organizations; more recently, groups are organized by patients, their relatives, or their friends to provide services for themselves, and hence are designated patient-member organizations.

The citizen-member organization is the familiar form of philanthropy. Its members are interested in community service and thus are motivated to give time, thought and money to accomplish an objective to promote the welfare of their community. Patient-member organizations are motivated by mutual aid. Those who have a disease for which there is now no known cure or have a disability that causes them to be different from, and even shunned by, other people often become isolated and withdrawn or seek the company of fellow sufferers. They are faced with anxieties and frustration from which they find some relief by uniting to fight their common enemy, the disease. The patients may be able to help themselves in specific ways (e.g., by organizing better treatment facilities) or they may hope to help other sufferers, including their families if the disease is hereditary. They gain support from the knowledge that they are not alone in facing their problems. Recently some groups have taken an advocacy role, such as AIDS groups.

Voluntary organizations are financed to a considerable extent, if not wholly, by fund-raising. The organization may conduct its own campaign for funds, or be a member of a federated fund. Many of the agencies also receive public grants.

11.1. OBJECTIVES AND ACTIVITIES

Generally, the objectives and activities of many of voluntary organizations include (28):

- *Education*: public education and dissemination of information to lay and professional people;
- *Advocacy*: social action, sometimes specified, sometimes implied;
- *Research*: collection of statistics, investigation of reported "cures", surveys of resources and needs, encouragement and support for basic and clinical research;
- *Direct patient services*: supply of diagnostic and treatment clinics, special equipment (e.g., wheelchairs, crutches, colostomy bags, hoists, inhalation tents, prosthetic appliances), transportation and accommodation for patient and family, home treatment, therapies, vocational assessment and workshops; some take on official functions (e.g., the Children's Aid Society) and provide many services needed by society, including eye banks, and first aid;
- *Prevention*: the prevention and eradication of the disease or disability;
- *Coordination of key players*: the coordination of public and private agencies with similar interests; and
- *Fund-raising*.

11.2. ROLE IN RELATION TO GOVERNMENT

Voluntary agencies continually identify new areas of need and provide for those needs to the limit of their capacity. This capacity relates directly to the agency's ability to raise money and, in some cases, needs are met only in a token fashion. Nevertheless, the organizations often are able to impress upon the public's mind the importance of the services they provide and occasionally change the public's sensitivity to needs (for example, the Canadian Mental Health Association's exposé of mental hospitals as tawdry, overcrowded, and desolate places for patients). With increasing affluence and heightened social conscience, our governments had recognized that many of these initiatives were universally needed for the care of citizen and hence government had funded or taken over the responsibilities of many volunteer organizations' services.

However, in recent years, there has been a reversal of this trend and increased reliance is being placed on the voluntary sector. In practice, the functions of voluntary organizations and the government in the health field intermingle to such an extent that at times there is little differentiation in function, which, may create tension between the government and voluntary organizations.

11.3. SCOPE OF WORK

Examples of national voluntary organizations are presented here.

The **Canadian Red Cross Society** was established to furnish volunteer aid to the sick and wounded of armies in time of war, in accordance with the Treaty of Geneva, and in times of peace or war to carry on and assist in the improvement of health, the prevention of disease, and the mitigation of suffering throughout the world. Activities include veterans' services, international relief, emergency services, water safety services, Red Cross Youth, and Red Cross Corps. (As of 1997, the Canadian Red Cross is no longer involved in the provision of blood transfusion services in Canada.)

The **Canadian Cancer Society** was established in 1938 to coordinate individuals and agencies to reduce the mortality from cancer in Canada, to disseminate information on cancer, and to research activities about cancer.

Local volunteer groups include local chapters of larger organizations, as well as volunteer organizations that meet special needs in the community. These include volunteer groups working in hospitals, nursing homes, and crisis centres.

Voluntary agencies have adapted to the changing needs of society. For example, what was once known as the Canadian Tuberculosis Association has changed its name and mandate, with the decreasing incidence of tuberculosis, to the **Canadian Tuberculosis and Respiratory Disease Association**; its Ontario chapter calls itself the **Ontario Lung Association** and focuses on all lung diseases. Voluntary health organizations fulfil an important role in shaping the health care system and will continue to do so.

12. SELF-HELP GROUPS

People join together in groups for companionship, mutual assistance, and the exchange of problem-solving skills. The most obvious example of the self-help concept is the family, a small group where socialization, identification, and support originate. Self-help efforts are also evident in collective enterprises such as food or housing cooperatives, tenants' associations, and civil rights groups. But groups also exist for those who have a common personal concern, such as a physical disability or an addiction. Romeder et al. (29) defines self-help groups as small, autonomous, open groups that meet regularly. Members share common experiences and meet each other as equals. The primary activity of these groups is personal mutual aid, a form of social support that focuses on sharing experiences, information, and ways of coping. In addition to personal change, members often engage in activities directed to social change. Group activities are voluntary and usually free. In some cases, there is already a national or international body of self-help groups focused on a given concern, and this may offer consultative and public relations support to new self-help groups or associations. Alcoholics Anonymous, established in 1935, has been the model for the development of other self-help groups (e.g., Narcotics Anonymous, Schizophrenics Anonymous).

Self-help groups usually attract members who are between 30 and 50 years of age, from the middle class or a common educational level or socioeconomic status. For many people with many types of difficulties, such groups can be very effective for coping with personal pressures. The major activities of these groups include group meetings, sponsorship of new members, educational activities for their members and the general public, and advocating for change. Apart from these general services, activities are as diverse as the groups themselves. They include home or hospital visits to the sufferer, hot lines, newsletters and brochures, public conferences, fairs, advocacy, recreational activities, and material aid (e.g., sitter services, transportation, exchange of goods). There are a number of support groups that help persons with specific health conditions, such as AIDS, breast cancer, and prostate cancer.

13. TELE-HEALTH

Already well-established in the U.S., tele-health is emerging rapidly as a new branch of health care in Canada. Tele-health uses telephones, ranging from conventional telephone service to sophisticated computerized call-data centres, to facilitate health care. It is especially useful in monitoring the health status of patients in rural, Northern and remote communities. It harnesses technology to support health care professionals in delivering health care. It helps patients to find their way around the health care system and to get the health information they need. Tele-health applications include hospital-based video conferencing, health information lines, telephone triage, Internet Nurses and tele-home care (home visits over distance). Canada has the world's longest-running tele-health service at the Memorial University of Newfoundland. Most provinces such as Quebec, New Brunswick, Nova Scotia, and Ontario have programs for telehealth to serve its rural and remote communities.

14. SUMMARY

Health care is delivered at the local level through a spectrum of services. These health services include primary care, secondary care, hospital care, home care, public health services, and private nursing homes. The funding sources for these services are varied. Although in every province, basic hospital and medical services are provided through the government health insurance plans, what is provided either through public or private insurance varies.

Primary health care is service provided at the first contact between the patient and the health care professional and is usually provided by general or family practitioners in their offices on a fee-for-service basis. Most physicians bill provincial health insurance plans for their services. Apart from the physician, there are a number of other health care professionals who provide primary health care (including dentists, nurses, chiropractors, optometrists, podiatrists, and physiotherapists). *Walk-in clinics* that offer primary care are becoming increasingly popular.

Secondary care is usually delivered by specialized practitioners using specialized resources. Patients usually receive secondary care after referral from a primary care provider. *Tertiary care* requires very specialized facilities and professional skills.

Today, *hospitals* are the major centre for health care services. They provide inpatient services, services for ambulatory patients in outpatient clinics, emergency rooms, and rehabilitation services. Hospitals are classified on the basis of the kind of the service they provide, and are paid by the provincial government. In most provinces they are governed by a regional board. Hospitals usually have a chief executive officer, president or administrator who is in charge of day-to-day operations and executes policies formulated by the regional board. Most physicians are considered "users" of hospitals via hospital privileges rather than as "employees" of the hospital.

Health units are semi-autonomous in nature and form liaisons with local hospitals, medical practitioners, and voluntary health agencies. Their functions depend on the mandate set out by the provincial public health act and funding, and include the control of communicable disease, maternal and child health services, health promotion, dental health, and environmental health.

Recently, there has been increasing emphasis on *home care*. The services delivered by the home care programs range from nursing services to an array of health and social services. There are three basic models for home care: the maintenance and preventive model, the long-term care substitution model, and the acute care substitution model. Most provincial home care programs are funded by the government, but some charge user fees, often based on the ability to pay.

Mental health activities represent one of the largest administrative areas in terms of expenditure and employees. Community mental health facilities are reaching beyond mental health institutions to provide greater continuity of care, deal with incipient breakdown, and rehabilitate patients in the community. Currently, funding is not adequate to meet the needs of de-institutionalized patients.

The availability of social and support *services in the community for people with disabilities* depends on the location of the community and the nature and type of disability. Most communities have home care programs available for people with disabilities.

Voluntary organizations have played and continue to play an important part in shaping our health, welfare, and educational systems. These non-profit organizations operate under boards of volunteers, with the primary or major objectives being the promotion of health, the prevention of illness or disability, and the identification, treatment or rehabilitation of people with disease or disability.

Self-help groups are small, autonomous, open groups that meet regularly. As a result of personal crisis or chronic problems, members share common experiences and meet each other as equals. The primary activity of these groups is personal mutual aid, a form of social support that focuses on the sharing of experiences, information, and ways of coping.

15. REFERENCES

1. Tonkin R. Primary Health Care. Canadian Journal of Public Health 1976;67(4):289-294.
2. Barnsley J, Williams AP. The Impact of Walk-in Clinics on Ontario's Health Care System. Toronto: Health Management Research Unit, Department of Health Administration, University of Toronto, 1996.
3. Personal Communication. Physician Remuneration in Canada. Ottawa: Canadian Institute for Health Information, Health Human Resources Division, 1997.
4. Strachan JPC. Physician Billings Database. Ottawa: Canadian Institute for Health Information, 1997.
5. Vayda E. Physicians in Health Care Management: 5. Payment of Physicians and Organization of Medical Services. Canadian Medical Association Journal 1995; 150(10):1583-1588.
6. Abelson J, Birch S. Alternative Funding and Delivery Models: Practice and Prospects in Ontario. Journal of Ambulatory Care Management 1993;16(3):19-29.
7. Health Canada. Canada Health Act Annual Report: 1994-95. Ottawa: Ministry of Supply and Services Canada, 1996.
8. Fleming SM. Midwifery in Canada. Midwives Chronicle 1992;105(1258):338-40.
9. Ontario Hospital Association. Midwifery: The Integration of Midwifery Services Into Hospitals. Ontario Hospital Association, 1994.
10. Relyea MJ. The Rebirth of Midwifery in Canada: An Historical Perspective. Midwifery 1992;8(4):159-169.
11. Millar WJ. Uses of Alternative Health Care Practitioners by Canadians. Canadian Journal of Public Health 1997;88(3):154-158.
12. Collège des médecins du Québec. ALDO Quebec: Legislative, Ethical and Organizational Aspects of Medical Practice in Quebec. Montreal: Collège des médecins du Québec, 1995.
13. Health Canada. Provincial Health System Reform in Canada. Ottawa: Ministry of Supply and Services Canada, 1995.

14. Reamy J. Health Service Regionalization in New Brunswick, Canada: A Bold Move. International Journal of Health Services 1995;25(2):271-282.
15. Leatt P, Lemieux-Charles L, Aird C, eds. Program Management and Beyond: Management Innovations in Ontario Hospitals. Ottawa: Canadian College of Health Services Executives, 1994.
16. Leatt P, Lemieux-Charles L, Aird C, Leggat SG. Strategic Alliances in Health Care. Ottawa: Canadian College of Health Services Executives, 1996.
17. Gray C. CMA-Cosponsored Conference Raises Many Questions About Future of Regionalized Health Care. Canadian Medical Association Journal 1995;153(5):642-645.
18. Leatt P, Vayda E, Williams JI, Barnsley J. Medical Staff Organization in Canadian Hospitals. Ottawa: Canadian Hospital Association Press, 1987.
19. Ontario Ministry of Health. Mandatory Health Programs and Services Guidelines. Toronto: Ministry of Health, 1989.
20. Federal/Provincial/Territorial Working Group on Home Care. Report on Home Care. Ottawa: Ministry of Supply and Services, Health and Welfare Canada, 1990.
21. Federal/Provincial/Territorial Subcommittee on Continuing Care. Description of Long-Term Care Services in Provinces and Territories of Canada. Ottawa: Health Services Directorate, Health Services and Promotion Branch, Health and Welfare Canada, 1991.
22. Vincent L, Dawson H, Trentowsky S, Muter M. Survey Underscores Challenge of Planning Palliative Care Services for Cancer Patients. Ontario Medical Review 1990;57(10):17-22.
23. Health Services Directorate. Palliative Care Service Guidelines: Report of the Subcommittee on Institutional Program Guidelines. Ottawa: Health Services and Promotion Branch, Health and Welfare Canada, 1989.
24. The Royal Victoria Hospital. Palliative Care Services, Royal Victoria Hospital. The R.V.H. Manual on Palliative Hospital Care. Montreal: 1980.
25. Mount B. The Problem of Caring for the Dying in a General Hospital: The Palliative Care Unit as a Possible Solution. Canadian Medical Association Journal 1976;115(2):119-21.
26. Scott J. Palliative Care 2000: What's Stopping Us? Journal of Palliative Care 1992;8(1):5-8.
27. Osoba D. Recommendations of the National Clearinghouse on Community Cancer Programs: A Vision for the Future. Canadian Medical Association Journal 1991;144(11):1433-1436.
28. Govan E. Royal Commission on Health Services, Voluntary Health Organizations in Canada. Ottawa: Ontario Queen's Printer, 1966.
29. Romeder JM. The Self-Help Way, Mutual Aid and Health. Ottawa: Canadian Council on Social Development, 1989.

Chapter
16
Regulation of Health Care Professionals

In 1992, *Health Personnel in Canada* (1) listed 31 health care occupations. The 1990 edition of the *Canadian Hospital Directory* (2) listed more than 50 specifically related to hospitals, and there are more than 130 separate fields of employment in the health care system.

     This chapter presents a discussion of those occupations directly involved with patient care. Before describing the various health care professions, para-professions, and allied occupations, however, it starts with a definition of professionalism and a brief history of the modern medical profession. The chapter ends with an explanation of the regulations of health care professions and future regulatory trends.

1.   PROFESSIONALISM

     The concept of professionalism is very difficult to define. Most writers list traits or characteristics normally attributed to the established professions, and the significance assigned to those traits varies widely. According to *Webster's Third International Dictionary* the meaning of the word "profession" is as follows: "a calling requiring specialized knowledge and often long and intensive preparation including instruction in skills and methods as well as in the scientific, historical or scholarly principles underlying such skills and methods, maintaining by force of organization or concerted opinion, high standards of achievement and conduct, and committing its members to continued study and to a kind of work which has for its prime purpose the rendering of a public service"(3). Most definitions emphasize the public service or altruistic aspect of professionalism. This type of description is an idealized one (4) and considering the influence wielded by the established professions, the above definition undoubtedly represents the image projected by the professions themselves. The following lists characteristics commonly attributed to an established profession.

Specialized Knowledge and Skill

There is a specific body of detailed knowledge and complex skills common and unique to the members of the profession, which require a lengthy period of training to acquire. Professionals' extensive education and the importance of their role in society entitle them to the confidence of their clients and to a position of prestige.

Autonomy

Professions are self-regulating, that is, they are governed by associations made up of members of the profession. The professional association sets standards for the practice of the profession, determines who is qualified to practise (licensing authority), and enforces uniformity of practice. A code of ethics is defined. Those who fail to meet the prescribed standard or who violate the code of ethics are disciplined by the professional association. Members are free to practice independently in the manner of their choice (within the aforementioned prescribed limits) and are not subject to bureaucratic control. Even those members who choose to be employed by institutions or corporations rather than practise privately are generally free to create their own roles (5).

Service Orientation

Professionals deal directly with their clients, and their prime concern is to provide good service rather than to pursue self-gain. This does not necessarily imply altruism, but simply that personal gain is secondary to service. The professional must be free of outside influence to be able to make unbiased decisions with only the client's welfare in mind.

Responsibility

The professional helps clients make informed decisions and also makes decisions on their behalf. In the case of medicine, these decisions may involve life or death. The clients trust the professional, and divulge confidential and privileged information. The professional must maintain an impersonal and objective approach.

Recognition

Members of established professions are recognized by the public as being "professional" and are accorded a certain degree of respect. In most cases, this recognition is also extended by government, so that the established professions are accorded formal status by statute.

However, non-professionals sometimes take exception to these characteristics of professions. The requirement of difficult and lengthy training, for example, is seen as an obstacle for entry into the profession that restricts membership to an elite group. Self-regulation, particularly with regard to licensing authority, is a means of establishing a monopoly (6). Licensed members of a profession practise under a protective cloak of presumed competence whether or not they actually are competent. Incompetence or unethical behaviour is rarely punished, and members of the profession are reluctant to criticize each other. Uniform norms of practice inhibit innovation.

Many people deny that there is any reliable evidence that professionals are more service oriented than non-professionals. There is a strong movement, particularly in people's dealing with the medical profession, toward accepting greater responsibility for oneself and surrendering less control to the professional. Many today question the power and prestige traditionally enjoyed by the established professions especially the dominant role played by medicine.

The truth must lie somewhere between, these opposite views of professionalism There is no question that established professions occupy positions of power and prestige in society. But social structure is dynamic. The medical profession in particular has not always enjoyed the pre-eminence that it does today, as is discussed in the next section. Furthermore, significant changes in both the status and the regulation of the professions are currently taking place.

2.   EVOLUTION OF THE MEDICAL PROFESSION

The practice of medicine is ancient, as evidenced by the trephined skulls of pre-historic human, and the recorded histories of Babylon, Egypt, India, and China. However, the profession of medicine as it exists in the western world today is relatively recent. Western medicine had its beginnings in ancient Greece with Hippocrates and Aristotle, and with the founding of a Greek medical school in Alexandria in 300 B.C., which continued to operate during the heyday of the Roman Empire. After the fall of Rome, although the knowledge of the Greeks was preserved and translated by monks, little progress was made until the late middle ages. The practice of medicine was a trade learned by apprenticeship, with much the same status as other trades.

The first medical school in Europe was founded at Salerno, Italy, in the 11th century. In 1221, the Holy Roman Emperor, Frederick II, decreed that no one could practise medicine unless he had attended the school at Salerno. This seems to have been one of the earliest attempts of regulation. Later in the middle ages, medical faculties were established at universities in the major cities of western Europe. The first medical faculty at a university in the United Kingdom was founded in Edinburgh in 1726, and the first medical school in the United States opened in Philadelphia in 1766.

With the establishment of medical faculties at the medieval universities of western Europe, medicine joined the more traditional professions of law and theology as one of the "learned professions", and thus achieved some status. Although the mainstream of the medical profession was now formally trained at universities and medical schools, there was still little scientific basis to the art of medicine. The rapid expansion of scientific knowledge and the tremendous growth of universities that occurred in the late 1800s and early 1900s dramatically changed the practice of medicine. The scientific basis of medicine was established by the great discoveries of men such as Pasteur, Lister, and Koch. Medicine became ever more closely connected with science, particularly following the Flexner report on medical education in the United States and

Canada published in 1910. Professional schools changed from institutions that had no prerequisites for admission to those that required high school graduation and then university training in the basic sciences. Professional courses lengthened from a few months of lectures to years of disciplined study. Concurrently, the effectiveness of treatment dramatically improved.

The physician became someone to be trusted and sought out in time of suffering, rather than one to be feared and avoided. At the same time, the great body of knowledge required to practise medicine increased the educational gulf between practitioners and patients, giving the profession an aura of mystique. All of these factors combined to enhance the prestige of the profession. The profession also achieved considerable influence with governments, so that by the early 20th century, all developed countries except the then newly founded Soviet Union, which purposefully sought to decrease physician autonomy and equalize the status and prestige of all health care workers, had enacted legislation to make the medical profession self-regulating with powers of licensure and discipline. This act indicates that the state recognized its own responsibility with regard to the regulation of the medical profession, but delegated this responsibility to the profession. Once the statutes were in place, most states adopted a policy of non-interference and, in a sense, abdicated responsibility. There were no government representatives on the governing councils of the professional associations. The medical profession achieved virtual autonomy.

The last two decades have seen the beginnings of a reversal in the evolution of medical dominance described above (7). The scientific knowledge upon which medicine is based and the effectiveness of medical treatment have both continued to grow. Nevertheless, the authority of the profession, particularly the monopoly over service delivery and the degree of autonomy enjoyed for at least the last half century, has been increasingly questioned. There are several reasons for this. First, the increasing democratization of western societies has resulted in less deference to all forms of authority. Second, the great increase in the general level of education, especially among the large numbers of individuals employed in scientific disciplines and social sciences, has removed the mystique once associated with the profession. Third, consumer demand has achieved the recognition of alternative forms of health services delivery even when the state was not yet prepared to sanction them (e.g., the legal recognition of midwifery).

In Canada, the most important de-professionalizing factor has undoubtedly been the establishment of government-sponsored universal medical insurance. Because the state pays for physician services, it has an obligation to its citizens to ensure that they receive good value for their tax money. The responsibility for regulating the practice of medicine, once delegated to the profession by the state, is now in the process of being taken back. Although the profession still enjoys considerable autonomy, it is becoming more accountable to government and consumers. The extent to which this has occurred and possible future developments are discussed in later sections.

3.   EVOLUTION OF OTHER HEALTH CARE PROFESSIONS

An industrializing society has been described as a "professionalizing" society. The rapid proliferation of knowledge in all fields of science and technology has, in recent decades, brought about the establishment of many new professions, some of which are in the health care field. In seeking professional status, these groups usually follow the model set by the older established professions. They develop complex technologies, establish lengthy periods of training, impose strict registration requirements, develop codes of ethics, and seek statutory recognition.

However, although many groups have been accorded professional status, it could be argued that few of them can be described in terms of the definition earlier quoted from *Webster's Dictionary*. The word "profession" seems to have become more narrowly associated with specialized knowledge, and there appears to be less emphasis on the characteristics of autonomy, service orientation, and responsibility. Most of the health-related non-physician groups have followed the same pattern established by medicine, but only dentistry has achieved a similar degree of autonomy. With the exception of nursing and midwifery, all have a much shorter history than medicine. For example, the world's first school of dentistry was established in Baltimore in 1840.

Medicine is the dominant profession in the health field. In achieving professional status, the mainstream of medicine either eliminated, absorbed, or controlled competing disciplines. Pharmacy and nursing, for example, achieved professional status by becoming subordinate to medicine (8). Osteopathy, naturopathy, and homeopathy have remained separate entities, on the "fringe" of medicine and, in most communities, in restricted forms of practice. Optometrists and chiropractors have an autonomous status, but also are subject to many restrictions (e.g., practitioners cannot prescribe drugs or perform surgery). Most of the other health care professions and allied technical trades have developed as auxiliaries to medicine and are a product of the expansion of the scientific basis of medicine and the resultant need for support trades. This is true, for example, of physiotherapy, laboratory technology, and radiation technology.

Perspectives on Health Occupations lists the educational and licensing requirements, function, future directions, and national professional associations for approximately 50 health occupations. The *Catalogue on Health Manpower Legislation* (10) provides the licensing and registration requirements for major health care providers for each province. (Recently, the legislation in Ontario has changed and this is discussed subsequently in this chapter). Similarly, a federal publication is available for certifying bodies, professional associations, and accrediting agencies for various health care occupations in Canada (11). The next section of this chapter provides examples of how some of these professions are regulated in Quebec and Ontario.

4.   REGULATION OF HEALTH CARE PROFESSIONS

The *Constitution Act of 1867* gave provincial governments the responsibility for health care. As discussed in earlier chapters, the federal government has recently acquired considerable influence in health care matters through various cost-sharing arrangements under which provinces must meet certain conditions before being eligible to receive federal funds. Nevertheless, the legislation that regulates the activities of the various health care occupations is provincial. It follows then that there are 12 different groups of legislation (ten provincial and two territorial). Although generally similar, there are important differences. As stated in the previous section, the medical profession (and some other health care professions) in Canada had achieved autonomy prior to the introduction of universal medical insurance. Since then, most provinces have enacted, or intend to enact, legislation to ensure greater public control of the professions. The earliest and most significant of these changes occurred in the provinces of Quebec and Ontario.

4.1. PROFESSIONAL CODE OF QUEBEC

The *Professional Code* of Quebec (12), enacted in 1973, places the regulation of all professions under one act. A total of 38 professions, 22 of them in the health care field, are included. The Code is unique in that it defines what a profession is and establishes formal criteria by which an occupation gains statutory recognition as a profession. Each recognized profession is governed by a professional "order" (previously called a professional "corporation"). The order is charged with the traditional functions of a licensing agency. It determines the qualifications necessary to enter practice, including setting the length of training, examines candidates' credentials, maintains a register of members of the profession, defines the scope of practice, regulates specialists' certificates, determines what acts may be delegated, collaborates with educational institutions, and handles disciplinary matters within the profession. Under each governing legislation, there are acts that are given exclusively to a profession which could delegate an act to other professions and these are known as "delegated acts".

In addition, because the order is first and foremost concerned with the protection of the public, it is responsible for the ongoing supervision of the practice of its profession and is given broad powers to supervise the practices of individual members. This is a significant innovation. Traditionally, professional regulatory bodies have only disciplined members whose unethical, improper behaviour, or incompetence has been reported by third parties. The Code requires each professional order to maintain ongoing surveillance of the quality of individual practices and take corrective measures, such as requiring refresher training. In addition, it ensures that the administration of any given profession is not conducted exclusively by the members of that profession. Non-members are appointed by the Quebec Professions Board and are there to represent the government and to protect the interests of the public. Disciplinary matters are handled by the disciplinary committee of each order. The committee is informed of and investigates every complaint made against a member. It consists of at least three members and chaired by a lawyer with at least ten years of practice and is appointed by the government. Professionals conducting the inquiry of their order into any complaint, as well as those testifying before a discipline committee hearing, are immune from prosecution.

The Code distinguishes between two categories of professionals: exclusive professions and professions with reserved titles. Exclusive professions reserve the right to practise the profession and bear the corresponding professional title (for example, nurses or physicians). Professions with reserved titles, on the other hand, give their members the right to use a particular title, while the activities of their profession are not limited exclusively to them (e.g., social workers or psychologists).

The Code also establishes two overall supervisory and regulatory bodies. The Quebec Professions Board is a governmental agency composed of five members appointed by the Lieutenant Governor-in-Council (the provincial Cabinet). It is responsible for ensuring that each order properly carries out its duty to protect the public. It monitors the performance of each order and takes corrective action when necessary. For example, it may require an order to issue a new regulation or revise an old one, and, if the order fails to do so, the board may act in its place. The Quebec Professions Board reports directly to Cabinet. The second body is the Quebec Interprofessional Council, made up of representatives from each of the professions covered by the Code. It coordinates the activities of the professional orders and deals with general issues encountered by all professional orders. It has no power to regulate, but can, of course, make recommendations to the Quebec Professions Board (13).

4.2. REGULATED HEALTH PROFESSIONS ACT OF ONTARIO (1991)

Ontario's *Regulated Health Professions Act* (RHPA) (14) was passed in 1991 and replaced the *Health Disciplines Act* (15), which had been enacted in 1974. The RHPA has been amended twice since passage (16) — first in 1993 to include regulations and sanctions for sexual abuse by health care professionals (discussed later in this chapter), and then in 1996 by the Omnibus legislation (*Ontario Act 26*) to allow the RHPA to comply with changes to the *Ontario Drug Benefit Act* and the *Prescription Drug Cost Regulation Act.* Like the Professional Code of Quebec, the RHPA was enacted to obtain greater public accountability in the regulation of the health care professions.

Many consider the RHPA to be progressive legislation. It increased the number of professions under its jurisdiction, including seven not previously covered (see Table 16.1 for professions included in the RHPA). The *Health Disciplines Act* had only licensed the five health care professions of physicians, dentists, nurses, pharmacists, and optometrists (the distinction between licensing and certification is discussed later).

A "template from which many future legislative efforts in health care will evolve" (17), the RHPA increases equity within the health care professions, reducing the role of the physician as gatekeeper and increasing direct consumer access to a wider variety of professionals. It allows for the growth of emerging health care professions, which can apply for regulation to raise their status. Regulation is a separate issue from funding, however; although 24 health care professions are officially recognized and regulated in the RHPA, they are not all funded by the provincial health insurance plan (see Chapters 13 and 14).

The most progressive aspect of the legislation is that the professions are not defined by the scope of their practice, but that professionals are licensed to perform various procedures, or "controlled acts", that are potentially dangerous. Only five of the professions — medicine, chiropractic, optometry, dentistry, and psychology — are licensed to "diagnose", and the title "doctor" is also limited to these professionals. Other professionals are licensed only to "assess" and not diagnose. Neither diagnosis nor assessment are defined in the legislation, and interpretations are left for courts to determine. Other controlled acts include, for example, performing a procedure beyond the dermis or below the surface of the cornea or below the surface of the teeth, administering a substance by injection or inhalation, and managing labour or conducting the delivery of babies. There are 13 controlled acts in total. None of the 24 regulated health professions is authorized to perform all of them (although physicians are authorized to perform 12 out of the 13), and some of them are not authorized to perform any of them (e.g., dieticians, speech and language pathologists, occupational therapists). Furthermore, the same controlled act can come under the purview of more than one profession. For example, physicians, physiotherapists, and chiropractors are all authorized to manipulate the joints of the spine. These multiple authorizations were legislated in order to help break the monopoly that medicine had over health services and allow people a greater range of health providers when making decisions concerning their personal health. Traditional Aboriginal healers and Aboriginal midwives are exempt from the RHPA. Uncontrolled acts are open to all, including unregulated workers.

The RHPA is structured so that individual acts regarding each profession's scope of practice and licensed acts follow a general section on legal and procedural provisions, which pertain to all the health professions included in the act. This allows for legislation to be coordinated instead of the previous patchwork of legislation. It gives the Minister of Health broad powers to supervise the regulation of all 24 disciplines, increasing their accountability and protecting the interests of the public. The emphasis is on the public good, rather than professional interests.

Each health care profession must constitute a college that is responsible for regulating the practice of the health care profession and governing its members in accordance with the RHPA. The college must maintain standards of entry, qualification, and practice, and establish and maintain standards of competence and ethics among its members. Each college must have a governing council that excludes members of health care professions. Public members are appointed to the council by the Lieutenant Governor-in-Council. Meetings of council, except in prescribed circumstances, are to be open to the public. In addition, a standard system of committees and a uniform method

Table 16.1:   Professions covered by the *Regulated Health Professions Act* of Ontario (1991)

Audiologists	Massage therapists	Osteopaths
Chiropodists	Medical lab technicians	Pharmacists
Chiropractors	Medical radiation technologist.	Physicians
Dental hygienists	Midwives	Physiotherapists
Dental technicians	Nurses	Podiatrists
Dentists	Occupational therapists	Psychologists
Denturists	Opticians	Respiratory therapists
Dieticians	Optometrists	Speech and language pathologists

of handling licensing, hearings, and discipline are established for all colleges.

The statutory committee structure for each of the 24 health care professions included in the legislation is identical. The committees are the: executive committee, registration committee, complaints committee, discipline committee, fitness to practice committee, continuing competence committee, quality assurance committee, and patient relations committee. The actual membership of each committee and quorums, however, differ; these are described under the specific profession.

The Health Disciplines Board established under the previous *Health Disciplines Act* continues as the Health Professions Board, an independent, appointed body of 12 to 20 members, none of whom is a health care professional. The Board acts as an appeals agency for decisions made by the Complaints Committees and the Registration Committees of each College. It does not hear appeals from the Disciplinary Committees; these are made directly to the Supreme Court of Ontario. The Disciplinary Committee Chairperson can assign a panel of three to five members for a hearing, one of whom must be a member of the public.

The Minister of Health is the designated member of Cabinet who is responsible for administering the RHPA. The Minister's duties, set out in the RHPA are to ensure that the regulatory system works, and to focus on both the professions (making sure that the professions are regulated and coordinated in the public interest, and making sure that standards of practice are kept) and on consumers (ensuring freedom of choice of health care provider, and making sure that consumers are treated fairly and sensitively). To this end, the Minister may conduct investigations into the operations of institutions or practices, may require reports to be submitted by the colleges, reviews proposed changes in college regulations, and can request that a college make, amend, or revoke regulations. If the college fails to do so, the Minister may act in the college's place (through Cabinet). In practice, however, these powers are rarely exercised. In Quebec, these functions are carried out by the Quebec Professions Board, rather than directly by Cabinet.

At this point, a distinction should be made between licensing and certification. Certain health care professionals are required to be licensed; that is, they must hold a licence in order to practice their profession, and all others are prohibited from such practise. Other professions and occupations are certified. In some instances, certification is controlled by government regulations, in which case individuals are prohibited from using the relevant title or claiming to be qualified in the occupation unless they are appropriately certified and registered. They are not necessarily prohibited from performing some functions of the occupation. In some occupations, certification (or registration) is granted by voluntary organizations. This type of certification has no legal status, but employers frequently hire only those who are certified by their national or provincial associations; an example is social workers, who are certified by the College of Social Workers.

4.2.1. Health Professions Regulatory Advisory Council

The Health Professions Regulatory Advisory Council (HPRAC) is an independent council, separate from both the Minister of Health and the professional colleges, and created by the RHPA in order to facilitate ongoing policy development concerning the health care professions. Specifically, the duties of the HPRAC include advising the Minister of Health on matters relating to regulating new health care professionals or deregulating existing ones, including changes in scope of practice and licensed acts, suggesting amendments to the Act and related regulations, and providing advice and policy guidance on any matter referred to it by the Minister of Health. Additionally, the HPRAC exercises supervisory functions, ensuring that the health care professionals (through their colleges) maintain good patient relations and effective quality assurance programs. The HPRAC is made up of five to seven lay persons appointed by the Lieutenant Governor in Council, and excludes registered health care professionals and Ontario public servants.

4.3. MAJOR HEALTH CARE PROFESSIONS

Several of the major health care professions are described here, as well as their regulatory organizations in Ontario where such exist.

4.3.1. Medicine

Physicians are required to be licensed in all provinces. Although each provincial college has its unique requirements for licensor, a certain standard of uniformity has been established. All provinces require the physician to pass the national examination of the Medical Council of Canada plus examination by the Royal College of Physicians and Surgeons of Canada for specialists, and examination by the College of Family Physicians of Canada for family practice. The example of Ontario is used here, as most provinces have similar structures.

In Ontario, the licensing agency is the College of Physicians and Surgeons of Ontario and is made up of the following bodies, as detailed in the *Regulated Health Professions Act*:

Council of the College. The College overall governing body and board of directors is made up of four members appointed by the medical faculties of four universities in Ontario, four to six lay members appointed by the Lieutenant Governor-in-Council, and 12 to 16 members elected by the membership at large. The Council's most important functions are the preparation of regulations for the profession as authorized by the act subject to approval by the Minister, and the appointment of members to the Executive Committeee, Registration Committee, Complaints Committee, Discipline Committee, Fitness to Practice Committee, and Continuing Competence Committee. All of these committees, with the exception of the Fitness to Practice Committee, have lay members.

Executive Committee. This committee is drawn from the Council and acts for the Council between Council meetings. Actions taken by the Executive Committee are subject to ratification at the next Council meeting.

Registration Committee. This committee determines eligibility for licensure. The Registrar of the College, who is appointed by the Council, performs this function on a daily basis, but refers any doubtful applications for licensure to the Registration Committee.

Complaints Committee. This body investigates complaints made by members of the public or the College about the conduct of any member of the College. Anyone can complain, regardless of whether the complainant was the patient involved in alleged poor treatment (in practice, however, complaints are most often made by patients or their families). The procedures followed ensure that the member against whom the complaint has been made is given a fair hearing. The Committee may refer its findings to the Discipline Committee or the Executive Committee, or may direct that the matter not be referred further.

Discipline Committee. The Discipline Committee considers allegations of professional misconduct or incompetence referred to it by the Council, the Executive Committee, or the Complaints Committee. If it determines that the allegations are correct and that a member of the College is guilty of professional misconduct or incompetence, it may take the following actions: revoke the license of the member, suspend the license for a stated period, impose restrictions on the license, reprimand the member, impose a fine to the maximum of $5,000, direct that any penalty above be suspended for a period of time, or any combination of these.

Fitness to Practice Committee. If the Registrar of the College has evidence that a member may be incapacitated, the Registrar reports this to the Executive Committee, who in turn may appoint a board of inquiry. The board of inquiry investigates the matter and reports back to the Executive Committee. If appropriate, the Executive Committee refers the matter to the Fitness to Practice Committee, which will hold a formal hearing. If the member is found to be incapacitated, the Fitness to Practice Committee may revoke the member's licence, suspend the licence for a stated period, or attach limits to the licence.

Continuing Competence Committee. This committee is a new statutory committee under the RHPA. Its purposes are to maintain and enhance the competence and standards of practice of members in the care of patients, and in record-keeping in relation to members' practices. The program established by the Committee may involve member participation in continuing education and remediation programs, written or oral tests of clinical knowledge, skill, or judgement, and other modalities.

Medical Review Committee. This committee was established not under the RHPA but rather under the *Health Insurance Act.* It is a committee of the College of Physicians and Surgeons composed of six members nominated by the College but appointed by the Minister, plus two lay members also appointed by the Minister. Its function is to review billing matters referred to it by the provincial health insurance plan. Such referrals would occur if it appeared that a physician had billed for services not rendered, for services that were not medically necessary, for services not provided in accordance with accepted professional standards, or where the nature of services provided is misinterpreted. The Medical Review Committee, after reviewing the matter, may recommend that the health insurance plan refuse payment, reduce the amount of the payment, or require reimbursement from the physician. Thus, the Medical Review Committee is a potent regulatory agency and functions in addition to the regular committees of the College as established by the RHPA. There is yet another way in which the practice of medicine is regulated, at least that part of the practice conducted within hospitals (see Chapter 13).

4.3.2. Dentistry

Dentists are required to be licensed in every province. Graduates of approved Canadian dental schools are not required to write a licensing examination. They may apply for a certificate from the National Dental Examining Board (NDEB). Graduates of other institutions must pass an NDEB examination to obtain the certificate. The NDEB examination is recognized by all provinces. Specialists are certified by provincial licensing agencies. Most dentists are in private practice and are reimbursed on a fee-for-service basis directly by their patients. Some provinces have prepaid dental plans for children and seniors, and many corporations have prepaid plans for their employees and their dependants. In Ontario, the dental profession is now regulated in a manner similar to physicians under the RHPA.

4.3.3. Nursing

Nurses perform many functions depending on their location, their employer, and their appointment. Hospital nurses may perform general bedside nursing care, or may be employed in very specialized units such as intensive care, coronary care, renal dialysis, or neurosurgical units. Public health nurses deal with the community in such matters as immunization and health education. Many nurses hold administrative positions within hospitals or other institutions. Nurses who work in frontier communities frequently perform many of the functions normally performed by physicians (these positions are generally held by nurse practitioners). In addition, nurses may be privately employed by physicians, chiropractors, private care institutions, and corporations.

Registered nurses and registered nursing assistants (now referred to as registered practical nurses, or RPNs) in Ontario are required to be certified and licensed by the College. Generally, this means that they have passed an examination prepared by the Canadian Nurses' Association (a national body). If their certification has expired or have been unemployed for a certain period, they may be required to take refresher training before being recertified. Quebec has a distinct and separate regulatory body for nurses. In Ontario, nurses are regulated by the RHPA as described above. In other provinces, regulation is delegated to the voluntary professional organizations. The increase in the status and importance of nursing in recent years is indicated by the fact that three provincial Ministries of Health (British Columbia, Alberta, and Manitoba) now have special ministerial positions for provincial nursing officers or provincial nursing advisory councils.

Recently, nurse practitioner (NP) programs have received increased attention. Currently, NP training programs exist in Ontario, Newfoundland, and Alberta. There are 250 NPs practising in Ontario, with an additional 400 anticipated by the end of the century. In urban settings, NPs usually practice in collaboration with physicians in a team environment; those in more remote areas frequently practise solo. Remuneration is usually either by salary or by capitation and comes out of Ministry budgets.

While medicine, dentistry, and nursing are three health care professions traditionally considered most important to the delivery of health services, chiropractic and midwifery are two of the health professions where consumer demand for alternative health delivery modalities helped create pressure for official recognition.

4.3.4. Chiropractic

The practice of chiropractic is defined as "the assessment of conditions related to the spine, nervous system and joints, and the diagnosis, prevention and treatment, primarily by adjustment of...the spine and joints" (17). In order to receive the legitimacy and official recognition of being one of the regulated health care professions, the practice of chiropractic moved much closer to mainstream medicine. Originally, in its historic development, it was seen as a direct alternative to medicine and was associated more closely with naturopathy. This association, as well as the broader scope of practice associated with earlier years of chiropractic, has been downplayed in recent years as chiropractors have become regulated and have come to comprise part of the primary health care delivery team (7).

Because chiropractors are considered one of the primary care providers in Ontario, they do not require referrals from other physicians. This status, together with their position as one of the five health care professionals authorized to diagnose, has been allowed because of the current "general-diagnosis" training of chiropractors, which is similar to that of physicians in medical schools. As indicated in Chapter 14, chiropractors generally practice in solo practices and bill patients on a fee-for-service basis. The costs of chiropractic services are partially covered by provincial health insurance plans in Ontario, Manitoba, Saskatchewan, Alberta, and British Columbia. The portion of the fee not covered through public insurance is covered either out-of-pocket by the individual or by private health insurance companies. In Ontario, chiropractors are regulated by the College of Chiropractors of Ontario.

4.3.5. Midwifery

The practice of midwifery is defined as "the assessment and monitoring of women during pregnancy, labour, and the post-partum period and of their newborn babies, the provision of care during normal pregnancy, labour and post-partum period and the conducting of spontaneous normal vaginal deliveries" (16). Although community midwives have been practising throughout Canada (especially in rural and northern regions) for more than a century, they have received little official recognition from the state. This has slowly started changing, largely due to ongoing consumer pressure to receive non-medical labour and delivery care. At the beginning of 1997, midwives were officially recognized as primary health care professionals and were licensed to practise only in Ontario and in British Columbia, while appropriate regulatory legislation was in various stages of development in Alberta, Manitoba, Quebec, and New Brunswick. Additionally, Saskatchewan has created a Midwifery Advisory Committee to review the possibility of using midwives instead of physicians to attend normal births, and Newfoundland is undergoing a similar exploratory phase in the official recognition and use of midwives.

5.   SEXUAL ABUSE OF PATIENTS

Sexual abuse of patients by members of health care professions, in particular, the medical profession, emerged as a prominent and distressing concern in some provinces, particularly Ontario, Alberta, and British Columbia in the early 1990s. Sexual abuse represents a transgression of the trust placed in a health care professional. Due to the position of power of the health care professional in relation to the patient, any suggestive or sexual behaviour or language in a clinical setting can be deemed inappropriate.

In Ontario, a task force on the sexual abuse of patients, which was an independent body commissioned by the College of Physicians and Surgeons, made a series of recommendations following the review of evidence from patients reporting sexual improprieties on the part of medical practitioners. These recommendations were reviewed and released by the Council of the College of Physicians and Surgeons in late 1992 (19), who recommended that the *Regulated Health Professions Act* be amended to include a new section regarding actions of professional misconduct of a sexual nature with different levels of offence and penalties, such as fines or revocation of licence for the more severe offences. The legislative amendments have included a requirement that any health care professional with reasonable grounds to believe a colleague had committed any of the sexual offences must report this offence. Sexual abuse in the RHPA is now defined as sexual intercourse or other forms of physical sexual relations between the practitioner and the patient, touching of a sexual nature of the patient by the practitioner, or behaviour or remarks of a sexual nature toward the patient. However, the legislation also states that the words "sexual nature" do not include touching, behaviour, or remarks of a clinical nature appropriate to the service provided. The RHPA includes procedures for awarding financial compensation to patients who have been sexually abused by health care professionals to cover costs of counselling and treatment for sexual abuse; financial compensation is not foreseen by the RHPA for any other patient complaints.

6. TRENDS AND ISSUES

Earlier, it was mentioned that a recent process of de-professionalization has begun. Legislation aimed at obtaining greater public control of the self-regulating professions has been enacted. This process is certain to continue. This section presents some of the issues involved and trends that may be expected.

Since governments now pay most medical bills, they are likely to become more interested in the value they receive for taxpayers' money, not only in terms of quantity, but also of quality. This could mean greater government involvement in the design of medical school curricula, in the licensing procedures of provincial colleges, and in the monitoring of individual practices. The result could be periodic re-examination for re-licensure, enforced continuing education, and similar measures for ensuring the competence of licensed physicians.

The medical profession is certain to see increased government regulation as a threat to its freedom and autonomy. The profession is likely to react by becoming more politicized; lobbying with governments may increase, as may efforts to enlist the aid of the public. Union-like activities (e.g., withholding of services) will probably become more common. It is also likely to react by improving its own regulation. Stricter requirements for re-licensure, continuing education, peer review, and evaluation of individual practices may be imposed to forestall government action in these areas. Some degree of confrontation seems inevitable, but it is to be hoped that those issues described will be resolved in a manner that will lead to better health care for Canadians and, in the long run, a stronger, if less autonomous, profession.

The new legislation in Ontario also throws some light on the future direction on the regulation of health care professionals (20). It states that "the sole purpose of professional regulation is to advance and protect the public interest. The public is the intended beneficiary of regulation, not the members of the professions. Thus, the purpose of granting self-regulation to a profession is not to enhance its status or increase the earning power of its members by giving the profession a monopoly over the delivery of particular health services".

Another major change is that an increasing number of health care occupations are demanding to be considered as professions and to participate in health insurance programs. This will create tension among the different health care providers. Definitions of health care professions will become restrictive, and professionals will be equated with individuals with specialized knowledge and skill but not necessarily those with responsibility, autonomy, or service orientation. Many more new problems will undoubtedly arise as both governments and consumers seek a greater voice in health care. One thing is certain: the 1990s have brought many changes and the next decade will bring more.

7. SUMMARY

This chapter examined the definition of professionalism, discussed the historical background of the modern medical professions, and listed and described the various health professions, para-professions and allied occupations, and discussed their regulation and future trends in regulation.

The concept of *professionalism* is very difficult to define, and hence most definitions consist of lists of characteristics commonly attributed to an established profession. These characteristics include specialized knowledge and skill, autonomy, service orientation, responsibility, and external recognition.

Medicine is the dominant profession in the health care field. In achieving this dominance, the mainstream of medicine either eliminated, absorbed, or controlled competing disciplines. Other health care professions have followed the same pattern established by medicine, but only dentistry has achieved a similar degree of autonomy.

Most provinces have enacted, or intend to enact, legislation to ensure greater public control of the professions. The earliest and most significant changes occurred in the provinces of Quebec and Ontario.

The *Professional Code of Quebec* defines what a profession is and establishes formal criteria by which an occupation gains statutory recognition as a profession. Furthermore, each profession is governed by a professional "order". This order maintains surveillance of the quality of individual practices, and is empowered to take corrective measures. The Code also establishes two overall supervisory and regulatory bodies: the Quebec Professions Board and the Quebec Interprofessional Council.

In Ontario, the *Regulated Health Professions Act* (RHPA) was enacted in 1991. One of the major aspects of the new legislation is the expansion of the number of professions under its jurisdiction to 24. The RHPA was enacted to obtain greater public accountability in the regulation of the health care professions, and is regarded as increasing equity among the health care professions, reducing the role of the physician as the gatekeeper and increasing direct access for the consumer to a wider variety of professionals. The most revolutionary aspect of the legislation is that the professions are not defined by the scope of practice but professionals are licensed to perform various procedures, or controlled acts, that are potentially dangerous.

The RHPA gives the Minister of Health broad powers to supervise the regulation of the 24 disciplines included, and increases the accountability and protection of the interests of the public. The emphasis is on the public good, rather than professional interests.

Each health care profession is required to constitute a *college* that is responsible for regulating the practice of profession and to govern its members in accordance with the RHPA.

Physicians are required to be licensed in all provinces by the College of Physicians and Surgeons. The licensing agency is made up of the council of the college, the executive committee, the registration committee, the complaints committee, the discipline committee, the fitness to practice committee, the continuing competence committee, and the medical review committee. Dentists, like physicians, are required to be licensed in every province. As well, in Ontario, the dental profession is regulated in a manner similar to physicians under the RHPA. Nurses perform many functions depending on their location, their employer, and their appointment. Registered nurses in Ontario must to be licensed by their college. Chiropractic and midwifery are two health care professions where consumer demand for alternative health care delivery modalities helped to create pressure for official recognition.

A recent process of *de-professionalization* has begun. Legislation aimed at obtaining greater public control of the self-regulating professions has been enacted and this process is certain to continue. The medical profession is certain to see increased government regulation as a threat to its freedom and autonomy. Reaction by the profession is likely to take two forms: the profession will become more politicized and may attempt to improve its own regulation.

8.   REFERENCES

1.   Minister of National Health and Welfare. Health Personnel in Canada 1992. Ottawa: Ministry of Supply and Services, 1994.
2.   Canadian Hospital Association. Canadian Hospital Directory 1989-1990. Ottawa: Canadian Hospital Association, 1989. vol 37.

3. Webster's Third New International Dictionary of the English Language, Unabridged. Springfield, Mass.: Mearriam-Webster, 1993.

4. Bohnen L. The Sociology of the Professions in Canada (Four Aspects of Professionalism in Canada). Ottawa: Consumer Research Council of Canada, 1977.

5. Bucher R, Stelling J. Characteristics of Professional Organizations. Journal of Health and Social Behaviour 1969;10(1):3-15.

6. Freidson E. Profession of Medicine. New York: Dodds, Mead, and Co., 1970.

7. Coburn D. State Authority, Medical Dominance, and Trends in the Regulation of the Health Professionals: The Ontario Case. Social Science and Medicine 1993;37(2):129-138.

8. Torrance G. Socio-Historical Overview: The Development of the Canadian Health System. In Coburn D, D'Arcy C, New P, eds. Health and Canadian Society. Toronto: Fitzhenry and Whiteside Ltd., 1981:17.

9. Canadian Medical Association. Perspectives on Health Occupations. Ottawa: Canadian Medical Association, 1986.

10. Federal-Provincial Advisory Committee on Health Manpower. Catalogue on Health Manpower Legislation, 1985. Ottawa: Health Human Resources Division, Health and Welfare Canada, 1985.

11. Canada Health and Welfare. Directory of National Certification Bodies, National Professional Associations and National Accreditation Agencies for Various Health Occupations in Canada. Ottawa: Health Human Resources Division, Health and Welfare Canada, 1990.

12. Government of Quebec. Professional Code. Statutes of Quebec, Chapter 43, 1973.

13. Collège des médecins du Quebec. ALDO-Quebec: Legislative, Ethical and Organizational Aspects of Medical Practice in Quebec. Montreal: Collège des médecins du Quèbec, 1995.

14. Government of Ontario. Regulated Health Professions Act (Ontario) 1993. Queen's Park, Toronto: Government of Ontario, 1993.

15. Government of Ontario. Health Disciplines Act (Ontario). Revised Statutes of Ontario, 1980. Chapter 196. Toronto: Queen's Printer for Ontario, 1981. (Gordon A, ed.).

16. Bohnen L. Regulated Health Professions Act: A Practical Guide. Aurora, Ontario: Canada Law Book Inc. 1994.

17. Pooley D. Regulated Health Professions Act, 1991. The New Benchmark for Future Health Care Legislation. Journal of Canadian Chiropractic Association 1992;36(3):161-164.

18. Health Disciplines Act (Ontario). Revised Statutes of Ontario, 1980. Chapter 197. Toronto: Queen's Printer for Ontario, 1981. (Gordon A, ed.)

19. College of Physicians and Surgeons of Ontario, McPhedran M. Task Force on Sexual Abuse of Patients. The Final Report. November 25 1991. Toronto: College of Physicians and Surgeons of Ontario, 1991.

20 Health Professions Legislation Review. Striking a New Balance: A Blueprint for the Regulation of Ontario's Health Professions. Toronto: Ministry of Health of Ontario, 1989.

Canadian Health Care into the 21st Century

Universal hospital and medical care insurance were introduced to Canada when health services were provided almost exclusively in hospital or in physicians' offices. Consequently, the current national health care system in Canada is a mixture of community-based, home care, and extended care services, roughly imposed onto a pre-existing system of hospitals and medical care. Furthermore, because provinces (and not the federal government) have an exclusive jurisdiction in most health care matters, regional variations and variable fiscal capabilities have led to ten provincial and two territorial government health insurance plans. While these are referred to as health care systems, their primary focus and funding mechanisms deal mainly with illness rather than health.

From an international perspective, in the last two decades health care systems in industrialized nations, including Canada, have been under considerable stress, leading to a universal re-examination of how to provide the most effective health care while limiting rising costs. These stressors include:

- Continually increasing costs to look after the sick and infirm;
- Questions about the appropriate role of government in society;
- Need for evidence-based care, resulting in conflicts between government and health care professionals;
- Rise of consumerism;
- Changing demographics, with greater numbers of the elderly and increased demand for expensive, high-technology medical care;
- Evidence of health-related inequities among people living in poverty;
- Need for disease prevention and health promotion; and
- The inappropriate use of resources by both patients and providers.

Since the late 1980s and into the early 1990s, every province in Canada, as well as the federal government, has appointed various task forces, commissions, boards of inquiry, and working groups to conduct their own fundamental reviews of the health care system (1-7). These provincial and federal reviews were conducted by panels of health system experts with considerable public consultation and participation. All recent task force and royal commission reports from different provinces have been summarized by Mhatre and Deber (8) and the *Angus Report* (9), while currently reform efforts are summarized in several key publications (10).

Perhaps the most influential of these commissions was the National Forum on Health. As briefly described in Chapter 13, the Forum was officially launched in 1994. It was created to address the reform of the Canadian health care system. Of main concerns were the need for increased efficiency and cost effectiveness, improved access, and high-quality care. Like its provincial predecessors, the Forum committees included representatives from government, health policy and health economics experts, health care professionals, and consumers. As with its provincial predecessors, public participation and consultation were central to the Forum's mandate and activities.

The Forum addressed the broad determinants of health, evidence-based decision making, Canadian values governing health and health care, and striking a balance between the public and private sectors. The final report of the National Forum on Health was published in February 1997, in which the members of the Forum concluded that "the health care system [of Canada] is fundamentally sound", that it receives an adequate amount of funding, and that there is room for improving certain aspects of its functioning (11). Its main recommendations were as follows.

- The current health care system of Canada must be preserved and protected. In order to achieve this, the following elements of the system should not be changed:
  - Public funding for medically necessary services;
  - The single-payer model of health services financing;
  - The five principles of the *Canada Health Act*; and
  - A strong federal/provincial/territorial relationship.
- Preserving a strong health care system also requires:
  - The expansion of publicly funded services to include home care and pharmaceuticals;
  - The reform of primary care delivery, funding, and organization;
  - The establishment of a multi-year transition fund to support evidence-based innovations.
- Health programs designed to improve the health of Canadians must focus on:
  - A broad, integrated child and family strategy consisting of both programs and income support, coordinated throughout government without limitation to ministry of health initiatives;
  - Aboriginal health programs, including the establishment of the Aboriginal Health Institute designed to help Aboriginal communities find solutions to their health problems;
  - Increased focus on evidence-based decision making, including the development of a nationwide population health information system and the development of a comprehensive research agenda designed to address knowledge gaps;
  - Increased collaboration between the public sector and the private sector in achieving improved outcomes and building community support.

A review of provincial commissions on health care reform reveals several issues that were similar across Canada (9, 12-20). Specifically, provincial review committees studied the questions of rising health care costs, a lack of responsiveness in the system, and health services efficacy in improving health status. Proposed solutions also converged: regionalize decision-making structures and decentralize decision-making authority, reform the health care system to prioritize primary care and the broad determinants of health, reform health human resources policies, and improve evaluation and research to allow for more effective decision making. Thus, as can be seen, the provincial reports did not depart radically from the Forum. They too set out to review primary care, the broad determinants of health, and cost effectiveness. They too were motivated to a large extent by economic issues, specifically cost containment within the health care sector and the improvement of cost effectiveness.

However, the Forum framed its recommendations on core Canadian values and how they should drive further changes in the health care system, rather than focus on strictly economic analyses. The fundamental values identified by the Forum's public consultation process include equity and access; compassion; dignity and respect for all individuals; quality, efficiency and effectiveness; personal responsibility for appropriate use of health resources; and public participation in health system decision making (21). These values should steer ongoing discussions about the health system of the next century and its reform within a uniquely Canadian hybrid that reflects unique Canadian concerns and needs.

This chapter discusses some of the stressors of the Canadian health care system today in the context of the fundamental values identified by the Forum. It first presents issues of equity and access to health services, particularly among certain vulnerable groups; it then turns to a discussion of ongoing measures to increase the efficiency, effectiveness, and quality of the health care system; and third, it examines the question of personal responsibility for health and consumer access to decision-making processes. The chapter ends with an overview of some of the reform efforts underway in all provinces aimed at helping Canadians revise and maintain an effective and responsive health care system.

1.   VALUE SET #1: EQUITY AND ACCESS, COMPASSION, DIGNITY, AND RESPECT

A review of recent provincial commissions concluded that Canada "wants to achieve equitable access to health" (8). Similarly, the Forum found that the values of fairness and equity of access to services should be given the highest priority in guiding the Canadian health care system of the future. Canadians do not want to see a health care system that treats the rich differently from the poor. The previous objective in Canada of ensuring equal access to medical care has largely been achieved by the universal system of hospital and medical insurance. It is now widely held that the development of medical care has reached its zenith in contributing to improved health status.

However, in the current situation in the Canadian political, economic, and social environment, citizens differ in the likelihood that they will achieve health as defined in its broadest sense of a resource for everyday living. The determinants of health are described in Chapter Four, and disparities particularly evident in the health status of special groups such as the elderly, children living in poverty, the homeless, Aboriginal peoples, and the disabled are reviewed in Chapter Six. There are also socioeconomic disparities in health status distributed throughout the population, such that life expectancy is five to six years shorter for those whose incomes fall into the lowest quintile, compared to those whose incomes fall into the highest (22).

Achieving equity in health so that income, geography, age, gender, or cultural background is not a limitation involves a re-ordering of priorities. It also underscores the other fundamental values of compassion, dignity, and respect for all individuals, which the Forum heard was so prized by the Canadian people. A number of strategies have been proposed to reduce inequities related to psychosocial determinants. Some, such as the integration of health and social services, would transform many aspects of the organization of health services if fully implemented. Others, such as cultural and racial sensitivity, would reduce barriers to care for Aboriginal peoples, recent immigrants, and other cultures. Attention to literacy in educational literature and treatment instructions would facilitate communication with those literacy limitations, which is a prevalent problem in Canada. These strategies are discussed below.

1.1. CULTURAL AND RACIAL SENSITIVITY

Multicultural health is used to refer to health care provided in a culturally and racially sensitive manner. A multicultural health care facility "reflects the contributions and interests of diverse cultural and social groups in its mission, operations and products or services" (23). In order for health care to become truly multicultural, health care providers must be aware of the cultural and ethnic determinants of health, the differing beliefs about health and medicine among ethnic communities, and the barriers faced by members of ethnic minorities in gaining access to health care.

1.1.1. Determinants of Health in Multicultural Communities
In general, mortality and morbidity rates are higher among members of cultural and racial minority groups. Contributing factors include assimilation to the culture of the host country in terms of diet and lifestyle, the degree to which the ethnic traditions are maintained, and the extent of support systems in the community of origin; these have a significant bearing on the incidence and prevalence of diseases such as elevated blood pressure and coronary heart disease.

The health problems of Canada's ethnic groups can be categorized as particular to people of certain ethnic origins because of biological factors, and those due to environmental factors. For example, the incidence of lactose intolerance is as high as 80% to

90% among African Canadians, Bantus, and Asians. Genetic differences also underlie the varying response that people of particular ethnic origins may have to certain medications (24).

Problems arising from environmental factors include the mental health problems experienced by many immigrants and refugees, especially those from visible minorities. Immigrants and refugees experience stress associated with migration, separation from family members and communities, loss of homes and possessions, possible inability to speak either French or English, difficulty in finding suitable employment, negative public attitudes toward immigrants and refugees, ethnocentrism and racism, and pressures of assimilation, which affect family relations. These experiences can lead to feelings of alienation, loss of self-esteem, and emotional disorders, placing immigrants to Canada at considerable risk for mental illness (25).

Cultural factors can also be included as determinants of health. For example, alcoholism is more prevalent among the French and Irish than among Jews and Italians, and some cultures consider obesity to be healthy. Wife abuse is also tolerated in some cultures more than others, which means a woman may be faced with the option of living with the abuse or being isolated from her community (26).

1.1.2. Inaccessibility of Health Care

Personal factors that contribute to the inaccessibility of health care services for members of ethnic minorities include their own cultural beliefs concerning health care and health care practitioners, language barriers, lack of knowledge about access to health services, and a fear of racism or ethnocentrism. Health care providers may be hindered by a lack of information about ethnic communities and health, lack of cross-cultural training and ethnically representative staffing, and an unwillingness to deliver health services in a culturally sensitive manner. Differing beliefs about health issues can significantly affect the approach to health care for members of some ethnic groups. For example, in many cultures birth control and open discussions of sex and sexuality are unacceptable. Reliance on herbal medicine or alternative treatment (e.g., acupuncture) can further complicate patient care. Although many cultural communities accept western medicinal practices, there are many that prefer their own forms of treatment and delivery. Many people prefer to discuss their health problems with someone from an ethnic organization or with an immigration services worker rather than with a trained health care practitioner, particularly when it comes to mental health. This highlights the need not only for cross-cultural training and increased ethnic representation in health care staff, but also the importance of outreach and liaison work with community organizations regarding health issues. Awareness of these differences is therefore vital to the implementation of multicultural health care practices.

1.1.3. Language Barriers

Demographic profiles indicate that approximately 1% of Canadians are unable to conduct a conversation in either official language. These people may be clustered in large urban areas (e.g., Toronto and Vancouver), or scattered sporadically across rural areas such as northern Canada. Without proper translation and interpretation services, this language barrier can affect members of ethnic minorities at every stage of the health care continuum. Educational materials provided only in French and English fail to inform members of linguistic minorities about health promotion, disease prevention, early recognition of certain health problems, and the availability of health care services and resources.

Ineffective translation and interpretation services prevent many people from seeking health care services, and may create problems for those who do. Many health care facilities make attempts at translation, asking kitchen or janitorial staff who speak the same language as the client to translate even though such people are not likely to be trained interpreters or health care practitioners. As a result, much vital information gets lost in the translation, particularly when the client may feel embarrassed having her or his health problems translated by someone who may inform the rest of the client's community, and inappropriate assessments and treatment may result. Thus, at every stage in the health care system, language barriers are detrimental to the health promotion, assessment, and treatment of members of ethnic minorities. Fortunately, many hospitals and community health care centres in cities with large immigrant populations such as Toronto and Vancouver are beginning to recognize this difficulty and are altering staffing patterns to include bilingual health care professionals for at least some of the more numerous ethnic clients being served (e.g., Cantonese speakers).

1.1.4. Racism and Ethnocentrism

Members of visible minorities and ethnic groups often experience racist or discriminatory treatment from health care practitioners. This behaviour may come in the form of negative comments or attitudes toward immigrants and refugees, a lack of respect or ignorance of the different health beliefs of ethnic communities, or stereotyping. The effects of this kind of treatment are twofold: the patient receives improper or inappropriate treatment and may therefore develop further health problems, and as a result of the poor treatment the patient and others from her or his community are discouraged from seeking future treatment.

It is important to realize that the real difficulties in accessing health care do not arise from the traditional health beliefs and practices of ethnic communities. Cultural insensitivity on the part of the health care providers is seen as the main obstacle for many members of ethnic minorities. For example, whereas 30% of mental health clinic patients in the general population withdraw from their programs after the first interview, 50% of the patients from ethnic minorities do so. The most frequent complaint is that the mental health therapists do not provide treatment that is culturally and linguistically appropriate (27).

1.1.5. Assimilation versus Accessibility

The reluctance of many health care professionals to develop multicultural structures and policies may be based on the belief that ethnic minorities should simply assimilate to the Canadian health culture, and that the health care system should not be responsible for ensuring the accessibility of services to members of cultural communities. This view is not only ethnocentric and unrealistic, but also ignores the health implications of forced assimilation. Individuals who identify strongly with their own ethnic communities have lower levels of suicide than those who did not consider themselves to be part of a cohesive ethnic community (27).

1.1.6. Organizational Barriers

Factors preventing health care organizations from successfully addressing multicultural health needs include an unwillingness to become culturally sensitive, a tendency to adopt superficial solutions such as translators from support staff, a lack of demographic and health data on ethnic communities, insufficient financial and human resources, a lack of training and skills development, an absence of monitoring and evaluative mechanisms, rigid, hierarchical, and competitive organizational climates not conducive to change, and a lack of commitment from senior management (27).

1.1.7. Human Resources and Education

Once a commitment to multicultural health has been made, significant changes to the organization must occur, starting with the staff. Health care practitioners usually receive no education concerning the health profiles and needs of ethnic minority groups. Therefore, extensive cross-cultural training must be provided to and made mandatory for health services workers and students. Emphasis should be placed on the fact that what may be seen by the health care provider as an accessibility or educational problem may often be interpreted by the consumer as evidence of racism or ethnocentrism.

The education and training of health services providers must be accompanied by a change in hiring practices. As well as ensuring that properly trained translators and interpreters are provided, health care facilities and educational organizations should also promote the education and hiring of health care providers who are members of ethnic minorities. This kind of affirmative action policy will reduce the need for translators and interpreters, and ensure understanding of the particular health problems of the community, as well as making the health care facility more welcome for members of the ethnic communities.

1.2.   LITERACY

1.2.1. Prevalence of Literacy Problems

The high prevalence of problems with reading both simple and more complex sentences in the Canadian population has already been highlighted in Chapter Four. One out of every four Canadians is functionally illiterate. This has serious implications in terms of people's ability to participate fully in society, especially in terms of obtaining access to information, using community services, and complying with medication and other health-related instructions. It is unlikely that remediation and upgrading reading programs will reach all those who could benefit. Therefore, increased awareness and the development of strategies to address illiteracy at the level of the patient and at the level of the community, especially in community-based health education and communication programs, are needed.

1.2.2. Readability and Health

The essential component of literacy awareness in health care is the critical analysis of printed material that is developed or distributed in terms of its readability. It is estimated that 50% of patients cannot read or have difficulty with instructions at the fifth-grade level. Changes to written material can increase its readability for its intended audience. They include keeping sentences to 20 words or less (although varying the length), using simple concepts, using words that can be pictured, using active verbs, using material related to the patient's experience, and avoiding unnecessary words (28). Pictorial cues, use of audiovisual media and stories using photographs or drawings can improve communication if there is a literacy problem (29).

1.2.3. Medication Compliance

It is estimated that 30%-80% of patients do not use their medication properly. It has been shown that compliance can be improved, for example with verbal reinforcement of instructions by a pharmacist. More effective reinforcement comes via brochures or written instructions, if these are understood. However, one study of patient education aids assessed the average reading level of the educational material at grade 11.8 ± 1.7 level, which was considered to be far too high for the average patient (30).

2. VALUE SET #2: EFFICIENCY, EFFECTIVENESS, AND QUALITY

The second group of core values was identified in the Canadian health care system as efficiency and effectiveness. To effect change and reform, these must be increased without sacrificing the quality of health care services.

2.1. HEALTH GOALS

The first step toward increasing the efficiency and effectiveness of health services in Canada is to determine exactly what the health system is trying to achieve. Yet, many commissions have pointed out a lack of formalized goals and objectives for the health system. **Goals** provide broad statements about the general direction of health programs, and **objectives** specify the desired results of programs. Objectives should be measurable targets for achievement in a certain period. It was recommended that provincial governments set health goals and implement systems to monitor their achievement. Ontario recently extended this principle of measurable goals and objectives to include business plans for all of its health divisions.

2.2. INFORMATION SYSTEMS AND EVIDENCE-BASED DECISION MAKING

An integral part of evaluating the effectiveness of the health system and monitoring the fulfilment of predetermined health goals must be the development of sound information systems. As described in Chapter 13, several provinces have been developing "smart" health identification cards that allow province-wide computerization of personal health information based on an individualized, unique identifier. There are still many issues concerning security of information access, privacy, and confidentiality that must be worked out, but such provincial information systems would permit the many diverse health care professionals who may be working with any given individual to understand his or her complete health picture. It is hoped that this sharing of service knowledge among providers will allow for better coordination of care, decrease unnecessary duplication of services or tests, and help identify when competing services may actually be harmful to the individual.

At the macro level, integrated information systems are used to help provincial policy makers identify areas of health service provision that need improvement. Questions such as the over- or under-utilization of services, gaps in service provision, or barriers to cost-effective service provision can be identified via information systems and programs targeted to correcting these gaps can then be developed. The Forum has recommended a national health information system integrating all provincial systems to allow for similar studies of service provision and cost effectiveness. The federal government is also committed to establishing a National Health Information Institute to study Canadian data from this information system and help develop best-practice policies (31). Ontario and Manitoba, for example have well-established provincial information systems being used in research institutes to help establish evidence-based decision making: the Institute of Clinical Evaluation Sciences (ICES) in Ontario and the Manitoba Centre for Health Policy and Evaluation.

2.3. INTEGRATION AND COORDINATION OF SERVICES

An additional step to improving the quality of services provided to Canadians, as well as increasing the overall efficiency of the system, is increased integration of services provided across societal sectors. For many special-needs groups, health and social needs go hand-in-hand. Thus, at the very minimum, increased coordination and integration of health and social services have long been a priority among provinces. Additionally, current knowledge about the very many broad determinants of health, of which health services are but one part, also makes increased coordination of policy efforts across sectors imperative. Housing, employment, education, environment, and recreation are just some of the other government sectors whose policies directly affect the health of Canadians.

2.3.1. Health and Social Services

There are many groups (such as people who are elderly and poor, disabled, and have multiple diagnoses), whose health problems dictate a need for a wide spectrum of health and social services. In many instances, the services available or provided are fragmented. Due to lack of correlation between boundaries for health services and social services, there is frequently poor coordination of services for the individual. Individuals may have to enter the system at multiple points and try to make their way through a haze of bureaucracy to receive services at a time when they are most vulnerable due to ill health. These difficulties are compounded by the disadvantaged social circumstances of many of these special groups.

One of the common themes in the recent provincial reports is the integration of health and social services. There is a desire for a broad policy framework that integrates the delivery of all human services better, i.e., health and social services (32). Community control of the planning and delivery of these services so that services are more responsive to local needs is a related objective and usually incorporated in integration.

Since 1970, Quebec has had an integrated system of health and social services as a result of the reorganization proposed by the Castonguay-Nepveu Commission. It is organized on a regional basis in the form of regional councils. These have recently been given responsibility for allocating funding according to regional and sub-regional priorities.

Six provinces (in addition to the long-standing system in Quebec) have proposed models for integration of health and social services in their recent provincial reports, but only British Columbia, Manitoba, New Brunswick, and the Yukon have succeeded in completing this merger. In these provinces funding and policy direction are still centralized at the provincial level. A different model of integration was strongly supported by the Premier's Council on Health, Equity, and Social Justice in Ontario. The recommendation was to decentralize delivery of health and social services and integrate some of the major elements of the ministries of health and social services. A number of barriers, however, were identified and the proposal has since been abandoned.

There are systemic barriers at the provincial level that frequently inhibit health and social services integration, namely lack of strategic planning across health and social services, fragmented program funding and policy development, incompatible structures of the ministries, and lack of consumer input and influence. At the local level, frequent barriers are different regional boundaries for each ministry, uneven service distribution across the province, and direct government delivery of services. Local areas also need a mix of services and resources tailored to their needs, and these differ among areas. With the regionalization of the health care system (and sometimes social services, as in New Brunswick), some of the barriers discussed below can be addressed, although it is still too early to evaluate success or failure.

As previously indicated, the integration of health and social services can occur at the executive level of both systems and devolve to a greater or less extent at the more peripheral levels. It may also occur at the level of local service delivery without the need for a total restructuring of health and social services. One model for the achievement of this objective is the community health centre (CHC), which has developed in Canada in the last 30 years, most notably in Quebec. Quebec has developed numerous local community health centres (CLSC), which are described in Chapter 15; these are community-oriented, multidisciplinary centres that offer a broad range of services on a non-fee-for-service basis. Staff, including medical staff, are salaried and the centres are run by their own community boards.

2.3.2. The Determinants of Health

There is a clear need to coordinate government policies more effectively across all sectors of society. As described in Chapter One, the health care sector is but one component of the many determinants of population health. General trends within the health and political sectors reflect growing national consensus on the need for greater system-wide integration of policies. For example, during the 1997 federal election the issue of child poverty featured prominently in candidates' discussions. In addition, Parliament had passed a resolution in 1989 to eliminate child poverty in Canada by the year 2000. Governments have also made a commitment to reform child tax benefits and increase money for the support of children by the end of this century. The final report of the National Forum on Health also emphasized the importance of integrating broad social policy in order to improve the health of Canadians: "We believe that the social and economic determinants of health merit particular attention. We are particularly concerned about the impact of poverty, unemployment, and cuts in social supports on the health of individuals, groups, and communities" (7). Chapter Six deals with some of the federal initiatives in the section on child poverty.

The report identified several high-risk groups with health needs particularly affected by social, employment, housing, and education issues. Specifically, the Forum highlighted Aboriginal peoples and also maternal and child health (the special health needs of these groups and some of the federal initiatives are discussed in Chapter Six). The federal government has committed itself to hosting a federal-provincial-territorial conference on Aboriginal health issues scheduled for 1998, followed by the establishment of the National Aboriginal Health Institute. The final report also emphasizes issues of family and child poverty and its detrimental effects on the health of this large segment of the Canadian population. The Forum calls for increased inter-sectorial coordination of policy to begin addressing this issue. These are issues already addressed by the Ottawa Charter on Health Promotion (see Chapter One), but continue to play a pivotal role for the health of Canadians.

2.4. HEALTH PROMOTION AND DISEASE PREVENTION

Conventional wisdom has long recognized that an ounce of prevention is worth a pound of cure, and the health care system is no exception. A vital step toward increasing the cost effectiveness of the Canadian health care system and improving its general effectiveness and quality is to focus on preventing ill-health and disease before they start. All provincial reports, as well as the final recommendations of the National Forum on Health, pointed to the need for a greater emphasis on the need for health promotion and illness prevention.

Currently, less than 5% of health care dollars is spent on activities related to disease prevention and health promotion. A reduction in health care costs could be achieved through health promotion and disease prevention strategies. It was recommended that a greater proportion of health care dollars should be spent on these programs. The common recommendation was for a shift from curative to preventive health and a corresponding increase in funding for research and development into health promotion and preventive medicine, typically to 1% of the annual health care expenditures. Regional health boards are also mandated to focus, as a priority, on health promotion and disease prevention. All provinces that have regionalized their health care system now include health promotion as a "core service" to which regional boards allocate resources. In spite of repeated calls for "increased emphasis" or "ongoing focus" in these areas, it remains difficult to monitor exactly what is being done. In a 1997 review of all health reforms throughout the provinces, the Canadian College of Health Services Executives noted that Alberta, Saskatchewan, and New Brunswick had increased their budgets specifically for health promotion initiatives. Other health promotion initiatives and programs are woven into provincial reforms of primary care, community care, and home care (12).

3.   VALUE SET #3:   PERSONAL RESPONSIBILITY

Another core value identified by the National Forum on Health and referred to in many recent provincial reform reports is personal responsibility for health and health choices. **Personal responsibility** is understood to be essential to individual health and to the population's health, and to the appropriate use of health care resources. In many instances, provinces tied in the value of personal responsibility for health together with recommendations for savings in health systems. Although this seems a laudable goal, the issue of personal responsibility must be carefully presented. Personal responsibility for health can be, and often is, misconstrued as a desire to deny medical coverage to those individuals whose health needs are deemed the result of personal lifestyle choices. The Forum's report specifically addresses this dilemma and underscores the fact that its public consultation process did not add this second interpretation to this value. On the contrary, Canadians indicated that denying health services to anyone regardless of their condition and its cause would deny the most fundamental of all Canadian health principles, namely that of equity and fairness. A secondary issue that was not addressed, however, is whether health services utilization choices are strictly in the hands of the consumer, or whether health providers can significantly influence consumer choices. This thorny issue remains to be analysed and addressed.

4.   VALUE SET #4: PUBLIC PARTICIPATION IN DECISION MAKING

Citizens have long been involved in organizing the delivery of health services to their peers. Over the last century, citizens have become more involved in the health care system through voluntary health agencies and, lately, through consumer advocacy movements. In the context of health care, the word "citizen" is often interchanged with the word consumer or client. The distinctions are difficult to differentiate because every citizen consumes some health care services (e.g., public health services such as immunization, water purification, sanitation).

4.1.1. Major Concerns of Consumers about Health Care

Citizens of developed countries now regard health as a basic human right, and governments have responded by providing health care. However, in recent years, consumers have expressed concerns about inconvenience, the availability of health services, difficulties in communication between practitioners and consumers, paternalism on the part of providers, lack of individual input into care plans, and inadequacy of health care for certain groups in society. Many people feel that the system is designed for the convenience of the health care practitioner rather than the client. Many would prefer to take a more active part in decisions regarding their own health care, be better equipped to give informed consent, and develop a more personal relationship with their practitioners than the harried atmosphere that office visits or hospital consultations allows.

In Canada, several aspects of women's health care are also being questioned (e.g., unnecessary surgery, particularly hysterectomies and cesarean sections). Women have expressed concern about the insufficient numbers of female practitioners in certain specialities, the medical monopoly on birth control and abortion, the over-prescription of drugs for female patients, and the paucity of home delivery and midwives. Women's advocacy groups have been at least partially successful in the last few years in obtaining official recognition of women's health issues as key policy priorities in several provinces. For example, British Columbia, Saskatchewan, Manitoba, Ontario, and Quebec now include women's health divisions or advisory councils as part of their ministries of health. Breast cancer screening programs have been strengthened in seven of the ten provinces, and two provinces now officially recognize midwives as a legitimate part of the primary care team for women, with an additional five preparing to do so in the near future (see Chapter 16).

4.1.2. Modes of Public Participation

Clearly, consumers wish to be more involved in health care. Their participation can be facilitated by:

- Sharing knowledge about the causation of diseases, since many of these relate to the lifestyle of the population (e.g., smoking and lung cancer, chronic bronchitis, heart disease). Individual citizens can decrease their risk after gaining health knowledge and modifying their behaviour.
- Participating in the formulation of health care policies, which usually involve formal and informal discussions with citizens. Citizen involvement can be achieved by the establishment of a royal commission, task force, or working group at the governmental level and by the initiation of studies by other health-related agencies.
- Creating citizens' voluntary groups, many have already changed the system (e.g., AIDS advocacy groups)

Citizens may also participate in the health care system through membership on hospital boards or committees and boards that are involved in the regulation of health professions.

4.1.3. Factors Inhibiting Public Participation
Consumer involvement in health care meets obstacles at two levels: at the level of the individual consultation with the physician, and at the level of community involvement in health policy formation and system planning. At the individual level, health care — particularly medical care — is dominated by technology and professional super-specialization. How can an individual know whether the care he or she receives is good? The supply is restricted by the professional bodies through their licensing requirements, creating a monopoly, and the suppliers of health services can generate the demand for their own services (e.g., a dentist can ask a patient to come back once or ten times for treatment of a dental disorder). In this context, the individual tends to do what the professional dictates. Health care is episodic and crisis-oriented and the consumer is often dissatisfied. However, once the crisis is over, the problems encountered by consumers become less important than other aspects of their life, and hence complaints are rarely made to providers.

At the systemic level, public participation studies have consistently shown that only the more affluent and the higher educated consumer is likely to participate in policy formation debates (33). Alternatively, only those individuals with a vested interest in a particular issue find the necessary time and energy for political activism. Conversely, health care professional associations are better organized and better funded for political activism, and frequently have privileged access to state policy makers through well-established government committees. In light of these barriers, consumers and small consumer organizations frequently do not have the voice in policy debates that is required for truly effective involvement.

4.1.4. Advantages and Disadvantages of Public Participation
Public participation should result in less disparity between the rich and the disadvantaged sections of population (i.e., overuse by the privileged and underuse by welfare recipients and rural residents). Increased interaction between the consumer

Table 17.1:   Consumer Rights in Health Care

I. Right to be informed

- About preventive health care including education on nutrition, birth control, drug use, appropriate exercise;

- About the health care system including the extent of government insurance coverage for services, supplementary insurance plans, the referral system to auxiliary health and social facilities and services in the community;

- About the individual's own diagnosis and specific treatment program including prescribed surgery and medication, options, effects and side effects;

- About the specific costs of procedures, services, and professional fees undertaken on behalf of the individual consumer.

II. Right to be respected as the individual with the major responsibility for his/her own health care

- Right that confidentiality of his or her health records be maintained;

- Right to refuse experimentation, undue painful prolongation of his or her life or participation in teaching programs, or right of adult to refuse treatment;

- Right to die with dignity.

III. Right to participate in decision making affecting his/her health

- Through consumer representation at each level of government in planning and evaluating the system of services, the types and qualities of service, and the conditions under which health services are delivered ;

- With the health care professionals and personnel involved in his or her direct health care.

IV. Right to equal access to health care (health education, prevention, treatment and rehabilitation) regardless of the individual's economic status, sex, age, creed, ethnic origin, and location

- Right of access to adequately qualified health care personnel, right to a second medical opinion, right to prompt response in emergencies.

Source: Consumers' Association of Canada.

and the health care professional at the individual level frequently accelerates lifestyle changes, such as the cessation of smoking. At the systemic level, consumer participation in planning health care policy may provide a sense of gratification and accomplishment, as well as aid in changing the traditional attitudes of people toward health care.

However, there are certain unavoidable disadvantages in consumer participation. Greater participation involves, at least initially, increased expenditure, as the consumer lacks knowledge about health care. Citizens need to be organized, which requires expenditures for public meetings, seminars and circulation of printed materials; newly established organizations also incur operational costs. Another disadvantage of consumer participation is that technological advances can make it increasingly difficult for the lay person to understand and evaluate the quality of the care received from the provider, which may lead to tension. The wide range of consumer interests and needs also makes it difficult to satisfy everyone.

4.1.5. The Future of the Public Participation Movement in Health Care

Several trends have developed as consumers become more vocal and aware of their rights. One is the consumers' bill of rights in health care. This describes explicitly the health care providers' responsibility toward the consumer (see Table 17.1), and is gaining widespread support. Citizens will likely be elected rather than appointed to public health and hospital boards and to regional and district health councils. There is a trend toward more programs for people who are elderly, dying, disabled, and socially disadvantaged that cater not only to the medical, but also to the psychosocial needs of these groups. Hospitals will be organized for the convenience of the consumers, and not only of the providers. Structural and legal changes such as those enshrined in Ontario's *Regulation Health Care Professionals Act* (see Chapter 16) will facilitate consumer involvement in the regulation of health care professionals; this may extend to the selection of students for admission to professional schools.

5.   REFORMING THE HEALTH CARE SYSTEM

To achieve the recommendations made by provincial review committees and the National Forum on Health, continuing emphasis on certain key reforms remains a priority. This section describes efforts to address all of the fundamental values identified by the Forum in a complementary and systematic way. For example, reforms related to regionalization and the devolution of decision making address the issues of increased responsiveness and effectiveness of the health care system, the most cost-effective allocation of scarce health care resources, and increased public participation in decision making. Similarly, the reform of specific program areas, such as primary care and long-term care, as well as mental health reform, addresses the fundamental Canadian health values already discussed.

5.1.   REGIONALIZATION AND DECENTRALIZATION

As discussed in greater detail in Chapter 13, regionalization emerged as a major theme in all the provincial reports and has been implemented in every province except Ontario. However, no consensus exists on a definition of regionalization, although one report on regionalization and health care policy in Canada defined as follows:

"[embodying] the selective application over time of concepts contained within its decentralization, geographic, *and* rationalization *dimensions by governments,*

agencies and pressure groups responsible for the planning, financing and delivery of health and related social services" (34).

The decentralization of administrative authority to regional units with local accountability results in resources centralized for a geographic area. The mandated requirement to provide services to those in a defined region implies that identical boundaries for health and social services would be a positive first step. Rationalization involves the efficient use of scarce resources. The issue of regionalization is complex and involves reorganizing of accountability and responsibility for the management and financing of health care services. There are contradictory federal policies in this area that provide the centralization inherent in the concept of universality and uniform standards in health services, and the decentralization of administrative authority in order to meet local needs.

5.2. PRIMARY CARE

Primary health care has been a priority of health care reform in industrialized and non-industrialized countries alike. It has been defined as:

"essential health care based on practical, scientifically sound and socially acceptable methods and technology made universally accessible to individuals and their families in the community through their full participation and at a cost that the community and country can afford to maintain at every stage of their development in the spirit of self-reliance and self-determination" (35).

Key to this notion is the idea no single system or set of conditions can describe primary health care. The type of care provided in each community or country must be relevant to that community or country. Thus, in order to determine what constitutes proper primary health care in a particular society, one must apply the relevant results of research into the social, biomedical, and health sciences aspects of the community as well as results of public health experience. The minimum requirements of a primary health care system, however, include education about the prevailing health problems of the community and methods to prevent and control those problems, and the promotion of a healthy food supply and proper nutrition.

Partly due to the regionalization of health services, all of the provinces have recently undertaken reforms of primary health care delivery. One of the main motivating factors driving regionalization was local regions' ability to respond to community health needs. Primary health care delivery is also a priority due to fiscal constraints on all the provinces, pressuring ministries to decrease dependence on expensive institutional care. Primary health care delivery models now being implemented include walk-in/urgent care clinics (every province), community health centres (Quebec, Saskatchewan, Ontario, New Brunswick, Prince Edward Island), nursing telephone hot-lines designed to decrease "inappropriate" use of emergency rooms (New Brunswick), health and community nursing resource centres (Manitoba) (10). Methods of delivery of primary medical care in Canada and some of the alternative delivery methods are described in greater detail in the section on organization of provincial health care delivery in Chapter 13.

5.3. LONG-TERM CARE

There is no identifiable Canadian policy, terminology, information system, or set of standards of care for long-term care (LTC). Each province has developed its own range of services and policies. There is a lack of standard jurisdiction; some provinces locate LTC in the purview of health, and others consider them social services. Even within a province, jurisdictional roles frequently change. The issue is further complicated by the fact that LTC can be provided by either the public or private sectors, and in institutions or through community- and home-based services, and it is not covered under by the *Canada Health Act.* As a result, it is very difficult to systematically gather information concerning the provision of long-term care. Furthermore, the family, especially women, provides most long-term care — approximately 80%. Significant changes to the structure and coherence of family units are reflected in the ability of family members to provide care.

LTC is required when an individual's health deficiencies impede independent functioning and help is required from formal service providers. The people who use such services are usually the elderly, people with disabilities, or people with a chronic or prolonged illness: there are also significant numbers of young people with disabilities in long-term institutions or supported by family and friends whom they may outlive and so become dependent on the publicly provided system.

Internationally and in most Canadian provinces there is an emphasis on community care (as opposed to institutional care) to encourage independence in the community for as long as possible. For the majority of elderly, this can be achieved through the provision of instrumental support services (such as home maintenance). Personal health care services (such as bathing) may also be required for people who are elderly or disabled, and may be provided in the community, although more usually in an institutional setting. A spectrum of care settings is desirable, with staged residential care that allows for some supervision and support as an option between community independence and institutionalization. The predictors of institutionalization are advanced age, lack of spouse in the household, hospital admission in the previous two years, cognitive impairment, and difficulty with taking care of personal care needs. Of these, cognitive impairment is a determining factor for many elderly. It has been estimated that up to 65% of the very elderly suffer cognitive impairment, and provisions must be met for the necessary care.

The issue of referral and access to LTC has become a major concern and has been addressed by a number of provincial strategies and reform initiatives. The issue is whether home care and chronic care beds should require a medical referral. Most LTC reform reports recommend that personal choice and consumer input in terms of preference be involved in placement decisions. Cultural sensitivity and appropriateness are also stressed. Of particular concern is the quality of life of residents in long-term care institutions.

Many provincial commissions have recommended a shift away from institution-alization of extended care patients, as well as a reduction of extended care or chronic care beds in acute care hospitals to no more than 10% of the hospital's total beds. However, in order for de-institutionalization to be successful, more home support is needed. And while home-supported LTC placements seem preferable to institutional-ized care in many respects, few provincial health plans can afford to cover the costs for families taking care of relatives at home. Some critics consider de-institutionalization of long-term care an attempt to shift health care costs out of government budgets and onto the private sector via the family.

In summary, the trend in long-term care is to maximize independence in the com-munity for people who are elderly, disabled, or chronically ill through the transfer of resources from the institutional sector to the community. Although LTC is deemed a high priority in every provincial health reform strategy, there is no national policy, and provinces are at different stages in adoption and development of more appropriate models of service delivery. There is need for leadership at top levels of governments of planning and policy for long-term care.

5.4. MENTAL HEALTH SERVICES

The recent trend in mental health services in Canada has been the development of community support services for those who are mentally ill and of appropriate community- and hospital-based health services to maintain former policies of de-institutionalization. De-institutionalization policies of the 1960s and 1970s, although undertaken with good intentions, had resulted in a concentration of the severely/criminally mentally ill people in psychiatric hospitals and the development of psychiatric units within general hospitals. This resulted in an unintended side effect: those with neuroses and mild mental health disorders received care while difficult patients were neglected. For this reason, the current priority continues to develop a network of community-based services.

Community mental health services have evolved in the last ten years, but con-tinue to be criticized in relation to lack of coordination and continuity of care, as well as lack of availability of some types of supportive services. Most recently the self-per-ceived needs of those with psychiatric illness have been recognized as often being at variance with the objectives of professionals and families. Families often push for a "cure" and further research, and professionals push for convenient modes of treatment and "containment", whereas consumer advocacy emphasizes the needs for employ-ment, nondiscriminatory housing, drop-in centres, and a humanization of psychiatric services (36).

5.4.1. De-institutionalization
In the 1960s, the U.S. began depopulating its mental institutions so that by 1975 the number of inpatients had been reduced by two-thirds. The intention was to promote

the integration and rehabilitation of inpatients in the community through a community mental health program. In Canada, 0.4% of the population was in mental institutions in 1960, and half had been hospitalized for more than seven years (37). In 1961, the report of the Canadian Mental Health Association and the 1964 *Report of the Royal Commission on Mental Health Services* reflected a commitment to the philosophy of de-institutionalization. There was a call for the integration of psychiatric services into the physical and personnel resources of the rest of medicine, regionalization of treatment services, decentralization of management of psychiatric services, and close cooperation and coordination among the psychiatric services in hospitals, clinics, and community agencies. Between 1960 and 1976, the numbers of beds in Canadian mental hospitals decreased by more than 32,000. The bed capacity of psychiatric units in general hospitals increased to almost 6,000, from less than 1,000. De-institutionalization occurred in all provinces and each adopted a different approach to the development of new delivery systems for services.

5.4.2. Two-Tiered System

The establishment of psychiatric units in general hospitals resulted in psychiatric professionals discovering a new group of patients with mild symptomatology who were more responsive to treatment than the severely intractable psychiatric patients. This new group included those with mild depression for whom group therapy was appropriate. As there were fewer resources in the psychiatric hospital sector, those who were severely disabled had no representation in the psychiatric services to respond to their needs. It soon became evident that the U.S. experience of a community-based mental health system that ineffectively cares for discharged patients was being reproduced in Canada. In addition to the removal of resources for specialized psychiatric care, there was inadequate follow-up in the community and lack of support for the mechanics of everyday living. The plight of the chronically disturbed ex-psychiatric patient frequently became homelessness or ghetto-type living, exacerbated of symptoms, despondency, suicidal tendencies, and alienation from the community. The effects of these well-intentioned but ultimately unproductive policies continue to reverberate.

5.4.3. Community Mental Health Program

All provinces have now developed community mental health programs that include case management, rehabilitation, housing programs, and other support services. With an emphasis on multidisciplinary care and flexible service delivery, community mental health programs have come a long way in striving to meet the individualized needs of those who are mentally ill. However, certain problems persist, such as fragmentation of care, poor accountability, ineffective case management, high readmission rates, and insufficient links between hospitals and the community (38). In the 1990s, there has been a universal re-examination of mental health services, as well as an ongoing strong financial commitment to mental health reform in virtually every province. With the advent of regionalization in all provinces except Ontario, the funding and delivery of mental health services is now the responsibility of regional health boards. However, most provinces have a central mental health advisory committee or council to help develop broader policies and strategic plans. In Ontario, the Ministry of Health continues to hold most responsibilities for mental health programs, with municipalities and local regions scheduled to take over this function in the near future.

5.4.4. Issues in Mental Health Reform

Issues that have recently arisen in strategic planning for mental health services include the following (39):

Target population. Whose needs are to be met and what are the priorities? Those with major mental disorders and those who are significantly disabled comprise 1% to 2% of the population who are most in need. Recent reform efforts in mental health services have focused on particular high-risk populations, including Aboriginal people, women, children and adolescents, and those who are elderly, or mentally or physically disabled.

Role of the General Hospital Psychiatric Unit. The functions of these units must be reviewed. There is a need for greater availability of different types of resources, such as holding beds, intensive care beds, day hospitals, and crisis intervention services. The interrelationship with community support systems is also paramount.

Role of Psychiatric Hospitals. There is no apparent justification for the current ratio of individual beds to population, especially if community services are developed. It is estimated that there is a prevalence of 15 per 100,000 population with major psychiatric disorders and conditions, which may be accompanied by severe behaviour disorders (e.g., dementia, mental retardation, brain damage, paranoid schizophrenia, schizophrenia with severe regression). It is estimated that possibly only half of all existing psychiatric hospital beds are currently required.

Continuity of Care. For continuity of care, it is necessary to have a range of services that are linked, monitored, and evaluated for their provision of ongoing coordinated and integrated community support. An example of an approach to continuity of care is case management, which is highly individualized in terms of assessment of need, planning, and monitoring of services appropriate for a client.

Co-morbidity. The presence of another condition such as substance abuse or disability increases the vulnerability of an individual with a psychiatric condition and must be addressed.

Service Integration. There is need for a single system with a coordinated structure that works for people. Most provinces have integrated central and local authority by giving regional health boards the flexibility to deliver mental health services according to local needs, while maintaining provincial mental health authorities or councils as centralized coordinating structures. Nova Scotia and Prince Edward Island have also initiated programs of cooperation and coordinated services between mental health services and the Ministry of Correctional Services.

Consumerism. As previously indicated, a strong consumer movement is developing and challenging the system to include its input into policy development and services. Some psychiatric patients who have had many dealings with the system of psychiatric care, including institutionalization, tend to regard themselves as "survivors" of an inhumane and stifling experience. Consumers or "survivors" of the system have expressed the need for income maintenance, adequate housing, social support, non-traditional services such as peer support and self-help groups, and more choices in life. These are not generally the focus of the traditional psychiatric care approach, which supports dependency rather than independence.

5.4.5. Future Canadian Initiatives

There has been a significant resurgence in planning and policy development for mental health services in Canada in recent times. Federal guidelines for review of policies and programs were developed following consultation with the provinces and released in 1988 in a document that identified the importance of mental health for Canadians in the achievement of overall health. Mental health was defined in a broad sense as:

"the capacity of the individual, the group and the environment to interact with one another in ways that promote subjective well-being, the optimal development and use of mental abilities (cognitive, affective and rational), the achievement of individual and collective goals consistent with justice and the attainment andpreservation of conditions of fundamental equality" (40).

Almost every province has implemented strategies to reform its mental health system, and existing services are briefly described in Chapter 13. A number of provincial policy initiatives in strategic reform of mental health have been proposed, giving an indication of future directions. Provincial reforms focus on the creation and maintenance of community-based mental health services that are integrated and interconnected with other components in order to reduce fragmentation, increase family and patient participation in planning, allocate resources appropriately, and deliver care for special-needs population. Reforms also focus on those who are seriously mentally ill and their families.

6.   FROM HERE TO THERE

The last few chapters of this book have addressed the evolution of the Canadian health care system into the system we know today. Canadian health care was, and continues to be, a matter of intense personal pride for Canadians — a modern-day social success program story that helps define the Canadian national identity (8). But since the early 1970s, Canada, together with all other industrialized nations of the world, has faced a series of systemic stressors that have led to the re-examination of the health care system — its goals, its organization, and the way it functions. As a result, the current health care system is in flux as each province and territory in Canada, and the federal government, strives to find that particular combination of health policies and reforms that will best meet the health needs of its population. This chapter has highlighted some of the common themes found in all Canadian health care reforms and the underlying values each is trying to address. The roads to reform are many, but the ultimate destination is the same — improving the health of Canadians.

As Canada turns to face the 21st century, many of the issues discussed in this chapter continue to dominate the policy agenda. Questions concerning cost effectiveness and cost control continue to play a lead role in all discussions. As a result, the possibility of creating more effective and cost-efficient models of health services delivery will need to be constantly re-evaluated. Integrated delivery systems based on patient rostering, capitation payments to health care providers, and vertically and horizontally integrated care are likely to evolve into the key models under consideration. The shift to community-based health centres away from institutions will continue, and the emphasis on primary care will grow. As the effects of the social sector on health continue to be understood, pressure will likely build to improve the coordination of government policies for the benefit of health, in particular for the most vulnerable population in Canada (children, women, people who are poor or homeless, Aboriginal peoples, and ethnic and cultural minorities). One component of this increased emphasis on the needs of special groups is the need for broader citizen representation and more widespread public participation in health care — both at the individual level and the systemic level. Currently, regionalization of health services and the accompanying devolution of policy making to the local level attempt to broaden the spectrum of public participation in health care and to democratize the policy-making process. These models are not without their problems, however, and it is possible that federal, provincial, and territorial reformers will continue to tinker with various organizational models as their health systems are fine-tuned.

What remains clearest in all of this debate about health care and health care reform in Canada is that concerns with cost containment and system effectiveness must not overshadow the fundamental Canadian beliefs in compassion, respect for others, and the value placed on human dignity. It is the combination of all these fundamental values that will shape reform in the years to come and the quest for that unique Canadian combination that embodies those traits and beliefs that will lead us into the next century.

7.   SUMMARY

Canada aims to achieve equitable access to health care for all Canadians. So far, equal access to medical care has been largely achieved by the universal system of hospital and medical insurance. However, during the last two decades there has been a series of trends that have placed significant stress on the health care system throughout the industrialized world, including Canada; this has led to a universal re-examination of how to provide the highest quality and most effective health care while decreasing health system costs. These stressors include continually increasing costs to look after the sick and infirm, questions concerning the appropriate role of the state in society, in particular resulting in conflicts between government and health care professionals, the rise of consumerism, changing demographic patterns leading to increased numbers of the elderly and increased demand for expensive, high-technology medical care, evidence of health inequities among particular high-risk population groups, awareness of the need for disease prevention and health promotion for achieving health for the population, the emergence of high-technology health care and its accompanying high price tag, and the inappropriate use of resources by both patients and providers. Since the late 1980s and early 1990s, every province in Canada, as well as the federal government, has undertaken a fundamental review of current health systems via task forces, commissions, boards of inquiry, and working groups to address these problems.

Perhaps the most influential of recent commissions that have reviewed the health care system was the National Forum on Health. The Forum was officially launched in 1994 in order to address the issues of reform of the Canadian health care system while maintaining a strong commitment to the five pillars of medicare. Of main concern were questions of increased efficiency and cost effectiveness, access, and high-quality care. Like its provincial predecessors, the Forum included representatives from government, health policy and health economics experts, health care professionals, and consumers. Public participation and consultation were central to its mandate and activities. Although the Forum was motivated largely by issues of costs and improving cost effectiveness through a variety of means, as were the provincial reviews, the Forum recommended a return to the question of core Canadian values and how they should drive further changes in the health care system. The fundamental values, which were identified through the Forum's public consultation process, are equity and fairness, compassion, dignity and respect for all individuals, quality, efficiency and effectiveness, personal responsibility for appropriate use of health resources, and public participation in health system decision making.

Equity, Compassion, Dignity, and Respect. In recent years, it has been increasingly evident that the health care sector must adapt to Canada's cultural diversity. Many health care facilities do not respond to the needs of the members of ethnic groups. This lack of responsiveness is due to cultural insensitivity; for example, the failure of many health care professionals to recognize and accommodate differences in language, values, or diet can discourage members of ethnocultural minorities from seeking effective health care. As well, the lack of responsiveness is due to the insufficient knowledge of the health care provider with respect to particular health needs of the ethnocultural group. In addition, the cultural beliefs of members of ethnic communities about health care and health care practitioners, language barriers, illiteracy, and fear of racism and ethnocentrism prevent them from gaining full accessibility to health care.

Equity and accessibility of health services in Canada must now focus on multicultural health. The term "multicultural health" refers to health care provided in a culturally and racially sensitive manner. Health care providers must become aware of cultural and ethnic determinants of health, the differing beliefs concerning health and medicine among ethnic communities, and the barriers faced by members of ethnic minorities in gaining access to health care. In order to achieve multicultural health, both community and professionals require education and awareness of the health status and concerns of ethnic communities in Canada.

Efficiency, Effectiveness, and Quality. The first step towards increasing the efficiency and effectiveness of health services in Canada is knowing exactly what the health system is trying to achieve. To this end, the Forum recommended that provincial governments set health goals and implement systems to monitor their achievement. An integral part of this monitoring must be the development of sound information systems that allow for better coordination of care, decrease unnecessary duplication of services and testing, and help identify when competing services may actually be harmful to the individual. Integrated information systems are also used to help provincial policy makers identify areas of health service provision that need improvement. Questions such as the over- or under-utilization of services, gaps in service provision or barriers to cost-effective service provision can be identified via information systems and programs targeted to correcting these gaps can be identified.

An additional step to improving the quality of services provided to Canadians, as well as increasing the overall efficiency of the system, is increased integration of services provided across societal sectors. For many special-needs groups, health and social needs go hand-in-hand. Thus, at the very minimum, increased coordination and integration of health care and social services have long been a priority among provinces. In addition, our current knowledge about the many broad determinants of health, of which health services are but one part, also makes increased coordination of policy efforts across sectors imperative. Housing, employment, education, environment, and recreation are just some of the other government sectors that make policies that directly affect the health of Canadians.

Consumer Participation and Access to Decision Making. Citizens of developed countries now regard health as a basic human right, and governments have responded by providing health care through various programs. However, in recent years consumers have expressed concerns about inconveniences, the unavailability of health services, difficulties in communication between practitioners and consumers, and inadequacy of health care for certain groups in society. Consumers wish to be involved in health care, and their participation can be facilitated by the provision of knowledge by health care authorities about disease causation, citizens' participation in the formulation of health care policies, and the creation of voluntary groups. Citizens may also participate in the health care system through membership on hospital boards or committees and boards involved in the regulation of health care professions.

Reforms. In order to achieve the recommendations made by provincial review committees, as well as by the National Forum on Health, emphasis on certain key reforms remains a priority. These reforms centre on some of the most major attempts at addressing all of the fundamental values identified by the Forum in a complementary and systematic way.

Regionalization and the devolution of decision making for health policy emerged as a major theme of all the provincial reports and has been implemented in every province with the exception of Ontario.

Primary health care is an issue of growing concern in the health care field. It is defined as essential health care based on practical, scientifically sound, and socially acceptable methods and technology made universally accessible to individuals and their families in the community, through their full participation and at a cost that the community and country can afford to maintain at every stage of their development in the spirit of self-reliance and self-determination. It should link seamlessly with secondary and tertiary care and be fully integrated with the community care.

Long-term care is required when an individual's health deficiencies impede independent functioning and help is required from formal service providers. Those using the long-term care services include the elderly, people with disabilities, or those with chronic or prolonged illness. The major issue in long-term care is community care that allows independence in the community to be maintained for as long as possible. The trend in long-term care is to move toward maximizing independence in the community for people who are elderly or disabled through the transfer of resources from the institutional sector to the community.

In mental health services, there has recently been the development of community support services as well as the development of appropriate community- and hospital-based health services to maintain former policies of de-institutionalization of people who are mentally ill. This philosophy calls for the integration of psychiatric services into the physical and personnel resources of the rest of medicine, regionalization of treatment services, and decentralization of management of psychiatric services in hospitals, clinics, and community agencies. Almost every province has undertaken strategies to reform its mental health system. The types of issues that have arisen in strategic planning for mental health services are target population, role of general hospital psychiatric unit, role of psychiatric hospitals, political will to provide community support services, continuity of care, co-morbidity, service integration, and consumerism.

As Canada turns to face the 21st century, many of the issues discussed in this chapter continue to dominate the policy agenda. Questions about cost effectiveness and cost control continue to play a lead role in all discussions. As a result, the possibility of creating more effective and cost-efficient models of health services delivery will be constantly re-evaluated. What remains most clear in all of this debate about health care and health care reform in Canada, however, is that concerns with cost containment and system effectiveness must not overshadow the fundamental Canadian beliefs in compassion, respect for others, and the value placed on human dignity. It is the combination of all these fundamental values that will shape reform in the years to come and the quest for that unique Canadian combination that embodies those traits and beliefs that will lead us into the next century.

8.   REFERENCES

1. National Forum on Health. Report on Dialogue with Canadians. Ottawa: National Forum on Health, 1996.

2. National Forum on Health. National Goals and the Federal Role in Health Care. Ottawa: National Forum on Health, 1995.

3. National Forum on Health. What Determines Health? Ottawa: National Forum on Health, 1996.

4. National Forum on Health. The Public and Private Financing of Canada's Health System. Ottawa: National Forum on Health, 1995.

5. National Forum on Health. Summary Report: Evidence-Based Decision Making; A Dialogue on Health Information. Ottawa: National Forum on Health, 1995.

6. National Forum on Health. Advancing the Dialogue on Health and Health Care: A Consultation Document. Ottawa: National Forum on Health, 1996.

7. National Forum on Health. Canada Health Action: Building on the Legacy, Vol. 1: The Final Report of the National Forum on Health. Ottawa: Minister of Public Works and Government Services, 1997.

8. Mhatre S, Deber R. From Equal Access to Equitable Access to Health: A Review of Canadian Provincial Health Commissions and Reports. International Journal of Health Services 1992;22(4):645-668.

9. Angus DE. Review of Significant Health Care Commissions and Task Forces in Canada Since 1983-84. Ottawa: Canadian Hospital Association, Canadian Medical Association and Canadian Nurses Association, 1991.

10. Health Canada. Provincial Health System Reform in Canada. Ottawa: Ministry of Supply and Services Canada, 1995.

11. Wanatabe M, Noseworthy T. National Forum on Health Speaks To and For Us All. Annals of the Royal College of Physicians and Surgeons of Canada 1997;30(3):135-136.

12. Health Reform Update (4th ed.). Ottawa: Canadian College of Health Services Executives, 1997.

13. Government of Newfoundland and Labrador. Report from the Royal Commission on Hospital and Nursing Home Costs to the Government of Newfoundland and Labrador. St. John's: Government of Newfoundland and Labrador, 1984.

14. Government of Newfoundland and Labrador. A Green Paper on Our Health Care System Expenditures and Funding. St. John's: Government of Newfoundland and Labrador, 1986.

15. Government of Nova Scotia. Towards a New Strategy. The Report of the Nova Scotia Royal Commission on Health Care. Halifax: Government of Nova Scotia, 1989.

16. Ministère de la Santé et des Services Sociaux. Improving Health and Wellbeing in Quebec: Orientations. Ste. Foy: Government of Quebec, 1989.

17. Ministère de la Santé et des Services Sociaux. A Reform Centred on the Citizen. Ste. Foy: Government of Quebec, 1990.

18. Ministry of Health. Health for All Ontario. Toronto: Government of Ontario, 1987.

19. Ontario Minister's Advisory Group on Health Promotion. Health Promotion Matters in Ontario. A Report of the Minister's Advisory Group on Health Promotion. Toronto: Advisory Group, 1987.

20. Premier's Commission on Future Health Care for Albertans. The Rainbow Report: Our Vision of Health. Edmonton: Government of Alberta, 1989.

21. Kenny NP. Values, Health and Health Care. Annals of Royal College of Physicians and Surgeons of Canada 1997;30(3):144-146.

22. Wilkins R, Adams O. Healthfulness of Life: A Unified View of Mortality, Institutionalization, and Non-Institutionalized Disability in Canada. Montreal: Institute for Research on Public Policy, 1983.

23. Doyle R, Rahi K. Organizational Change Toward Multiculturalism. Toronto: Social Planning Council of Metropolitan Toronto, 1990.

24. Masi R. Multiculturalism, Medicine and Health, Part 4: Individual Considerations. Canadian Family Physician 1989;35(1):251-254.

25. Ministry of Supply and Services. After the Door Has Been Opened: Mental Health Issues Affecting Immigrants and Refugees in Canada. Ottawa: Government of Canada, 1988.

26. Masi R. Multiculturalism, Medicine and Health, Part 5: Community Considerations. Canadian Family Physician 1989;35(2):251-254.

27. Tator C. Strategy for Fostering Participation and Equity in the Human Services Delivery. In Doyle R, Rahi K, eds. Organization Change Towards Multiculturalism. Toronto: Access Action Council, 1990.

28. Berg A, Hammitt K. Assessing the Psychiatric Patient's Ability to Meet the Literacy Demands of Hospitalization. Hospital Community Psychiatry 1980;31(4):266-268.

29. Dunn M, Buckwalter K, Weistein L, Palti H. Innovations in Family and Community Health. Family Community Health 1985;8(3):76-87.

30. Mallet L, Spruill WJ. Readability Evaluation of Nine Patient Drug Education Sources. American Pharmacy 1988; NS28(11):33-36.

31. Wanatabe M, Noseworthy T. Creating a Culture of Evidence-based Decision-Making in Health. Annals of Royal College of Physicians and Surgeons of Canada 1997;20(3):137-139.

32. Working Group on Rationalization and Decentralization. The Language of Health System Reform. Ottawa: Canadian Medical Association, 1993.

33. Alford R. Health Care Politics: Ideological and Interest Group Barriers to Reform. Chicago: University of Chicago Press, 1975.

34. Carrothers L, Macdonald S, Home J, Fish D, Silver M. Rationalization and Health Care Policy in Canada: A National Survey and Manitoba Case Study. Winnipeg: Department of Community Health, Faculty of Medicine, University of Manitoba, 1991.

35. Report of the International Conference on Primary Health Care. Primary Health Care. Alma-Alta, U.S.S.R.: World Health Organization, 1978:6-12.

36. Metropolitan Toronto District Health Council. Metropolitan Toronto Mental Health Reform: Final Report. System Design and Implementation Recommendations. Toronto: Metropolitan Toronto District Health Council, 1996.

37. Richman A, Harris P. Mental Hospital Deinstitutionalization in Canada. A National Perspective with Some Regional Examples. International Journal of Mental Health 1989;11(4):64-83.

38. Wasylenki D, Goering P, Lancee W, Fischer L, Freeman S. Psychiatric Aftercare in a Metropolitan Setting. Canadian Journal of Psychiatry 1985;30(5):329-336.

39. Wasylenki D, Goering P, MacNaughton E. Planning Mental Health Services: 1. Background and Key Issues. Canadian Journal of Psychiatry 1992;37(3):199-205.

40. Health and Welfare Canada. Mental Health for Canadians: Striking a Balance. Ottawa: Ministry of Supply and Services, 1988.

Appendices and Index

Appendix

A
Manoeuvres to Be Included in Clinical Preventive Health Care*

Classified by Age, Strength of Evidence, Target Population, and Burden of Suffering

These tables summarize manoeuvres reviewed by the Canadian Task Force on the Periodic Health Examination (PHE) in this book, for which the medical evidence documents benefits that outweigh potential harm. They deal with screening and counselling for the asymptomatic individual that would be offered in a clinical setting by physicians, nurses, or associated health care workers. The tables exclude evaluation of interventions such legislation, school-based programs, and care provided by dentists. Therapeutic recommendations for individuals who have previously identified conditions (e.g., hypertension) are also not included.

Recommendations are summarized by age and gender into sub-groups such as prenatal/perinatal. The information is displayed with "A Recommendations" for the general population at the top (manoeuvres for which there is good evidence for inclusion in a periodic health examination). Conditions with a higher burden of suffering are listed first.

The second grouping on each page are "B Recommendations" for the general population (manoeuvres for which there is fair evidence for inclusion in a periodic health examination). Within this category, conditions with a high burden of suffering are again listed first. A sub-section of each group of recommendations specially addresses high-risk populations. For the details, readers are advised to consult web site listed at the end of the book.

*Source: Canadian Task Force on Periodic Health Examination. *The Canadian Guide to Clinical Preventive Health Care*. Pages xxxix - xlix, 1994. Printed with permission of Health Canada and Minister of Public Works and Government Services Canada, 1998.

1. Perinatal Care

CONDITION	MANOEUVRE	POPULATION
GOOD EVIDENCE TO INCLUDE IN PHE (A RECOMMENDATIONS):[1]		
Low birth weight/cognitive ability of child	Smoking cessation interventions	Pregnant women
Gastrointestinal and respiratory infection in the newborn	Counselling on breastfeeding; peripartum interventions to increase frequency of breast-feeding	Pregnant women (or women in the peripartum period)
D (Rh) sensitization	D (Rh) antibody screening and immunoglobulin (D Ig) administration after delivery of D-positive infant	Pregnant women
Neural tube defects	Folic acid supplementation	Women capable of becoming pregnant
Bacteriuria in pregnancy	Urine culture	Pregnant women
FAIR EVIDENCE TO INCLUDE IN PHE (B RECOMMENDATIONS):[1]		
Congenital rubella syndrome	Screen, counsel, and vaccinate post partum	Pregnant women
Preeclampsia	Blood pressure measurement	Pregnant women
Fetal alcohol syndrome	Screen and counsel	Pregnant women
Chlamydial infection	Smear, culture, or analysis	Pregnant or high-risk women
Perinatal morbidity and mortality	Single prenatal ultrasound	Pregnant women
Neural tube defects	Maternal serum alpha-fetoprotein/ultrasound, amniocentesis	Pregnant women
Down's syndrome	Triple screening and counselling	Pregnant women <35 yrs
Iron deficiency anemia in infants	Counselling parents on breastfeeding	Pregnant women (or women in the peripartum period)

High-Risk Populations		
D (Rh) sensitization	Repeat D (Rh) antibody screening and immunoglobulin (D Ig) administration	Pregnant women and women undergoing induced abortion or amniocentesis who are antibody negative
D (Rh) sensitization	D (Rh) antibody screening and immunoglobulin (D Ig) administration	After delivery of D-positive infant
Down's syndrome	Genetic screening and counselling	High-risk pregnant women
Hemoglobinopathies	1) Screen for carrier status (complete blood count and hemoglobin electrophoresis) 2) DNA analysis, fetal-tissue sample/counselling	1) High-risk pregnant women; 2) Families, parents, confirmed carriers

2. Neonatal and Well-Baby Care

CONDITION	MANOEUVRE	POPULATION
GOOD EVIDENCE TO INCLUDE IN PHE (A RECOMMENDATIONS):[1]		
Immunizable infectious disease	Immunizations, childhood	Infants and children
Hepatitis B	Immunization	Infants and children
Phenylketonuria	Serum phenylalanine screening	Newborns
Unintentional injury	Counselling on home risk factors, poison control	Parents of infants
Infection	Counselling on breast feeding; peripartum interventions to increase frequency of breastfeeding	Pregnant women (or women in the peripartum period)
Congenital hip dislocation	Physical exam, hips	Infants
Ophthalmia neonatorum	Ocular prophylaxis	Newborns
Amblyopia	Eye exam	Infants
Hearing impairment	Hearing exam	Infants

CONDITION	MANOEUVRE	POPULATION
GOOD EVIDENCE TO INCLUDE IN PHE (A RECOMMENDATION):[1]		
Congenital hypothyroidism	Thyroid-stimulating hormone (TSH) test	Neonates
Night-time crying	Anticipatory guidance on systematic ignoring	Parents of infants distressed by crying
High-Risk Populations		
Hemoglobinopathies	Hemoglobin electrophoresis	High-risk neonates
FAIR EVIDENCE TO INCLUDE IN PHE (B RECOMMENDATIONS):[1]		
Iron-deficiency anemia in infants	Counselling parents on breastfeeding, iron-fortified formula, cereal, supplements	Infants
Disorders of physical growth	Serial height, weight, head circumference measurement	Infants
Delayed mental development	Inquire about developmental milestones	Parents of infants
Iron-deficiency anemia	Routine hemoglobin 6-12 months	High-risk infants
HIV/AIDS	Voluntary HIV antibody screening	Infants of HIV-positive women

3. Preventive Health Care for Children and Adolescents

CONDITION	MANOEUVRE	POPULATION
GOOD EVIDENCE TO INCLUDE IN PHE (A RECOMMENDATIONS):[1]		
Tobacco-caused disease	Counselling on smoking cessation	Smokers
Dental caries, periodontal disease	Fluoride, toothpaste, or supplement; brushing teeth	General population
Hearing impairment	Noise control and hearing protection	General population
Hepatitis B	Immunization	Children and adolescents

High-Risk Populations		
All-cause morbidity and mortality	Referral to day care or preschool programs	Disadvantaged children
Child maltreatment	Home visits	High-risk families
Influenza	Amantadine chemoprophylaxis case	High-risk or unvaccinated individuals exposed to index
Tuberculosis	INH prophylaxis	Household contacts and skin test converters
HIV/AIDS, gonorrhea, chlamydia	Screening for sexually transmitted disease	High-risk populations

FAIR EVIDENCE TO INCLUDE IN PHE (B RECOMMENDATIONS):[1]

Motor vehicle accidents	Counselling on restraint use and avoidance drinking and driving	General population
Tobacco-related diseases	Counselling to prevent smoking initiation	Children and adolescents
Tobacco-related diseases	Referral to validated cessation program	Smokers
Household and recreational injury	Counselling on home risk factors, poisoning	Children, parents
Vision problems	Visual acuity testing	Preschool children
Unintended pregnancy; sexually transmitted diseases	Counselling, sexual activity, contraception	Adolescents
Congenital rubella syndrome	Screen and vaccinate or universal vaccination	Non-pregnant women of child-bearing age
All-cause mortality and morbidity	Moderate physical activity	General population
Problem drinking	Case finding and counselling	General population
Adverse consequences, children of alcoholics	Children of Alcoholics Screening Test (CAST)	General population
Skin cancer	Counselling on sun exposure, clothing	General population

High-Risk Populations		
Iron-deficiency anemia	Routine hemoglobin	Disadvantaged children
Cystic fibrosis (CF)	Sweat test	Siblings of children with CF
Cystic fibrosis	DNA analysis for carrier status	Siblings of children with CF
Lead exposure	Blood lead screening	High-risk children

4. Preventive Health Care for Adults

CONDITION	MANOEUVRE	POPULATION
GOOD EVIDENCE TO INCLUDE IN PHE (A RECOMMENDATIONS):[1]		
Tobacco-related diseases	Counselling on smoking cessation and offer of nicotine replacement therapy	Smokers
Neural tube defects	Folic acid supplementation	Women capable of becoming pregnant
Hearing impairment	Noise control and hearing protection	General population
Breast cancer	Mammography and clinical exam	Women aged 50-69
Dental caries, periodontal disease	Fluoride, toothpaste or supplement, brushing and flossing teeth	General population
High-Risk Populations		
HIV/AIDS	Voluntary HIV-antibody screening	High-risk populations
Child maltreatment	Home visits	High-risk families
Progressive renal disease	Urine dipstick	Adults with IDDM
Gonorrhea	Gram stain/culture cervical or urethral smear	High-risk groups
Influenza	Amantadine chemoprophylaxis	Individuals exposed to index case

Influenza	Outreach strategies to reach high-risk groups	Specific sub-groups (e.g., diabetics, chronic heart disease)
Tuberculosis	Mantoux tuberculin skin test	High-risk groups
Tuberculosis	INH prophylaxis	Household contacts and skin test converters

FAIR EVIDENCE TO INCLUDE IN PHE (B RECOMMENDATIONS):[1]

Hypertension	Blood pressure measurement	Adults
Motor vehicle accidents	Counsel, use of restraint	General population
All-cause mortality and morbidity	Moderate physical activity	General population
Tobacco-related diseases	Refer to validated cessation programs after cessation advice	Smokers
Diet-related illness	Counselling on adverse nutritional habits	Adults
Problem drinking	Case finding and counselling	General population
Coronary heart disease	General dietary advice on fat and cholesterol	Males aged 30-69
Cervical cancer	Papanicolaou test	Women
Congenital rubella syndrome	Screen and vaccinate or universal vaccination	Non-pregnant women of child-bearing age
Osteoporotic fractures (and side effects)	Counselling, hormone replacement therapy	Perimenopausal women
Gonorrhea	Counselling, educational materials	General population
Skin cancer	Counselling on sun exposure, clothing	General population
High-Risk Populations		
Chlamydial infection	Smear, culture, or analysis	High-risk women

Tuberculosis	INH prophylaxis	High-risk sub-groups
Influenza	Immunization, annual	High-risk groups
Colorectal cancer	Colonoscopy	Those with cancer
Diabetic retinopathy	Funduscopy or retinal photography	Diabetics
Lung cancer	Dietary advice on leafy green vegetables and fruit	Smokers
Skin cancer	Physical exam, skin	First-degree relatives with melanoma

5. Additional[2] Preventive Health Care for the Elderly

CONDITION	MANOEUVRE	POPULATION
GOOD EVIDENCE TO INCLUDE IN PHE (A RECOMMENDATIONS):[1]		
Influenza	Outreach strategies for vaccination	Elderly
	High-Risk Populations	
Falls/injury	Multidisciplinary post-fall assessment	Elderly
Pneumococcal pneumonia	Immunization	Specific sub-groups
FAIR EVIDENCE TO INCLUDE IN PHE (B RECOMMENDATIONS):[1]		
Hypertension	Blood pressure measurement	Elderly
Influenza	Immunization, annual	Elderly
Hearing impairment	Enquiry, whispered voice test or audioscope	Elderly
Diminished visual acuity	Snellen sight card	Elderly

1 See Appendix B for recommendations not updated since 1979 (www.hc-sc.gc.ca/hppb/healthcare/pubs/clinical_preventive/index.html).
2 Continue appropriate interventions from adult tables.

B
Useful Web Sites

This appendix list several useful Web sites for retrieving current information on the subjects discussed in the book. While the accuracy of the addresses was checked, at the time of publication, experience suggests that from time to time, addresses for the Web site change, or some may no longer exist.

1. General

Health Canada <www.hc-sc.gc.ca>
Information and data on all aspects of health and health care in Canada, plus extensive sets of links to many national and provincial agencies such as the Canadian Institute for Health Information, provincial departments of health and international organizations such as the U.S. Centers for Disease Control in Atlanta. Sites are listed in following categories: Index (which provides details on most subject headings dealt in this book), Search, Links, News, Health Care, Public Health, Health Factors, Regulated Products, Health Research, and Regulation and Policy.

Statistics Canada <www.statcan.ca:80/start.html>
This site contains useful data on many aspects of demographic data, census data, health status, and other determinants of health, e.g., economics, unemployment, poverty.

Public Health and Preventive Medicine in Canada <phs.med.utoronto.ca/faculty/cshah.htm>
A resource for periodic updates of relevant Internet-based information.

2. Web Sites by Chapter

Chapter 1: Concepts, Determinants, and Promotion of Health
Health Promotion Online (Health Canada) <www.hc-sc.gc.ca/hppb/hpoe.htm>
Ontario Prevention Clearinghouse (OPC) <www.opc.on.ca/idxeng.html>
OPC is a non-profit organization with a multidisciplinary focus on health promotion and prevention activities across the province.

Chapter 2: Measurement and Investigation
Epidemiology textbook: Epidemiology for Uninitiated <www.bmj.com/epidem/epid.html>
Electronic statistical textbook <www.statsoft.com/textbook/stathome.html>

Chapter 3: Health Indicators and Data Sources
Chapter 4: Determinants of Health and Disease

Statistics Canada (population data) <www.statcan.ca/english/Pgdb/People/popula.htm>
Demographic data, population counts, projections, and growth for various areas, as well as information on age, sex, births and deaths, immigration, language, ethnic origin and religion.
U.S. Centers for Disease Control and Prevention <www.cdc.gov/scientific.htm>
Scientific data, surveillance, health statistics, and laboratory information.
Improving the accuracy of death certificate <www.ca/cmaj/vol-158/issue-10/1317.htm>

Chapter 5: Health Status and Consequences

British Columbia Archives <www.bcarchives.gov.bc.ca/textual/governmt/vstats/v_events.htm>
In addition to Health Canada Online, visit the sites of the provincial governments. The Web site for the British Columbia Archives is just one example of the vital statistics that can be retrieved online.
Sympatico "Health Links" on disability <www.mb.sympatico.ca/healthyway/DIRECTORY/B11.html>
Links to sites with patient information and some research data.

Chapter 7: Chronic Diseases and Injuries

Statistics Canada <www.statcan.ca/english/Pgdb/People/health.htm>
Ontario Prevention Clearinghouse (OPC) <www.opc.on.ca/idxeng.html>
Canadian Cancer Statistics <www.cancer.ca/stats/>
Canadian Centre on Substance Abuse
Canadian Health Network (Health Canada) <www.hc-sc.gc.ca/english/>
Canadian Council for Tobacco Council <www.cctc.ca/ncth/>
Addiction Research Foundation of Ontario
Web of Addictions <www.well.com/www/woa/>
Laboratory Centre for Disease Control <hwcweb.hwc.ca/hpb/lcdc/hp_eng.html>
Information on individual diseases.
Clinical Practice Guidelines (CPG) <www.cma.ca/cpgs>
Published by the Canadian Medical Association.

Chapter 8: Communicable Diseases

Laboratory Centre for Disease Control <www.hc-sc.gc.ca/hpb/lcdc/dpg_e.html>
Information and guidelines about vaccine-preventable diseases, STDs, and HIV.
U.S. National Center for Infectious Diseases <www.cdc.gov/ncidod/ncid.htm>

Chapter 9: Environmental Health

Environmental Studies Association of Canada (ESAC) <www.yorku.ca/faculty/academic/meisner/esac/links.htm>
Data on the environment and the major diseases related to it, plus a list of links.
Environmental Health Directorate (Health Canada's Health Protection Branch) <www.hc-sc.gc.ca/datahpb/dataehd/English/opening.htm>

Chapter 10: Occupational Health and Disease

Canadian Centre for Occupational Health and Safety (CCOHS)

Chapter 11: Periodic Health Examinations

Canadian Task Force on the Periodic Health Examination <www.hc-sc.gc.ca/
hppb/healthcare/pubs/clinical_preventive/index.html>
> *The entire text of the Task Force report.*

Guide to Clinical Preventive Services (U.S.) <text.nlm.nih.gov/ftrs/tocview>
> *The complete text of the second edition, with search engine.*

Guidelines Appraisal Project (GAP) <hiru.mcmaster.ca/cpg/>
> *Clinical practice guidelines, worked on by health services researchers, policy makers, and practitioners.*

Clinical Practice Guidelines (CPG) <www.cma.ca/cpgs>
> *Published by the Canadian Medical Association.*

Chapter 12: Evolution of National Health Insurance

Health Canada (health insurance) <www.hc-sc.gc.ca/medicare/index-e.html>
U.S. National Institutes of Health <www.nih.gov/health/>
U.K. Department of Health <www.open.gov.uk/doh/dhhome.htm>
U.K. Clearing House on Health Outcomes <www.leeds.ac.uk/nuffield/infoservices/UKCH/>
Australia Health Department
New Zealand Ministry of Health <www.moh.govt.nz/default.htm>
Organization for Economic and Community Development (OECD) Statistics
<www.oecd.org/std/> and <www.oecd.org/els/health/hc97data.htm>

Chapter 13: Federal and Provincial Health Organizations
Chapter 15: Community Health Services
Chapter 16: Regulation of Health Care Professionals

Canadian Government Information on the Internet <library.uwaterloo.ca:80/discipline/
Government/CanGuide>
National Health Research and Development Program (NHRDP) <www.hc-sc.gc.ca/hppb/nhrdp/indexe.html>
Alberta Health
British Columbia Ministry of Health and Seniors
Manitoba Health <www.gov.mb.ca/health/index.html>
Government of Ontario <www.gov.on.ca/MBS/english/index>
Ontario Ministry of Health <www.gov.on.ca/health/index>
Government of Quebec (in English) <www.gouv.qc.ca/introa.htm>
Ministère de la Santé et des Services sociaux (in English) <www.gouv.qc.ca/sante/indexa.htm>
New Brunswick Ministry of Health <inter.gov.nb.ca/hcs/>
Government of Newfoundland <www.gov.nf.ca/default.htm>
Newfoundland Ministry of Health <www.gov.nf.ca/health/>
Government of Northwest Territories <siksik.learnnet.nt.ca/ECE/default.html>
Nova Scotia Health <www.gov.ns.ca/heal/>
Prince Edward Island Health <www.gov.pe.ca/hss/index.asp>
Saskatchewan Health <www.gov.sk.ca/health/>

Chapter 14: Funding, Expenditures, and Resources
Chapter 15: Community Health Services
Chapter 16: Regulation of Health Care Professionals

Canadian Institute for Health Information
C.D. Howe Institute <www.cdhowe.org/eng/pro/about.html>
Caledon Institute of Social Policy <www.cyberplus.ca/~caledon/>

Centre for Health Evaluation and Outcome Sciences (University of British Columbia)
Cochrane Collaboration <hiru.mcmaster.ca/COCHRANE/>
Centre for Health Economics and Policy Analysis (McMaster University) <hiru.mcmaster.ca/chepa/>
Canadian Health Economic Research Association (CHERA) <qhp.queensu.ca/chera/>
HealNet <hiru.mcmaster.ca/nce/>
Health Information Sciences (University of Victoria) <www.hsd.uvic.ca/HIS/his.htm>
Health Information Research Unit at McMaster University (evidence-based medicine)
Health Services Utilization and Research Commission (HSURC Saskatchewan)
<www.sdh.sk.ca/hsurc/index.htm>
Institute for Clinical Evaluative Sciences (Ontario) <www.ices.on.ca/ices.htm>
KPMG Virtual Library <www.kpmg.ca/vl/main.htm>
Manitoba Centre <www.umanitoba.ca/centres/mchpe/1mchpe.htm>
Nursing Effectiveness Research Unit, McMaster University
<www-fhs.mcmaster.ca/nursing/unitver.htm>
Ontario Health Care Evaluation Network (OHCLEN)
<hiru.mcmaster.ca/ohcen/default.htm>
Queen's University Health Policy <qhp.queensu.ca/default.htm>
University of British Columbia Centre Health Services and Policy Research

Chapter 17: Canadian Health Care into the 21st Century

National Forum on Health

3. Other Useful Sites

U.S. National Institutes of Health (NIH)
National Library of Medicine (Medline, etc.)
United Nations Educational, Scientific and Cultural Organization (UNESCO)
World Health Organization (WHO)
U.S. National Center for Bioethics Literature <guweb.georgetown.edu/nrcbl/>

4. General Public Health Sites

Hardin MD Public Health and Preventive Medicine <www.lib.uiowa.edu/hardin/
md/publ.html>
Community Medicine Residence <www.library.utoronto.ca/www/cmres/index.html>

1. CRITICAL APPRAISAL

i) Characteristics of study design including sources of bias
(a) RCT
(b) Cohort
(c) Case-control
(d) Cross-sectional
ii) Measurements
(a) Characteristics of measurement, distributions, error, reliability, terminology
(b) Measurement of central tendency, dispersion, variability
(c) Test validation: sensitivity, specificity, pre-/post-test likelihood, predictive value
(d) Measurement of health and disease in a population
• specific rates (e.g., age/sex):
• incidence, prevalence
• standardization
• odds ratio
• relative risk
• attributable risk
• case fatality ratio
• primary/secondary attack rates
iii) Sampling, including sources of bias
iv) Analysis
Tests of significance
• statistical vs. clinical
• sample size
• p value, confidence intervals
• common tests (e.g., t-test, x^2)
• intro to multivariate analysis
v) Efficacy, effectiveness, efficiency, compliance

2. CONCEPTS OF DISEASE AND INJURY PREVENTION AND CONTROL

i) Concept of natural history of disease
ii) Models of causation
iii) Approaches and limitations to classification of health, function and disease
iv) Levels of prevention
(a) Primary (e.g., immunization, lifestyle)
(b) Secondary (e.g., screening, periodic health examination)
(c) Tertiary (e.g., disability, rehabilitation)
v) Screening, surveillance, case-finding, contact tracing
vi) Strategies for control
Points of intervention:
• host/agent/environment
vii) Prevention in clinical setting
Periodic health examination:
• conceptual approach
• protection packages
• updates of protection packages

3. DATABASE, VITAL STATISTICS, DEMOGRAPHY, HEALTH STATUS

i) Uses and limitations of Canadian data sources
(a) Census
(b) Statistics Canada
(c) Registries
(d) Medical examiners, autopsy
(e) Health surveys
(f) Birth certificates
(g) Death certificates
(h) Hospital, medical services data

* Source: Adapted from the Medical Council of Canada, *Objectives for the Qualifying Examination,* ed. Baumber J.S., 1992.

(i) Workers' compensation data
ii) Demographic characteristics of the
population
(a) Age/sex/structure
(b) Compression of morbidity
(c) Mortality
(d) Fertility
(e) Implications to the health care system
iii) Health indices and health status
(a) Direct
• Infant mortality rate
• Crude mortality rate
• Life expectancy
• Causes of death
• Specific health surveys
• Potential years of life lost
• Survivorship
• Age/sex specific distribution of mortality
• Disability days
• Activities of daily living
• Prevalence of disability
(b) Indirect
• Percentage of low birth-weight neonates
• Percentage of communities with potable
water
• Risk factor distribution
(c) Correlates
• Morbidity and utilization data
• Gross national product
• Socioeconomic status of individual
(d) Descriptive epidemiology of diseases
and injuries in Canada
• Motor vehicle injuries
• Cardiovascular disease
• Major cancers
• Respiratory diseases
• Common infectious diseases
• Substance abuse

4A. HEALTH CARE SYSTEM
i) Historical development and principles of
health services
(a) British North America Act
(b) Hospital Insurance and Diagnostic
Services Act
(c) Medicare
(d) Principles of b and c
(e) Established Programs Financing Act
(f) Canada Health Act

(g) International comparisons
(h) Trends and issues in the evolving health
system
ii) Organization of health services:
federal vs. provincial
iii) Self-regulation of professions
(a) Peer review
(b) Audit
iv) Professional organization
v) Methods of physician payment
vi) Distribution and projections of health
manpower
vii) Health resource allocation
viii) Institutional organization
(a) Structure
(b) Accreditation
(c) Audit
ix) Role of voluntary organizations
x) Alternate delivery systems
xi) Women's health movement

4B. PUBLIC HEALTH SYSTEM
i) Role of public health system in
(a) Maternal and child health
(b) Home care
(c) School health
(d) Sexually transmitted diseases
(e) Inspection
(f) Disease surveillance
(g) Mental health
(h) Health promotion
(i) Biological
ii) Role of physicians in public health
(a) Medical health officer
(b) Epidemiologist
(c) Occupational health
(d) Role of the practising physician
iii) Statutory responsibilities of the
practising physician
Reportable disease notification
iv) Outbreak investigation
v) National and international health
networks as relevant to the public health
system
vi) Product regulation
(a) Biologicals
(b) Drugs and pharmaceuticals
(c) Medical devices

5. OCCUPATIONAL AND ENVIRONMENTAL HEALTH

i) Exposure
(a) Long-term/low-dose
(b) Multiple
(c) Mechanisms of toxic action
• Cancer
• Reproductive hazards
• Respiratory diseases
(d) Routes of entry
(e) Types of exposures
ii) Standard setting
(a) Physical
(b) Chemical
(c) Biological
(d) Psychological
iii) Occupational diseases and injuries
iv) Occupational history taking
v) Risk assessment
vi) Ethics and occupational medicine
vii) Workers' compensation board functions
viii) Environmental health
• food, air, water

6. GROUPS WITH SPECIAL HEALTH CARE NEEDS

i) Characteristics and health status
(a) Canadian Indian/Inuit/Mètis
(b) Immigrants
(c) Low income/unemployed
(d) Elderly
(e) Disabled
ii) Service needs and availability

7. PSYCHOSOCIAL ASPECTS OF HEALTH

i) Health and illness behaviour and risk perception
ii) Compliance
(a) Barriers to individual
(b) Environmental and behavioural factors in compliance
iii) Family, social network and peer group alternatives to kinship
iv) Biopsychosocial, culture, gender, and age effects on health
(a) Health beliefs
(b) Patients and providers
v) Health education and health promotion
• Individual behaviour vs. social change
(a) healthy public policy
vi) Lifestyle and the environment
vii) Modalities of health education
(a) Behavioural diagnosis and modification
(b) Health marketing
viii) Blaming the victim
• Stigmatization
ix) Professional vs. consumer control of health-related initiatives

Index